# Handbook of Reproductive Medicine

# Handbook of Reproductive Medicine

Editor: Lorenza Campbell

AMERICAN
MEDICAL PUBLISHERS
www.americanmedicalpublishers.com

AMERICAN
MEDICAL PUBLISHERS
www.americanmedicalpublishers.com

**Cataloging-in-Publication Data**

Handbook of reproductive medicine / edited by Lorenza Campbell.
p. cm.
Includes bibliographical references and index.
ISBN 979-8-88740-160-7
1. Reproductive health. 2. Human reproduction. 3. Fertility, Human.
4. Embryology, Human. 5. Birth control. I. Campbell, Lorenza.
RG133 .H36 2023
613.9--dc23



American Medical Publishers,
41 Flatbush Avenue,
1st Floor, New York,
NY 11217, USA

ISBN 979-8-88740-160-7 (Hardback)

# Contents

# Preface

The world is advancing at a fast pace like never before. Therefore, the need is to keep up with the latest developments. This book was an idea that came to fruition when the specialists in the area realized the need to coordinate together and document essential themes in the subject. That's when I was requested to be the editor. Editing this book has been an honour as it brings together diverse authors researching on different streams of the field. The book collates essential materials contributed by veterans in the area which can be utilized by students and researchers alike.

Reproductive medicine refers to a subspecialty of medicine that focuses on the diagnosis and treatment of infertility, as well as other reproductive issues. It deals with issues associated with family planning, sexual dysfunction, sexual education and reproductive system disease. It also addresses difficulties linked with contraception, puberty and menopause. Reproductive medicine has enabled the growth of artificial reproductive techniques (ARTs), which have helped in overcoming the issue of human infertility, and these techniques are also being utilized in wildlife conservation and agriculture. Artificial insemination, embryo transfer, IVF and genome resource banking are a few types of ARTs. The evaluation and treatment of reproductive conditions is an important aspect of reproductive medicine. Congenital disorders, infectious diseases, endocrine disorders and benign tumors are among the most common medical conditions that have an impact on reproductive medicine. This book elucidates the innovative models around prospective developments with respect to reproductive medicine. Different approaches, evaluations, methodologies and advanced studies on reproductive health have been included herein. Researchers and students in this field will be assisted by this book.

Each chapter is a sole-standing publication that reflects each author´s interpretation. Thus, the book displays a multi-facetted picture of our current understanding of application, resources and aspects of the field. I would like to thank the contributors of this book and my family for their endless support.

**Editor**

# 1

# Predictors of unmet need for family planning among all women of reproductive age in Ethiopia

Afework Tadele[1*], Dessie Abebaw[2†] and Rahma Ali[1†]

**Abstract**

**Introduction:** Contraception is a good indicator of the extent to which couples have access to reproductive health services. Survey data on unmet need can provide overall direction by helping to pinpoint the obstacles in society and weaknesses in services that need to be overcome. This study is significant as it provides strong policy recommendations for the design and implementation of economic and non-economic interventions into family planning utilization by all eligible women.

**Objective:** To Identify Predictors of Unmet Need of Family Planning in Ethiopia.

**Methods:** A national level survey by performance monitoring and accountability (PMA 2020), which conducted between March and April 2016 among 7552 all women of 15–49 years were utilized. Stata® version13 were used for survey data for analysis using weighted frequency to give equal chances for enumeration areas represented. Binary and multivariate logistic regression employed. *P*-value < 0.05 were used to declare independent predictors of unmet need for family planning in Ethiopia.

**Result:** 7494 women responded to the interview giving response rate of 99.2%. Overall unmet need for family planning was 1, 214 (16.2%) of which 772 (10.3%) was for spacing and 450 (6.0%) for limiting. Overall unmet need was 540 (7.2%) in urban and 1431(19.1%) in rural areas of the Ethiopia. Statistically significant predictors with this were found to be women's age 0.73 AOR [95% C.I 0.6–0.9], being lower wealth 0.22 AOR [95% C.I 0.07–0.6] as compared to lowest, parity 2.1 AOR [95% C.I 1.4–2.9], number of children at first use of contraceptive 1.1 AOR [95% C.I 1.03–1.19], having final say with provider 0.03 AOR [95% C.I 0.003–0.23] as compared with own decision making.

**Conclusion:** Unmet need of family planning in Ethiopia was generally high especially with significant disparity in residence and regional states. Socio-demographic factors (age and wealth status) and obstetric factor (parity) were found to be significant factor. Informed decision making for provision of contraceptives and enhancing women's awareness starting their childbearing life with family planning were recommended.

**Keywords:** Unmet need, Family planning, Ethiopia, PMA2020

* Correspondence: afatadele@gmail.com
[†]Dessie Abebaw and Rahma Ali contributed equally to this work.
[1]Population and family health, Jimma University, Jimma, Ethiopia

## Plain English summary

This study examines the multiple predictors of unmet need for family planning. Through structured interviews of women in the reproductive age group in Ethiopia, the study seeks to determine socio-demographic, socio-economic and reproductive health factors how much eligible women for contraception received family planning to meet their need. The study finds more than 16 % of the women surveyed were unmet need for family planning. The factors that most predict this were found to be the age of women, household wealth status, parity, number of children at first use of contraceptive and having final say with provider to use contraceptive. We believe that our study makes a significant contribution to the literature because it provides a multivariate analysis of the complex set of factors whose predict meeting the need of family planning has been studied in an isolated fashion thus far. This study is also significant as it provides cogent policy recommendations for the design and implementation of economic and non-economic interventions into realize women's need for family planning.

## Article summary

### Strength of the study

The study was a secondary analysis of population level data about sociodemographic and belief/behavioral factors associated with unmet need for family planning. In their multivariable regression, they noted that unmet need was associated with age, number of living children at first use of family planning, wealth quintile, decisional autonomy, and parity.

### Limitations of the study

Being a survey, it is difficult to establish cause effect relationship.

## Introduction

Unmet need to family planning means when a married women who are able to give birth and want to stop or delay childbearing but are not using any method of contraception to prevent pregnancy [1]. One in ten married women face unmet need for family planning worldwide whereas, as many as one in five women in Africa. In 2017 met need of family planning among married or in-union women of reproductive age was 78% Worldwide. There is a difference in met need across different regions is lowest in Africa as 56% and above 75% in all other regions [2].

In Ethiopia despite family planning (FP) interventions of the Ethiopian federal ministry of health (EFMOH), including the Health Extension Program have significantly improved access to FP services [3], 22% of currently married women have an unmet need for family planning according to Ethiopian demographic health survey (EDHS) 2016 [4].

Unmet need for family planning is a valuable concept that is widely used for advocacy, the development of family planning policies, and the implementation and monitoring of family planning programs worldwide [5].

In each country, understanding the size of unmet need and the characteristics of women with unmet need can help planners strengthen programs. Survey data on unmet need can provide overall direction by helping to pinpoint the obstacles in society and weaknesses in services that need to be overcome [6].

Contraceptive utilization rate is a good indicator of the extent to which couples have access to reproductive health services [7]. The gap between women's reproductive intentions and their contraceptive behavior can be revealed by unmet need for family planning. The indicator is useful for tracking progress towards the target of achieving universal access to reproductive health. Information on contraceptive prevalence complements the indicator of unmet need for family planning [8]. The odds of unintended pregnancy were about 16 fold among women who reported facing unmet need for contraception compared to those who did not [9].

The projected unmet need for family planning is to remain above 10% worldwide up to 2030 despite the reductions anticipated for some regions. The largest declines are expected in Eastern Africa, where unmet need is projected to fall from 22% in 2017 to 16% in 2030. Living up to the commitment of the international community to achieve universal access to reproductive health by 2030 will require intensified support for family planning, including through the implementation of effective government policies and program. Access to health care services and the realization of reproductive rights for all people will be essential to fulfil the pledge of the 2030 Agenda for Sustainable Development that "no one will be left behind" [2].

Different literatures agree that different factors influencing unmet need of family planning were older age, high-parity, non-Muslim women to have an unmet need to limit fertility [10]. Knowledge of contraceptive method and discussion with partner and health extension workers [11]. A visit to a health facility, exposure to family planning from media, and an educational difference between a husband and wife Rural residence [12], contraception related factors like availability, accessibility, affordability, side effects as a cause for unmet need [13], partner attitude towards family planning services utilization, current menstrual status, healthcare providers visit and discussion about family planning issues [14], high for young married women in the richest wealth quintile and among unmarried women [15], Women who were housewife/farmers were more likely to have unmet need than those employed women [16]. Number of living children, ever use of contraceptive methods [17], social pressures, and provider bias limit knowledge about available options and access to appropriate methods, leading to higher rates of contraceptive failure and discontinuation after short periods. Addressing these barriers will improve maternal and child health, increase educational attainment and improve economic opportunities for young women [18].

The major reasons for not using contraceptives was inaccessibility of family planning methods, lack of knowledge, religious belief, fear of side effects of contraceptives they had suffered in the past, and opposition by husband [19], discontinuation due to health concerns and pressure from the surroundings were the most common cited reasons for non-use [20], less perceived risk of pregnancy due to breast feeding, religious prohibition [16].

## Methods and materials

**Population**: All women of reproductive age women in Ethiopia.

This is an analysis of cross-sectional data from the performance, monitoring and accountability (PMA)2020, obtained via phone survey of a representative sample of women in Ethiopia, divided into enumeration areas, with responses weighted according to Central Statistical Authority (CSA) probabilities to ensure generalizability.

### Sample design

PMA2020 Ethiopia uses a two-stage cluster design with residential area (urban and rural) and sub-regions as strata, sampling across all 11 geographic regions in Ethiopia. 95% of the target population, women of reproductive age 15–49 years, reside in five regions (Addis Ababa, Amhara, Oromia, SNNP and Tigray). Other regions with a total of less than 5% of the target population are allocated to a sixth synthetic region (referred to as "other"). Given the uneven population distribution and resource limitation, regional representative samples are only taken in the five regions (Addis Ababa, Amhara, Oromia, SNNP and Tigray). The fourth round sample of 221 EAs and 7651 households is designed to estimate modern contraceptive prevalence among all women at less than 2% margin of error at the national level, less than 3% for urban and rural estimates, and less than 5% at each of the five regional levels.

### Questionnaires

The PMA2020 is a comprehensive questionnaire that includes among other subjects, family planning. The field supervisors themselves administered the service delivery points(SDP) questionnaire at an additional three public SDPs that serve each enumeration areas(EA); the lowest, second lowest and third lowest-level public health SDPs (health post, health center, and district hospital) designated to serve each EA population.

Once listed, 35 households were randomly selected by field supervisors using a phone-based random number -generating application. All occupants in selected households were enumerated and from this list, all eligible women age 15–49 were approached and asked to give informed consent to participate in the study.

PMA2020 used standardized questionnaires for households, females and service delivery points (SDPs) to gather data about households, individual females and SDPs that are comparable across program countries and consistent with existing national surveys. Prior to launching the survey in each country, public health experts from Addis Ababa University review and modify these questionnaires to ensure all questions are appropriate to each setting. The questionnaires were translated into three local languages.

The household questionnaire gathers basic information about the household, such as ownership of durable goods, as well as characteristics of the dwelling unit, including wall, floor, and roof material, water sources and sanitation facilities. This information is used to construct a wealth quintile. The first section of the household questionnaire, the household roster, lists basic demographic information about all usual members of the household and visitors who stayed with the household the night before the interview. This roster is used to identify eligible respondents for the female questionnaire. In addition to the roster, the household questionnaire also gathers data that are used to measure key water, sanitation and hygiene (WASH) indicators, including regular sources and uses of WASH facilities and prevalence of open defecation by household members. The female questionnaire is used to collect information from all women age 15 to 49 who were listed on the household roster at selected households. The female questionnaire gathers specific information on education; fertility and fertility preferences; family planning access, choice and use; quality of family planning services; exposure to family planning messaging in the media; and the burden of collection water on women. The SDP questionnaire is used to collect information about the provision and quality of reproductive health services and products, integration of health services, and water and sanitation within the SDP.

### Data collection and processing

Fieldwork training started with a two-week training of new 30 new field staff, followed by a three-day refresher training for returning field staff before actual data collection. Data was collected from March to April 2016. Unlike traditional paper and-pencil surveys, PMA2020 uses Open Data Kit (ODK) Collect, an open-source software application, to collect data on mobile phones. All the questionnaires were programmed using this software and installed onto all project smartphones. The ODK questionnaire forms are programmed with automatic skip-patterns and built-in response constraints to reduce data entry errors.

This instantaneous aggregation of data also allowed for concurrent data processing and course corrections while PMA2020 was still active in the field. Throughout data collection, central staff at Addis Ababa University in Ethiopia and the data manager from the Gates Institute in Baltimore, Maryland routinely monitored the incoming data and notified field staff of any potential errors, missing data or problems found with form submissions on the central server. The use of mobile phones combined data collection and data entry into one step; therefore, data entry was completed when the last interview form was uploaded at the end of data collection in June, 2017. Once all data were on the server, data analysts cleaned and de-identified the data, applied survey weights, and prepared the final data set for analysis using Stata® version 14 software.

### Measurement

Women's unmet need for contraception were measured by asking questions all eligible women (all non-pregnant women's of reproductive age group) whether they are currently using any form of contraceptives or not. Those currently not using any form of contraceptive further asked whether they do not wish to become pregnant at all (unmet need for limiting) or within the next two years (unmet need for spacing). Finally, Percentage of fertile, sexually active women ages 15–49 who are not using contraception both for spacing and limiting were computed to get unmet need for contraceptives.

### Statistical analysis

Stata® version 13.0 were used to for analysis. The data were also explored again for inconsistencies and missing values. Variables having *p*-value less than 0.25 in binary logistic regression and variables of interest by investigators were selected as candidate for multivariable logistic regression. Multi-collinearities were checked among candidate variables if they have linear association among each other before entering them into multivariate logistic regression model for. Backward stepwise regression method was run by using entering at 0.1 and removal at 0.05. Finally, Odds ratio with 95% confidence interval and *P*-value less than 0.05 computed to assess the presence and degree of association and statistical significance independent predictors. The model fitness was checked using Hosmer and lameshaw test.

### Operational definitions

#### *Unmet need for family planning*

Proportion of women who [1] are not pregnant and not postpartum amenorrhoeic and are considered fecund and want to postpone their next birth for 2 or more years or stop childbearing altogether but are not using a contraceptive method, or [2] have a mistimed or unwanted current pregnancy, or [3] are postpartum amenorrhoeic and their last birth in the last 2 years was mistimed or unwanted Percentage of fertile, sexually active women aged 15–49 who are not using contraception and do not wish to become pregnant at all (unmet need for limiting) or within the next two years (unmet need for spacing) [4].

#### *Utilization of family planning*

Use of modern family planning method to prevent or postpone pregnancy.

#### *Reasons for non-use*

Reasons for non-use of contraceptive methods among married women who express a desire to postpone their next birth by two or more years.

#### *Method chosen by self or jointly*

Percentage of women ages 15–49 currently using a modern contraceptive method, reporting they decided on method themselves or jointly with a partner or provider.

#### *Number of living children at first contraceptive use*

Average number of living children at first contraceptive use among women ages 15–49 who have ever used contraception.

## Result

### Socio-demographic characteristics of women of reproductive age in Ethiopia, 2017

Seven thousand four hundred and ninety-four all women of reproductive age were interviewed yield response rate of 99.2%. The mean ($\pm$ standard deviation) age of the women was 27.8 ($\pm$ 0.14). Four thousand six hundred seventy-one (62.3%) of the women were married. Three thousand one hundred eighteen (41.6%) of the respondent never attended formal education. Two thousand four hundred and sixty-one (32.8%) of the women were nulliparous see Table 1.

### All women of reproductive age unmet need for family planning, in Ethiopia

Overall unmet need for family planning among all women was 1214 (16.2%) of which 772 (10.3%) was for spacing and 450 (6.0%) for limiting while 1799 (24.0%) among married women. It was 540 (7.2%) in urban and 1431(19.1%) in rural areas of Ethiopia. There is a regional disparity which

**Table 1** Socio demographic characteristics of women of reproductive age in Ethiopia, 2017

| Variables | categories | Weighted Percentage of sample | Weighted number | Unweighted number |
|---|---|---|---|---|
| Age | 15–19 | 23.6 | 1771 | 1735 |
| | 20–24 | 17.5 | 1308 | 1449 |
| | 25–29 | 18.2 | 1368 | 1447 |
| | 30–34 | 14.0 | 1053 | 1008 |
| | 35–39 | 11.6 | 871 | 824 |
| | 40–44 | 8.2 | 612 | 562 |
| | 45–49 | 6.8 | 512 | 456 |
| Marital status | Married | 62.3 | 4671 | 4224 |
| | Living together | 1.5 | 112 | 122 |
| | Divorced | 6.9 | 515 | 590 |
| | Widowed | 2.7 | 200 | 190 |
| | Never married | 26.6 | 1994 | 2351 |
| Parity | None[a] | 32.8 | 2461 | 2827 |
| | 1–2 | 23.8 | 1784 | 2019 |
| | 3–4 | 16.1 | 1209 | 1151 |
| | 5 or more | 27.2 | 2039 | 1480 |
| Education | Never attended | 41.6 | 3118 | 2443 |
| | Primary | 38.5 | 2885 | 2692 |
| | Secondary | 15.6 | 1168 | 1683 |
| | Technical/Vocational | 2.7 | 202 | 393 |
| | University | 1.5 | 116 | 26 |
| Wealth quintile | Lowest | 19.3 | 1449 | 923 |
| | Lower | 19.3 | 1445 | 963 |
| | Middle | 19.2 | 1440 | 972 |
| | Higher | 19.6 | 1471 | 1253 |
| | Highest | 22.6 | 1690 | 3370 |
| Region | Addis | 5.0 | 378 | 891 |
| | Amhara | 22.7 | 1702 | 1285 |
| | Oromiya | 38.4 | 2877 | 1736 |
| | SNNP | 22.4 | 1681 | 1594 |
| | Tigray | 6.7 | 499 | 1134 |
| | Other | 4.8 | 357 | 841 |
| | **Total** | **100.0** | **7494** | **7481** |

[a]stands for those never gave birth

is 22.4% in Oromia region while only 3.3% in Addis Ababa of all women have unmet need to family planning see Fig. 1.

### Reasons for not using family planning in Ethiopia

The most common reason for non-use of contraceptives among married women were four hundred sixty-one (20.88%) no menses since last birth, three hundred seven (13.90%) women says it is up to god and/or fatalistic, two hundred eighty-six (12.95%), two hundred thirty-two (10.51%) were health concerns, one hundred eighty-seven (8.47%) fear of side effects and one hundred eighty-five (8.38%) not having sex see Fig. 2.

### Predictors of unmet need for family planning in Ethiopia in 2107

Multivariate logistic regression model revealed that being younger age, having a final say jointly with family planning provider, having less number of living children at first use of contraceptive mothers, being in second wealth quintile as compared with first wealth quintile,

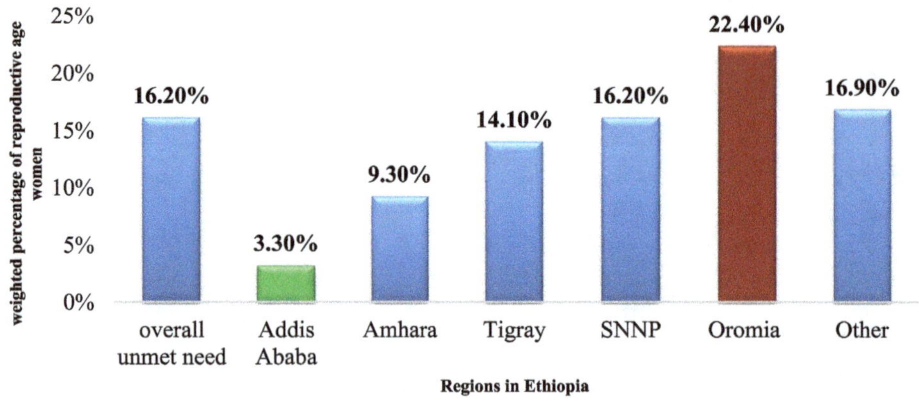


**Fig. 1** Regional status of all woman of reproductive age Unmet Need for family planning, in Ethiopia, 2017

having less parity were found to be significant predictors unmet need for contraception.

After controlling for potential confounders in the multivariate analysis revealed that as age of women's increase by one year the odds of being unmet need for family planning 20% less likely (AOR 0.8 [95% C.I 0.75–0.9]), having a final say jointly with family planning provider were 96% less likely as compared women's own final decision to be unmet need of family planning (AOR 0.04 [95% C.I 0.005–0.300]), as the number of living children at first use of contraceptive increases by one the odds being unmet for family planning 1.1 more likely (AOR 1.1 [95% C.I 1.01–1.2]), mothers in lower wealth quintile were 80% (AOR 0.2 [95% C.I 0.06–0.60]) less likely to be unmet need for family planning as compared to those in lowest wealth quintile, As parity increase with one birth the odds of being unmet need for family planning were twice more likely (AOR 2.1 [95% C.I 1.4–2.8]) see Table 2.

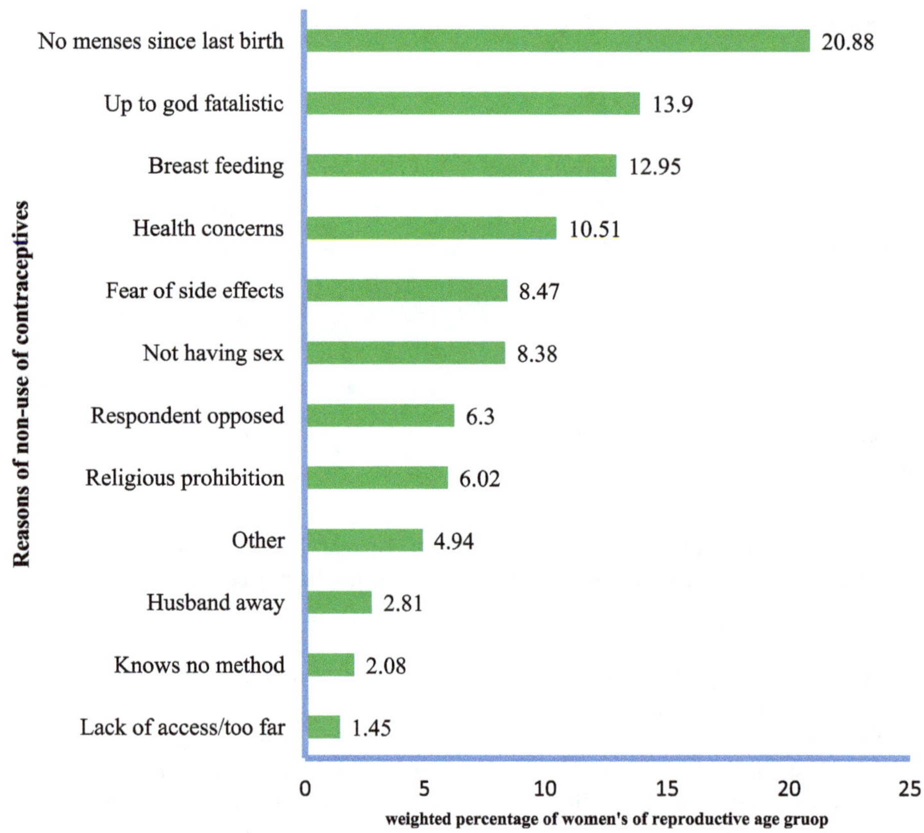


**Fig. 2** Reasons for non-use of contraception among women's of reproductive age group in Ethiopia, 2017

**Table 2** Multivariate logistic regression model of unmet need for family planning in Ethiopia in 2017

| Variables | Unmet need for family planning | | COR (CI 95%) | AOR (CI 95%) |
|---|---|---|---|---|
| | Yes (%) | No (%) | | |
| Age[a] | 1217(16.2) | 6277(83.8) | 1.02(1.01–1.03)** | **0.80(0.75–0.90)**** |
| Final decision | | | | |
| You alone | 70(43.5) | 930 (39.8) | 1.0 | 1.0 |
| Provider | 0.21(0.1) | 63(2.7) | 0.04 (0.01–0.33)* | 0.08 (0.006–1.2) |
| Partner | 15(9.3) | 222(9.5) | 0.86(0.36–2.01) | 1.20(0.30–4.0) |
| You and provider | 5(3.1) | 110(4.7) | 0.60(0.09–9.95) | **0.04(0.01–0.26)**** |
| You and partner | 71(44.1) | 1009(43.2) | 0.93(0.60–1.40) | 1.98(0.95–4.12) |
| Number of children at first use [a] | 1217(16.2) | 6277(83.8) | 1.05(1.01–1.09)* | **1.10(1.01–1.20)*** |
| Wealth quintile | | | | |
| Lowest | 349(28.6) | 1099 (17.5) | 1.0 | 1.0 |
| Lower | 284(23.3) | 1161(18.5) | 0.76 (0.59–0.98)* | **0.20(0.06–0.58)**** |
| Middle | 268(22.0) | 1172(18.6) | 0.72 (0.55–0.92)* | 0.580(0.20–1.89) |
| Higher | 203(16.7) | 1268(20.2) | 0.50 (0.38–0.65)** | 0.57(.20–1.90) |
| Highest | 113(9.3) | 1577(25.1) | 0.22 (0.17–0.29)** | 0.89(0.18–4.20) |
| Parity [a] | 1217(16.2) | 6277(83.8) | 1.92(1.79–2.06)** | **2.10(1.39–2.78)**** |

[a]Continuous variable,*Statistically significant at *P*-value < 0.05, ** statistically significant at *P*-value < 0.001, *COR* crude odds ratio, *AOR* adjusted odds ratio, 1.0 reference category. *NB* frequencies were weighted

## Discussion

The gap between women's reproductive intentions and their contraceptive behavior can be revealed by unmet need for family planning. Unmet need for contraception is useful for tracking progress towards the target of achieving universal access to reproductive health. The level of unmet need of family planning needs to be assessed periodically and identifying effective intervention areas has of great implication.

This study shows that unmet need of family planning in Ethiopia was among all women was 16.2%. It shows a little increment as compared with Ethiopian demographic health surveys (EDHS) in 2016 which is 15.2% among all women. This may be due to changes seen within a year for different levels of interventions and EDHS data a five year history while PMA2020 data collected annually [4].

This study also showed there were disparities among different regions of Ethiopia for instance unmet need of family planning among reproductive age married women in Addis Ababa were 6.9, 13.4% in Amhara region, 31.0% in Oromia region and 24.0% in southern nations, nationalities and peoples (SNNP) of Ethiopia. A cross sectional study in Enemay District, in 2013 and West Belessa district in 2015 both North western Ethiopia showed 25.6 and 39.5% unmet need for contraceptives respectively, which were higher as compared to this study finding in Amhara region. This shows that unmet need for contraception varies from place to place with sociocultural diversity, differentials in geographic and economic accessibility of reproductive health services for the women's [14, 17].

The main reasons for unmet need for contraceptives were found to be no menses since last birth, it is up to god and/or fatalistic, health concerns, fear of side effects and not having sex. This were supported with different cross-sectional studies in Saudi Arabia in 2018 found fear of side effect, in Egypt in 2017 discontinuation due to health concerns and in Dangila town, Awi Zone, Amhara regional state of Ethiopia in 2015 identified religious prohibition as main reasons for non-use of contraception [16, 19, 20].

In this study age of women were statistically significant that an increase by one year of age of the women, the odds of being unmet need for family planning would be 20% less likely. Similarly a demographic health survey comparative reports 34 in developing countries in 2014 reveals that unmet need to family planning was higher among younger women (age 15–19) than older women (age 20–24) and also another cross sectional study in 2015 in West Belessa District, North Western Ethiopia, among married women with 35 years and above were 70% less likely to have unmet need than women with 15–19 age group [14, 15]. This might be younger age groups have no adequate information regarding contraception and comprehensive education of sexuality and also majority of Ethiopians reside in rural areas in which contraceptive use among adolescent age groups believed to be shameful.

The study found that mothers in lower wealth quintile were 80% less likely to be unmet need for family planning as compared to those in lowest wealth quintile. Likewise, a comparative reports of the demographic health survey in

34 of developing countries in 2014 showed high unmet need for contraception among young married women in the richest wealth quintile [14]. This indicates that being in high wealth index doesn't guarantee for met need for family planning.

Parity was also found to be significant predictor of unmet need for contraception. As parity increase with one birth the odds of being unmet need for family planning were twice more likely. West Belessa district in 2015, revealed that, the odds of having unmet need for contraception increase as the number of living children increases [17]. This shows that having children in Ethiopia is unplanned and that is why maternal mortality and morbidity were high in the country. There would be no planned family can be without met-need of contraception.

The study revealed that having a final say jointly with family planning provider were 96% less likely as compared women's own final decision to be unmet need of family planning. This finding was supported with a cross sectional study in Misha district, Southern Ethiopia, in 2014 which revealed that having knowledge of contraceptive method and discussion with health extension workers were helpful for met need [11]. Decision regarding contraception was better if made with provider as informed decision was helpful for continuous use of contraceptive method of their choice as different women have different health problems and reproductive health goals choice of contraceptive individually. This study utilized country level data which is more representative and up to date than demographic health survey as the data were collected on annual bases. Being a survey, it is difficult to establish cause effect relationship.

## Conclusion

More than 16 % of women were responded that their need for contraception still not met. There was also great disparity regarding unmet need for family planning among urban and rural and also a regionally. The major reason for non-use of contraception were found to be no menses since last birth, it is up to god and/or fatalistic, health concerns, fear of side effects and not having sex.

Having a final say jointly with family planning provider, being younger age, having less number of living children at first use of contraceptive mothers, being in second wealth quintile as compared with first wealth quintile, having less parity were found to be significant predictors unmet need for family planning.

## Recommendation

- The disparities between urban and rural difference in unmet need for contraception regional difference should resolved strengthening the health systems and more advocacy through different information, education and communication making an agenda.
- Public health interventions on meeting the need for contraception among women should promote women to make informed decision regarding contraceptive use. Priorities should be given for younger age, those in second wealth quintile, having more child before starting contraception use and multi-parous women.

### Abbreviations

CSA: Central statistical agency; EA: Enumeration areas; EDHS: Ethiopian demographic health survey; EFMOH: Ethiopian federal ministry of health; FP: Family planning; ODK: Open Data Kit; PMA: Performance monitoring and accountability; SDPs: Service delivery points

### Acknowledgements

Performance Monitoring and Accountability 2020 (PMA2020) and Addis Ababa University school of public health.

### Authors' contributions

**AT** made substantial contributions to conception and design, or acquisition of data, or analysis and interpretation of data. **DA** involved analysis and interpretation of data. **RA** been involved in drafting the manuscript or revising it critically for important intellectual content. All authors read and approved the final manuscript.

### Author details

[1]Population and family health, Jimma University, Jimma, Ethiopia.
[2]Epidemiology, Jimma University, Jimma, Ethiopia.

### References

1. Bongaarts J. The impact of family planning programs on unmet need and demand for contraception; 2014. p. 247–62.
2. United Nations Department of Economic and Social Affairs, World Family Planning Highlights, NewYork, ST/ESA/SER.A/414, 2017.
3. fhi360. Family planning situation analysis in Ethiopia. Prog Fam Plan 2012;
4. CSA. Ethiopia Demographic and health survey. 2016.
5. Bradley SEK, Croft TN, Fishel JD, Westoff CF. Revising Unmet Need For Family Planning Dhs Analytical Studies 25. 2012;(January).
6. Prb. Unmet Need For Family Planning : Recent Trends and Their Implications for Programs. 2003.
7. UNFPA. Ethiopia situation analysis of population, reproductive health and gender. 2005.
8. United Nations. Department of Economic and Social Affairs, Population Division (2014).World. World Contracept use. 2014;POP(DB/CP/rev2014).
9. Bishwajit G, Tang S, Yaya S, Feng Z. Unmet need for contraception and its association with unintended pregnancy in Bangladesh. BMC Pregnancy Childbirth. 2017;17(186):1–9.
10. Austin A. Unmet contraceptive need among married Nigerian women : an examination of trends and drivers. Contraception. 2015;91(1):31–8 Available from: https://doi.org/10.1016/j.contraception.2014.10.002.
11. Chafo K, Doyore F. Unmet need for family planning and associated factors among married women in Misha District, Southern Ethiopia. J Women's Health Care. 2014;3(4).
12. Gebreselassie T, Govindasamy P. Levels and trends in unmet need for family planning among adolescents and young women in Ethiopia; 2013.
13. Sulthana B, Shewade HD, Sunderamurthy B, Manoharan K. Unmet need for contraception among married women in an urban area of Puducherry, India. 2015;3(January):115–118.
14. Dejenu G, Ayichiluhm M, Abajobir AA. Prevalence and associated factors of unmet need for family planning among married women in Enemay District, Northwest Ethiopia: a comparative cross-sectional study, vol. 13; 2013. p. 4.
15. Macquarrie K. Unmet need for family planning among young women : levels and trends Dhs comparative reports 34; 2014.
16. Genet E, Abeje G, Ejigu T. Determinants of unmet need for family planning among currently married women in Dangila town administration , Awi zone , Amhara regional state ; a cross sectional study. Reprod Health [Internet]. 2015;12(14):1–5. Available from: ???

17. Mihret N. Magnitude and associated factors of unmet need for contraceptive methods among currently married women in west Belessa District, North Western Ethiopia 2015;4(10):164–169.
18. PRB. 2017 World Population Data Sheet with a special focus on youth 2017;
19. Nahar S, Mohammed M, Farheen A. Unmet need and demand for family planning among married women of Abha, Aseer region in Saudi Arabia. Middle East Fertil Soc J. 2018;23(1):31–6. Available from. https://doi.org/10.1016/j.mefs.2017.07.004.
20. Mahmoud H, Elweshahi T, Ismail G, Saad S, Sadek E, El-sharkawy OG. Unmet need for postpartum family planning in Alexandria , Egypt. Alexandria J Med [Internet]. 2017:0–4. Available from. https://doi.org/10.1016/j.ajme.2017.03.003.

# 2

# Association between media exposure and family planning in Myanmar and Philippines: Evidence from nationally representative survey data

Pranta Das[1], Nandeeta Samad[2], Hasan Al Banna[3], Temitayo Eniola Sodunke[4], John Elvis Hagan Jr[5,6], Bright Opoku Ahinkorah[7] and Abdul-Aziz Seidu[8,9*]

## Abstract

**Background:** Although women in South Asia and South-east Asia have developed their knowledge regarding modern contraceptive and other family planning techniques, limited information exists on the influence of mass media exposure on the utilization of contraceptives and family planning. The current study examined the association between media exposure and family planning in Myanmar and Philippines.

**Methods:** The study analyzed data from the 2017 Philippines National Demographic and Health Survey (NDHS) and 2015–16 Myanmar Demographic and Health Survey (MDHS). Three family planning indicators were considered in this study (i.e., contraceptive use, demand satisfied regarding family planning and unmet need for family planning). A binary logistic regression model was fitted to see the effect of media exposure on each family planning indicator in the presence of covariates such as age group, residence, education level, partner education level, socio-economic status, number of living children, age at first marriage, and working status.

**Results:** The prevalence of contraception use was 57.2% in the Philippines and 55.7% in Myanmar. The prevalence of demand satisfied regarding family planning was 70.5 and 67.1% in the Philippines and Myanmar respectively. Unmet need regarding family planning was 16.6% and 19.9% in the Philippines and Myanmar respectively. After adjusting for the covariates, the results showed that women who were exposed to media were more likely to use contraception in Philippines (aOR = 2.24, 95% CI = 1.42–3.54) and Myanmar (aOR 1.39, 95% CI = 1.15–1.67). Media exposure also had a significant positive effect on demand satisfaction regarding family planning in the Philippines (aOR = 2.19, 95% CI = 1.42–3.37) and Myanmar (aOR = 1.34, 95% CI = 1.09–1.64). However, there was no significant association between media exposure and unmet need in both countries.

(Continued on next page)

* Correspondence: abdul-aziz.seidu@stu.ucc.edu.gh
[8]Department of Population and Health, University of Cape Coast, Cape Coast, Ghana
[9]College of Public Health, Medical and Veterinary Sciences, James Cook University, Townsville, Queensland, Australia

(Continued from previous page)

**Conclusions:** The study established a strong association between mass media exposure and the use and demand satisfaction for family planning among married and cohabiting women in Philippines and Myanmar. Using mass media exposure (e.g., local radio, television- electronic; newspapers) to increase both access and usage of contraceptives as well as other family planning methods in these countries could be pivotal towards the attainment of United Nations Sustainable Development Goal 3 (SDG 3) of improving maternal health.

**Keywords:** DHS, Family planning, Media exposure, Myanmar, Philippines, Women's health

## Background

Globally, it has been observed that family planning issues are highly influenced by the scientific use of mass media, especially television, radio, newspaper, and internet [1]. Similarly, the last three decades have shown that indicators of family planning such as contraceptive use, unmet need for family planning, and demand satisfied regarding family planning have significant association with media exposure [1, 2]. Furthermore, the world has noticed an increased trend regarding these indicators of family planning. For example, worldwide data in 2017 indicates that the rate of contraceptive use among married or in-union women of reproductive age rose to 63% from 35% in 1970. Likewise, an increased trend (78% from 75% in 2000) has also been observed concerning the demand for family planning satisfied by modern methods among married or in-union women. However, 12% of women have an unmet need for family planning, which has declined from 22% in 1970 [3, 4]. A study suggests that the SMS-based communication coverage regarding family planning is higher in Africa than Asia [5]. However, the percentage in terms of contraceptive use in Central and West Africa is very low (25%) and in Asia, the rate is 66.4%, which is considered low compared to Thailand, Vietnam, and Singapore [6–8].

It is evident that women in South Asia and South-East Asia have developed their knowledge regarding modern contraceptive techniques through the proper utilization of mass media [9, 10]. For instance, in India, Pakistan, and Philippines, women who own TV at their homes are more likely to get access in the coverage of contraceptives than women who do not have TV [11–13]. Similarly, exposure of mass media in Myanmar is associated with the age of women at first marriage [14, 15]. A study conducted from 47 DHS data of sub-Saharan Africa indicates that overall, 44.3% family planning related information is available from mass media [16]. Furthermore, in Nigeria, in terms of getting family planning related messages, people with higher socio-economic status have more opportunity of getting access to mass media, especially television and radio, than people with lower socio-economic status [17, 18]. In Indonesia, the exposure of television has increased than radio and print media regarding family planning [19]. Also, in Ethiopia, women's access to mass media, especially radio, television and newspaper has a significant impact on unmet need for child spacing and limiting births. For instance, data from the year 2005 in Ethiopia proved that women with no access to mass media had higher rate (38.1%) of unmet need for family planning than women with access to mass media (35.8%) [20]. In addition, some covariates like education, partner education, residence, and occupation also had significant impact on family planning. Specifically, urban women were more likely to utilize knowledge about contraceptive use from mass media than rural women. Similarly, educated women were more likely to obtain health related messages through mass media at their homes than healthcare centers [21].

Despite the numerous studies on family planning issues worldwide, these studies have paid more attention to the impact of basic socio-demographic status such as education, economic condition, and decision-making power on family planning rather than recognizing the importance of mass media for awareness building regarding family planning [19, 22–29]. Hence, the literature in Asia regarding media exposure and family planning is sparse. Although there is limited scholarly information on this issue, the influence of media exposure on family planning remains unclear [30, 31]. By utilizing the current DHS data, it is possible to present a valid outcome regarding this prevailing issue. Myanmar and Philippines were targeted for this study because in Myanmar, the contraceptive prevalence rate (CPR) was lower (41.0%) than other Southeast Asian countries (average rate of this region was 62.2% in 2007) [32]. Although the CPR increased at 52.2% in 2016, the rate was lower than a projected target of 60% by 2020 [33]. Rapid population growth, short life expectancy, low level of education, and poor healthcare system are the major loopholes in the process of achieving the goal of population control and ensure a sound maternal and child health by preventing unwanted pregnancies and encouraging birth spacing [14, 34]. Moreover, the rate of unmet need for family planning in Myanmar was very high (19%) than their nearest country, Thailand (3%) [34, 35]. Likewise, the population growth rate was highest in Philippines among the South-East Asia, along with the third highest total fertility rate (TFR) in the region. UN 2015 data indicated that the rate of unmet need of FP was 17.8%, which was higher than other Asian countries [36].

Furthermore, the overall contraceptive prevalence was only 40% among married women in 2017 in Philippines, where the rate of modern contraceptive prevalence increased by only 2% between 2013 and 2017 [37]. Therefore, evidence suggests these countries have challenges to increase the prevalence of contraceptive use and reduce the TFR [38]. This study, therefore, examines the association between media exposure and family planning in both Myanmar and Philippines. By making this assessment between these two countries, researchers and policy makers could get updated view on reproductive health issues for making proper guidelines and efficient programs.

## Materials and methods

### Data source and study settings

The study analyzed the 2017 Philippines National Demographic and Health Survey (NDHS) dataset, which took place from August 14 to October 27, 2017, and 2015–16 Myanmar Demographic and Health Survey (MDHS) dataset, which took place from December 7, 2015 to July 7, 2016. These two datasets were selected because they were the most recent dataset available for both countries.

### Study design

The 2017 Philippines National Demographic and Health Survey (NDHS), implemented by the Philippine Statistics Authority (PSA), was based on two-stage stratified sample design. It used the Master Sample Frame (MSF) which was designed as well as compiled by the PSA. In the first stage, 1250 primary sampling units (PSUs), distributed by province, were systematically selected. Systematic random sampling from each sampled PSU 20 or 26 housing units were selected at the second stage. Then, from each housing unit, women aged 15–49 were interviewed. To prevent bias replacement, changes in the pre-specified housing units were not allowed. After the data collection, information of 25,074 women were obtained.

The 2015–16 Myanmar Demographic and Health Survey (MDHS) was implemented by the Ministry of Health and Sports (MoHS). This survey followed a two-stage stratified sample design. From the master sample, 442 clusters (123 urban and 319 rural) were selected at the first. At the second stage, by using equal probability systematic sampling from each selected clusters (i.e., a total of 13,260 households), 30 households were selected. Then, from each household, women aged 15–49 were interviewed. After the data collection, data of total 12, 885 women were obtained.

The data of women who were married or currently in union and were usual residents and not pregnant, and with education level, including partner's education level were filtered out from the raw dataset of both countries. This filtered dataset was subsequently analyzed.

### Dependent variables

The indicators of family planning selected were contraception use, unmet need for family planning and demand satisfied regarding family planning. The variable contraception use was coded as "Yes" for a woman who was currently using any kind of contraception method, otherwise coded as "No" and the variable unmet need for family planning was coded as "Yes" for a woman who had an unmet need for spacing or unmet need for limiting otherwise "No". For a woman who had met the need for spacing or met the need for limiting, the indicator demand satisfied regarding family planning was coded as "Yes" otherwise "No".

### Independent variable

The variable media exposure was recoded as 'Yes' for a woman who was exposed to either newspaper, radio, television or the internet otherwise "No" for both the countries (Philippines, Myanmar).

A number of covariates were selected for this study based on previous literature [36–46]. These are age group (15–24, 25–29, 30–34, 35–39, 40–49), residence (urban, rural), education level (no education, primary, secondary, higher), partner education level (no education, primary, secondary, higher), socio-economic status (poorest, poorer, middle, richer, richest), number of living children (no children, 1–3, more than 3), age at first marriage (below 20, 20–25, more than 25), and working status (employed, unemployed).

### Statistical analysis

After the required filtration of the dataset, chi-square was performed between the confounders and the family planning indicators. The binary logistic regression model was fitted to see the association between media exposure with each family planning indicators in the presence of covariates age group, residence, educational level, partner's educational level, socio-economic status, number of living children, age at first marriage, and working status. In each model, the covariates were kept regardless of their $p$-value. Each model was assessed by calculating the area under the ROC curve and were found satisfactory. The analysis was done after considering the sample weight and the complex survey design. All the $p$-values less than 0.05 were considered significant. The analysis was conducted using software R version 3.6.0.

## Results

### Sample characteristics

The weighted sample size for Philippines and Myanmar was 4497 and 7047 respectively. For both countries, most of the women were in the age group 40–49 years (see Table 1). For Philippines, 60.2% of the women were from urban areas whereas 26.3% of the women in Myanmar were from urban areas. The sample from Philippines comprised 46.4% of women with a secondary level of education and 41.1% women with partner having secondary level of education whereas the sample of Myanmar comprised 29% women with a secondary level of education and 38.2% women with partner having secondary level of education. The socio-economic status of the women of Philippines was mostly in the richest quintile whereas women from Myanmar have socio-economic status mostly in the middle and poorer quintile. Most of the women of Philippines had age at first marriage within 20–25 while most of the women of Myanmar had age at first marriage below 20. For both countries, most of the women had 1–3 living children. Also, majority of the women from Philippines were employed whereas most of the women of Myanmar were unemployed.

**Table 1** General characteristics of the respondents

| Variable | Philippines (4497) | | Myanmar (7047) | |
|---|---|---|---|---|
| | N | Percent | N | Percent |
| Age group | | | | |
| • 15–24 | 543 | 12.1 | 860 | 12.2 |
| • 25–29 | 750 | 16.7 | 1057 | 15 |
| • 30–34 | 765 | 17 | 1353 | 19.2 |
| • 35–39 | 851 | 18.9 | 1395 | 19.8 |
| • 40–49 | 1588 | 35.3 | 2382 | 33.8 |
| Residence | | | | |
| • Urban | 2706 | 60.2 | 1854 | 26.3 |
| • Rural | 1791 | 39.8 | 5193 | 73.7 |
| Education level | | | | |
| • No education | 51 | 1.1 | 1097 | 15.6 |
| • Primary | 693 | 15.4 | 3348 | 47.4 |
| • Secondary | 2087 | 46.4 | 2041 | 29 |
| • Higher | 1666 | 37.1 | 561 | 8 |
| Partner education level | | | | |
| • No education | 59 | 1.3 | 1063 | 15.1 |
| • Primary | 934 | 20.8 | 2850 | 40.4 |
| • Secondary | 1849 | 41.1 | 2689 | 38.2 |
| • Higher | 1655 | 36.8 | 445 | 6.3 |
| Socio-economic status | | | | |
| • Poorest | 780 | 17.3 | 1423 | 20.2 |
| • Poorer | 775 | 17.2 | 1446 | 20.5 |
| • Middle | 880 | 19.6 | 1442 | 20.5 |
| • Richer | 1022 | 22.7 | 1373 | 19.5 |
| • Richest | 1040 | 23.2 | 1363 | 19.3 |
| Number of living children | | | | |
| • No children | 341 | 7.6 | 496 | 9.9 |
| • 1–3 | 3025 | 67.3 | 5022 | 71.3 |
| • More than 3 | 1131 | 25.2 | 1328 | 18.8 |
| Age at first marriage | | | | |
| • Below 20 | 1763 | 39.2 | 3322 | 47.2 |
| • 20–25 | 1909 | 42.5 | 2674 | 37.9 |
| • Above 25 | 825 | 18.3 | 1051 | 14.9 |
| Working status | | | | |
| • Employed | 2300 | 51.1 | 2458 | 34.9 |
| • Unemployed | 2197 | 48.9 | 4588 | 65.1 |

The family planning indicator contraception use prevalence was 57.2% in the Philippines and 55.7% in Myanmar (see Fig. 1). The prevalence of demand satisfied regarding family planning was 70.5 and 67.1% in the Philippines and Myanmar respectively. Unmet need regarding family planning was 16.6% and 19.9% in the Philippines and Myanmar respectively.

### Chi-square test between the confounding variables and family planning indicators

The results of the chi-square test and the distribution of the family planning indicators across the confounding variables are presented in the Tables 2, 3, 4.

### Binary logistic regression models between family planning indicators and media exposure

After adjusting for the covariates, the results showed that media exposure has a significant effect on contraception use for both Philippines and Myanmar (see Table 5). In Philippines, media exposed women are significantly 1.27 times more likely to use any contraception method than women who are not media exposed. Similarly, in Myanmar, media exposed women are significantly 39% more likely to use any contraception method than women who are not media exposed.

Media exposure also has a significant effect on family planning indicator demand satisfied in the presence of all the covariates for both countries (see Table 6). In Philippines media exposed women are significantly 1.15 times more likely to have demand satisfied regarding family planning than the women who are not media exposed. Similarly, in Myanmar media exposed women are 34% more likely to have demand satisfied regarding family planning than the women who are not media exposed.

But in the presence of all the covariates, the result shows that media exposure has no significant effect on

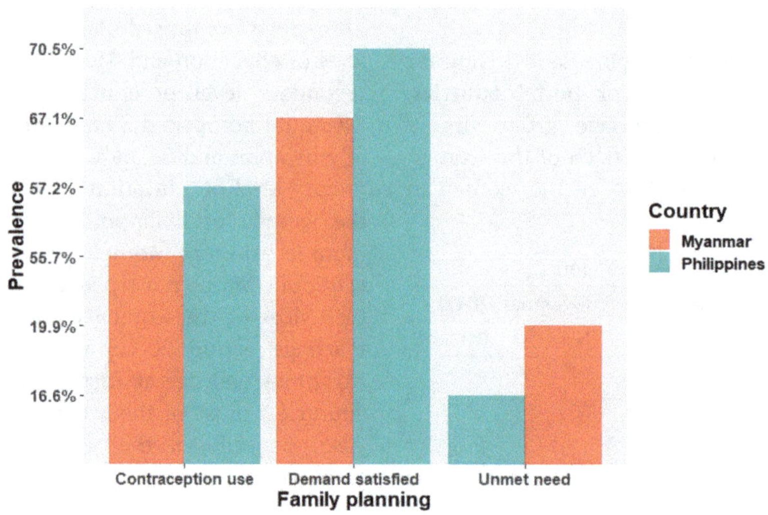


**Fig. 1** Prevalence of family planning indicators

family planning indicator unmet need for both countries (see Table 7).

## Discussion

We examined the association between mass media exposure and family planning and compared the assessment in both countries so that researchers and policy makers could get an utter view for making proper guidelines and efficient programs. Using data from the Demographic and Health Survey in Philippines and Myanmar, the regression analysis was fitted to show the effect of mass media exposure on the various family planning indicators. After adjusting for covariates, the study revealed that mass media exposure has a significant effect on contraception use in both countries. In the Philippines, the results indicate that women who had media exposure were approximately 2 times more likely to use any contraceptive methods as opposed to their counterparts who were not exposed to mass media. Similarly, in Myanmar, mass media exposed women were 39% more likely to use any contraceptive method than women who were not exposed to mass media. This finding supports other studies that have documented the influence of mass media communication interventions on contraceptive use [2–9]. Additionally, studies [10–12] have claimed that mass media remains a vital source of information and has the capacity to raise awareness, increase knowledge level, and influence attitudes towards family planning. This same evidence aligns with another work [13] in Kenya that revealed that access to media messages influences the use of contraceptives, intention to use contraceptives, and even desire for future births.

Other studies have demonstrated that mass media impacts women empowerment, including their ability to take household decisions on contraception [47–51]. For example, sexual partners who access diverse media platforms (e.g., television, radio, newspapers), communicate more about safer sexual practices and subsequently use contraceptives (e.g., condoms), and/or other family planning methods. Thus, exposure to media could improve knowledge and attitudes through behaviour modification associated with consistent use of some contraceptives and other family planning methods. Some behaviours and communication change models emphasize that knowledge is one key prerequisite for a positive behavioural change [14–17, 52].

Another important finding in our study is the effect of mass media exposure on demand satisfied regarding family planning. Surprisingly, there is little published data on this aspect and its association with mass media. The current study reveals that mass media exposure also has a significant effect on satisfaction of demands in the presence of all the covariates for both countries. For both countries, geographical disparities or heterogeneity (e.g., population density, ageing pattern) in attitudes and norms, differentials in employment, and other socioeconomic parameters (e.g., household wealth index) might mirror the accessibility of media platforms relative to information or messages on general and reproductive health care, including contraception and family planning methods toward demand satisfaction [53–55]. For instance, the regional groups in Myanmar show geographic inequalities in access to modern contraception or accessibility and quality of family planning services [53]. It is more likely that indicators such as physical distance, staying in hilly areas, and network access and/ or availability of media outlets might limit appropriate information or messages related to reproductive healthcare and services. This limitation could influence the demand satisfaction of the populace towards contraception and

**Table 2** Chi-square test of the association between contraception use and confounders

| Variable | Philippines | | | Myanmar | | |
|---|---|---|---|---|---|---|
| | Contraception use | | p-value | Contraception use | | p-value |
| | Yes | No | | Yes | No | |
| Age group | | | | | | < 0.01 |
| • 15–24 | 339 | 203 | | 580 | 280 | |
| • 25–29 | 454 | 297 | | 710 | 330 | |
| • 30–34 | 486 | 280 | < 0.01 | 834 | 522 | |
| • 35–39 | 530 | 320 | | 923 | 469 | |
| • 40–49 | 765 | 824 | | 880 | 1498 | |
| Residence | | | | | | |
| • Urban | 1564 | 1142 | 0.529 | 1170 | 684 | < 0.01 |
| • Rural | 1009 | 782 | | 2757 | 2433 | |
| Education level | | | | | | < 0.01 |
| • No education | 10 | 41 | | 443 | 633 | |
| • Primary | 355 | 337 | < 0.01 | 1820 | 1527 | |
| • Secondary | 1313 | 774 | | 1298 | 743 | |
| • Higher | 895 | 772 | | 366 | 194 | |
| Partner education level | | | | | | < 0.01 |
| • No education | 10 | 41 | | 429 | 634 | |
| • Primary | 355 | 337 | < 0.01 | 1595 | 1255 | |
| • Secondary | 1313 | 774 | | 1621 | 1068 | |
| • Higher | 895 | 772 | | 283 | 162 | |
| Socio-economic status | | | | | | < 0.01 |
| • Poorest | 398 | 381 | | 732 | 467 | |
| • Poorer | 494 | 281 | | 774 | 412 | |
| • Middle | 534 | 346 | < 0.01 | 765 | 391 | |
| • Richer | 610 | 412 | | 802 | 339 | |
| • Richest | 537 | 504 | | 854 | 314 | |
| Number of living children | | | | | | < 0.01 |
| • No children | 39 | 302 | | 266 | 430 | |
| • 1–3 | 1870 | 1154 | < 0.01 | 3088 | 1934 | |
| • More than 3 | 663 | 468 | | 573 | 755 | |
| Age at first marriage | | | | | | < 0.01 |
| • Below 20 | 1064 | 698 | | 1872 | 1450 | |
| • 20–25 | 1134 | 775 | < 0.01 | 1552 | 1122 | |
| • Above 25 | 374 | 451 | | 503 | 548 | |
| Working status | | | | | | 0.66 |
| • Employed | 1241 | 956 | 0.57 | 1381 | 1077 | |
| • Unemployed | 1332 | 968 | | 2546 | 2042 | |

other family planning methods in the country [56]. Further, media information related concerns about the side effects, health consequences, and inconvenience of methods might negatively influence demand and satisfaction on contraceptive usage. The unpleasant thoughts of side effects, method-related and health concerns might be reasons that may account for low patronage or possibly discontinuation of use [57, 58].

Although extensive research has been carried out on family planning, little or no study emphasizes the satisfied demands of women who have been exposed to mass media. However, few studies [18, 19] have documented

**Table 3** Chi-square test of the association between demand satisfied and confounders

| Variable | Philippines | | | Myanmar | | |
|---|---|---|---|---|---|---|
| | Demand satisfied | | *p*-value | Demand satisfied | | *p*-value |
| | Yes | No | | Yes | No | |
| Age group | | | | | | < 0.01 |
| • 15–24 | 339 | 190 | | 580 | 268 | |
| • 25–29 | 454 | 240 | | 710 | 313 | |
| • 30–34 | 486 | 188 | 0.04 | 834 | 414 | |
| • 35–39 | 530 | 172 | | 923 | 334 | |
| • 40–49 | 765 | 287 | | 880 | 594 | |
| Residence | | | | | | < 0.01 |
| • Urban | 1564 | 601 | 0.07 | 1170 | 403 | |
| • Rural | 1009 | 476 | | 2757 | 1520 | |
| Education level | | | | | | < 0.01 |
| • No education | 10 | 13 | | 443 | 375 | |
| • Primary | 355 | 200 | < 0.01 | 1820 | 895 | |
| • Secondary | 1313 | 438 | | 1298 | 515 | |
| • Higher | 895 | 426 | | 366 | 138 | |
| Partner education level | | | | | | < 0.01 |
| • No education | 23 | 22 | | 429 | 393 | |
| • Primary | 494 | 260 | < 0.01 | 1593 | 748 | |
| • Secondary | 1138 | 387 | | 1621 | 677 | |
| • Higher | 918 | 408 | | 283 | 106 | |
| Socio-economic status | | | | | | < 0.01 |
| • Poorest | 398 | 238 | | 732 | 467 | |
| • Poorer | 494 | 174 | | 774 | 412 | |
| • Middle | 534 | 203 | < 0.01 | 765 | 391 | |
| • Richer | 610 | 199 | | 802 | 339 | |
| • Richest | 537 | 263 | | 854 | 314 | |
| Number of living children | | | | | | < 0.01 |
| • No children | 39 | 165 | | 266 | 282 | |
| • 1-3 | 1870 | 663 | < 0.01 | 3088 | 1236 | |
| • More than 3 | 663 | 249 | | 573 | 405 | |
| Age at first marriage | | | | | | < 0.01 |
| • Below 20 | 1064 | 431 | | 1872 | 914 | |
| • 20–25 | 1134 | 415 | < 0.01 | 1552 | 676 | |
| • Above 25 | 374 | 230 | | 503 | 333 | |
| Working status | | | | | | 0.37 |
| • Employed | 1241 | 572 | 0.06 | 1381 | 704 | |
| • Unemployed | 1332 | 505 | | 2546 | 1219 | |

that women's exposure to media is one of the two important factors that influence contraceptive use and promote health-related behaviour such as reproductive preferences. Other studies that hold a similar view with the current study are earlier works of Hailemariam [20] at an individual level and those of Abulmageed [21] at a national level, which found a relationship between mass media exposure and reduction in fertility levels. Ultimately, this narrative holds the view that the use of mass media positively increases the awareness about the need for fertility control [59].

**Table 4** Chi-square test of the association between unmet need and confounders

| Variable | Philippines | | | Myanmar | | |
|---|---|---|---|---|---|---|
| | Unmet need | | p-value | Unmet need | | p-value |
| | Yes | No | | Yes | No | |
| Age group | | | | | | < 0.01 |
| • 15–24 | 89 | 439 | | 125 | 723 | |
| • 25–29 | 100 | 594 | | 156 | 867 | |
| • 30–34 | 97 | 577 | < 0.01 | 202 | 1046 | |
| • 35–39 | 87 | 615 | | 184 | 1073 | |
| • 40–49 | 233 | 818 | | 498 | 976 | |
| Residence | | | | | | < 0.01 |
| • Urban | 337 | 1829 | 0.20 | 246 | 1326 | |
| • Rural | 270 | 1214 | | 919 | 3359 | |
| Education level | | | | | | < 0.01 |
| • No education | 7 | 16 | | 261 | 557 | |
| • Primary | 128 | 427 | 0.01 | 570 | 2146 | |
| • Secondary | 261 | 1490 | | 283 | 1529 | |
| • Higher | 211 | 1110 | | 51 | 453 | |
| Partner education level | | | | | | < 0.01 |
| • No education | 13 | 31 | | 263 | 558 | |
| • Primary | 151 | 603 | 0.07 | 484 | 1858 | |
| • Secondary | 227 | 1298 | | 371 | 1926 | |
| • Higher | 216 | 1110 | | 47 | 342 | |
| Socio-economic status | | | | | | < 0.01 |
| • Poorest | 134 | 501 | | 292 | 907 | |
| • Poorer | 107 | 560 | | 247 | 939 | |
| • Middle | 122 | 615 | 0.08 | 232 | 924 | |
| • Richer | 104 | 705 | | 218 | 923 | |
| • Richest | 139 | 661 | | 176 | 992 | |
| Number of living children | | | | | | < 0.01 |
| • No children | 15 | 189 | | 59 | 489 | |
| • 1-3 | 385 | 2148 | < 0.01 | 778 | 3546 | |
| • More than 3 | 207 | 706 | | 328 | 650 | |
| Age at first marriage | | | | | | 0.001 |
| • Below 20 | 278 | 1217 | | 616 | 2170 | |
| • 20–25 | 231 | 1318 | 0.32 | 417 | 1811 | |
| • Above 25 | 97 | 508 | | 133 | 703 | |
| Working status | | | | | | 0.50 |
| • Employed | 324 | 1489 | 0.18 | 404 | 1681 | |
| • Unemployed | 283 | 1554 | | 762 | 3003 | |

This pioneering investigation of the effect of media exposure and family planning as an indicator of unmet needs for both Philippines and Myanmar, after adjusting for all the covariates, shows that media exposure has no significant effect on the unmet needs for both countries. However, this finding contradicts previous research [22, 23] that reported that exposure to newspaper/ magazine had a significant effect on unmet needs for family planning whereas those who had no information had a higher likelihood of their needs being unmet. The current finding is surprising because unmet needs for contraceptive and family planning methods is relatively higher in low-income developing countries like Philippines and Myanmar with low socio-economic indicators (e.g., poverty, low education) [60]. Therefore, in relatively low-income countries, the likelihood of few media establishments could restrict young people's capacity because of low media education or information related to accessing contraceptives or seeking sexual and reproductive health services [61, 62]. Besides, the growing trend of premarital sexual relationship and unintended pregnancies noted in many South-East Asian countries (e.g., Indonesia, Myanmar, Nepal, Pakistan, Philippines) requires a greater need for contraceptives among the sexually active population [41, 63]. Methodological variations and the type of media exposure studied in previous studies might account for the inconsistencies. The theoretical implication is that mass media communication campaigns are highly capable of influencing family planning methods in both countries.

### Strength and limitations

This study is the first to investigate the effect of mass media exposure on family planning indicators in Philippines and Myanmar. It also provides insights into the effects of media exposure on demand satisfaction on family planning methods and on unmet needs for both countries that previous studies have ignored. The study is not without some limitations. First, the use of the large DHS dataset from cross-sectional perspective restricts causality from the noted outcomes. Second, because of the research design used, the possibility of social desirability associated with self-reporting and recall bias from the respondents cannot be ruled out. Also, the effects of the type of mass media exposure of the sample were not captured in the current study. Other limitations might include the alterations in the coding of the study variables, which could potentially generate data extraction errors. However, no substantial modifications were done during coding and extraction within the current study [47]. Despite these limitations, the sample size allows for generalizability of findings in the studied countries because data used were nationally representative.

**Table 5** Association between media exposure and contraceptive use after adjusting for the covariates

| Variable | Philippines | | | | Myanmar | | | |
|---|---|---|---|---|---|---|---|---|
| | aOR | 95% CI | *P*-value | ROC curve | aOR | 95% CI | *P*-value | ROC curve |
| Media Exposure | | | | | | | | |
| • Yes | 2.27 | 1.45 -3.56 | < 0.001* | 68.2% | 1.39 | 1.15–1.67 | 0.001* | 69.7% |
| • No | Ref. | | | | Ref. | | | |

Note: Reference category of contraception use is 'No'
*CI* Confidence interval, *aOR* Adjusted odds ratio
*significant

**Table 6** Association between media exposure and demand satisfied regarding family planning after adjusting for covariates

| Variable | Philippines | | | | Myanmar | | | |
|---|---|---|---|---|---|---|---|---|
| | aOR | 95% CI | *P*-value | ROC curve | aOR | 95% CI | *P*-value | ROC curve |
| Media Exposure | | | | | | | | |
| • Yes | 2.15 | 1.41 -3.27 | < 0.001* | 65.5% | 1.34 | 1.09 –1.64 | 0.006* | 64.4% |
| • No | Ref. | | | | Ref. | | | |

Note: Reference category of demand satisfied is 'No'
*CI* Confidence interval, *aOR* Adjusted odds ratio
*significant

**Table 7** Association between media exposure and unmet need for family planning after adjusting for the covariates

| Variable | Philippines | | | | Myanmar | | | |
|---|---|---|---|---|---|---|---|---|
| | aOR | 95% CI | *P*-value | ROC curve | aOR | 95% CI | *P*-value | ROC curve |
| Media Exposure | | | | | | | | |
| • Yes | 0.79 | 0.55–1.15 | $0.23^{ns}$ | 60.6% | 0.87 | 0.72 –1.06 | $0.18^{ns}$ | 65.4% |
| • No | Ref. | | | | Ref. | | | |

Note: Reference category of unmet need is 'No'
*CI* Confidence interval, *aOR* Adjusted odds ratio, *ns* not significant

## Conclusions

The study established a strong association between mass media exposure and the use of contraceptive and family planning as well as demand satisfaction among the sexually active population in Philippines and Myanmar. Using mass media exposure (e.g., local radio, television-electronic; newspapers) to increase both access and usage of contraceptives as well as other family planning methods in these countries could be pivotal towards the attainment of United Nations Sustainable Development Goal 3 (MDG 3) of improving maternal health. Therefore, the dissemination of contraceptive use and other family planning information through media channels could help minimize neonatal and infant deaths, unsafe abortions, and maternal deaths often noticed in low-income countries like Philippines and Myanmar. Continuous education or advocacy on reproductive health matters (i.e., on contraception/ family planning) using the mass media could serve as a public health strategy for health-promoting behaviours. Public-private-sector partnership for the establishment of media houses in these countries is encouraged. Future studies could target the influence of the type of media exposure on contraception and/ or family planning methods possibly through longitudinal designs to establish clear patterns or trends for effective reproductive health interventions and policy direction.

### Abbreviations

NDHS: National Demographic and Health Survey; MDHS: Demographic and Health Survey; aOR: Adjusted odds ratio; CI: Confidence interval; SDG: Sustainable Development Goal; PSA: Philippine Statistics Authority

### Acknowledgments

We are grateful to MEASURE DHS for granting us free access to use the data for our study. We also appreciate the effort of Mr. Ebenezer Agbaglo, a budding linguist in the Department of English, University of Cape Coast, who took the pain to copyedit this manuscript.

### Authors' contributions

Conception and design of study: PD; analysis and/or interpretation of data: PD; drafting the manuscript: PD, NS, HA, TES, JEH, BOA and AS; revising the manuscript critically for important intellectual content; PD, NS, HA, TES, JEH, BOA and AS. All authors have read and approved the final manuscript.

### Authors' information

Department of Statistics, University of Dhaka, Bangladesh (PD); Department of Public Health, North South University, Bangladesh (NS); Institute of Social Welfare and Research, University of Dhaka, Bangladesh (HA); Bachelor of Science in Anatomy, University of Ilorin, Nigeria (TE); Department of Health, Physical Education, and Recreation, University of Cape Coast, Cape Coast, Ghana (JEH); Neurocognition and Action-Biomechanics-Research Group, Faculty of Psychology and Sport Sciences, Bielefeld University, Bielefeld-Germany (JEH), School of Public Health, Faculty of Health, University of Technology Sydney, Australia (BOA); Department of Population and Health, University of Cape Coast, Cape Coast, Ghana (AS); College of Public Health, Medical and Veterinary Sciences, James Cook University, Townsville, Queensland, Australia (AS).

### Author details

[1]Department of Statistics, University of Dhaka, Dhaka, Bangladesh. [2]Department of Public Health, North South University, Dhaka, Bangladesh. [3]Institute of Social Welfare and Research, University of Dhaka, Dhaka, Bangladesh. [4]Bachelor of Science in Anatomy, University of Ilorin, Ilorin, Nigeria. [5]Department of Health, Physical Education, and Recreation, University of Cape Coast, Cape Coast, Ghana. [6]Neurocognition and Action-Biomechanics-Research Group, Faculty of Psychology and Sport Sciences, Bielefeld University, Bielefeld, Germany. [7]School of Public Health, Faculty of Health, University of Technology Sydney, Ultimo, Australia. [8]Department of Population and Health, University of Cape Coast, Cape Coast, Ghana. [9]College of Public Health, Medical and Veterinary Sciences, James Cook University, Townsville, Queensland, Australia.

### References

1. Vijaykumar S. Communicating safe motherhood: strategic messaging in a globalized world. J Marriage Fam. 2008;44:2–3, 173-199. https://doi.org/10.1080/01494920802177378.
2. Naugle DA, Hornik RC. Systematic review of the effectiveness of mass media interventions for child survival in low- and middle-income countries. J Health Commun. 2014;19(sup1):190–215. https://doi.org/10.1080/10810730.2014.918217 PMID: 25207453; PMCID: PMC4205927.
3. World Family Planning Report. Department of Economic and Social Affairs. United Nations. 2017. Available at: un.org/en/development/desa/population/publications/pdf/family/WFP2017_Highlights.pdf
4. Alkema L, Kantorova V, Menozzi C, Biddlecom A. National, regional, and global rates and trends in contraceptive prevalence and unmet need for family planning between 1990 and 2015: a systematic and comprehensive analysis. Lancet. 2013;381(9878):1642–52. https://doi.org/10.1016/S0140-6736(12)62204-1 Epub 2013 Mar 12. PMID: 23489750.
5. Hu Y, Huang R, Ghose B, Tang S. SMS-based family planning communication and its association with modern contraception and maternal healthcare use in selected low-middle-income countries. BMC Med Inform Decis Mak. 2020;20(1):218. https://doi.org/10.1186/s12911-020-01228-5 PMID: 32912201; PMCID: PMC7488127.
6. Utami Ds NKAD, Wirawan DN, Ani LS. Sociodemographic factors and current contraceptive use among ever-married women of reproductive age: Analysis of the 2017 Indonesia Demographic and Health Survey data. J Prev Med Public Health. 2019;7(2):95–102. https://doi.org/10.15562/phpma.v7i2.211.
7. Ogini AB, Ahonsi BA, Adebajo S. Trend and determinants of unmet need for family planning services among currently married women and sexually active unmarried women aged 15–49 in Nigeria (2003—2013). Afr Popul Stud. 2015;29(1) Available at: http://aps.journals.ac.za/pub/article/view/694.
8. Chakraborty NM, Murphy C, Paudel M, Sharma S. Knowledge and perceptions of the intrauterine device among family planning providers in Nepal: a cross-sectional analysis by cadre and sector. BMC Health Serv Res. 2015;15:39. https://doi.org/10.1186/s12913-015-0701-y PMID: 25627578; PMCID: PMC4.
9. Majumder N, Ram F. Contraceptive use among poor and non-poor in Asian countries: a comparative study. Soc Sci Spectr. 2015;1(2):87–105 Available at: http://socialspectrum.in/index.php/sp/article/viewFile/13/10.
10. Ayanore MA, Pavlova M, Groot W. Unmet reproductive health needs among women in some West African countries: a systematic review of outcome measures and determinants. Reprod Health. 2016;13:–5. https://doi.org/10.1186/s12978-015-0104-x PMID: 26774502; PMCID: PMC4715869.
11. Bakht MB, Arif Z, Zafar S, Nawaz MA. Influence of media on contraceptive use: a cross-sectional study in four Asian countries. J Ayub Med Coll Abbottabad. 2013;25(3–4):3–8 PMID: 25226727.
12. Ansary R, Anisujjaman M. Factors determining pattern of unmet need for family planning in Uttar Pradesh, India. Int Res J Social Sci. 2012;1(4):16–23 Available at: http://researchgate.net/profile/Rabiul_Ansary/publication/299391064_Factors_Determining_Pattern_of_Unmet_Need_for_Family_Planning_in_Uttar_Pradesh_India/links/56f37c8908ae95e8b6cb5630/Factors-Determining-Pattern-of-Unmet-Need-for-Family-Planning-in-Uttar-Pradesh-India.pdf.
13. Khandeparkar K, Roy P, Motiani M. The effect of media exposure on contraceptive adoption across "poverty line". Int J Pharm Healthc Mark. 2015;9(3):219–36. https://doi.org/10.1108/IJPHM-06-2014-0034.

14. Chan N, Sawangdee Y, Pattaravanich U, et al. Birth cohorts, marriage patterns, and contraceptive methods used among women in contemporary Myanmar. J Health Res. 2020;34(3):209–19. https://doi.org/10.1108/JHR-06-2019-0127.
15. Thein SS, Thepthien B. Unmet need for family planning among Myanmar migrant women in Bangkok, Thailand. Br J Midwifery. 2020;28(3). https://doi.org/10.12968/bjom.2020.28.3.182.
16. Babalola S, Figueroa ME, Krenn S. Association of mass media communication with contraceptive use in sub-Saharan Africa: a meta-analysis of demographic and health surveys. J Health Commun. 2017;22(11): 885–95. https://doi.org/10.1080/10810730.2017.1373874 Epub 2017 Nov 10. PMID: 29.
17. Ajaero CK, Odimegwu C, Ajaero ID, Nwachukwu CA. Access to mass media messages, and use of family planning in Nigeria: a spatio-demographic analysis from the 2013 DHS. BMC Public Health. 2016;16: 427. https://doi.org/10.1186/s12889-016-2979-z PMID: 27220416; PMCID: PMC4877816.
18. Konkor I, Sano Y, Antabe R, Kansanga M, Luginaah I. Exposure to mass media family planning messages among post-delivery women in Nigeria: testing the structural influence model of health communication. Eur J Contracept Reprod Health Care. 2019;24(1):18–23. https://doi.org/10.1080/13625187.2018.1563679 Epub 2019 Feb 12. PMID: 30747544.
19. Ardiansyah B. Effect of mass media on family planning choices in Indonesia. Capstone Projects. 243. 2016. Available at: http://uknowledge.uky.edu/mpampp_etds/243.
20. Hailemariam A, Haddis F. Factors affecting unmet need for family planning in southern nations, nationalities and peoples region, Ethiopia. Ethiop J Health Sci. 2011;21(2):77–89. https://doi.org/10.4314/ejhs.v21i2.69048 PMID: 22434988; PMCID: PMC3275860.
21. Abulmageed SS, Elnimeiri MK. Sociodemographic and cultural determinants of seeking family planning knowledge and practice among a Sudanese community. Int J Community Med Public Health. 2018;5(8):3248–56. https://doi.org/10.18203/2394-6040.ijcmph20183053.
22. Min K T, Bhula R. Socioeconomic and demographic determinants of contraceptive use among currently married women in Myanmar. 2019. Available at: https://app.gs.kku.ac.th/gs/th/publicationfile/item/20th-ngrc-2019/HMO9/HMO9.pdf
23. Islam AZ, Mostofa MG, Islam MA. Factors affecting unmet need for contraception among currently married fecund young women in Bangladesh. Eur J Contracept Reprod Health Care. 2016;21(6):443–8. https://doi.org/10.1080/13625187.2016.1234034 Epub 2016 Sep 27. PMID: 27676285.
24. Lwin MM, Munsawaengsub C, Nanthamongkokchai S. Factors influencing family planning practice among reproductive age married women in Hlaing township, Myanmar. J Med Assoc Thail. 2013;96(Suppl 5):S98–106 PMID: 24851579.
25. Jirapongsuwan A, Latt KT, Siri S, Munsawaengsub C. Family planning practice among rural reproductive-age married women in Myanmar. Asia Pac J Public Health. 2016;28(4):303–12. https://doi.org/10.1177/1010539516645159 Epub 2016 Apr 27. PMID: 27122625.
26. Wai KM, Shibanuma A, Oo NN, Fillman TJ, Saw YM, Jimba M. Are husbands involving in their spouses' utilization of maternal care services?: A cross-sectional study in Yangon, Myanmar. PLoS One. 2015;10(12):e0144135. https://doi.org/10.1371/journal.pone.0144135 Erratum in: PLoS One. 2016; 11(3):e0151295. PMID: 26641891; PMCID: PMC4671588.
27. Kamal SM. Socioeconomic factors associated with contraceptive use and method choice in urban slums of Bangladesh. Asia Pac J Public Health. 2015;27(2):NP2661–76. https://doi.org/10.1177/1010539511421194 Epub 2011 Sep 13. PMID: 21914707.
28. Mon MM, Liabsuetrakul T. Predictors of contraceptive use among married youths and their husbands in a rural area of Myanmar. Asia Pac J Public Health. 2012;24(1):151–60. https://doi.org/10.1177/1010539510381918 Epub 2010 Sep 9. PMID: 20829275.
29. Colleran H, Mace R. Social network- and community-level influences on contraceptive use: evidence from rural Poland. Proc Biol Sci. 2015;282(1807): 20150398. https://doi.org/10.1098/rspb.2015.0398 PMID: 25904669; PMCID: PMC4424654.
30. Mutumba M, Wekesa E, Stephenson R. Community influences on modern contraceptive use among young women in low and middle-income countries: a cross-sectional multi-country analysis. BMC Public Health. 2018; 18(1):430. https://doi.org/10.1186/s12889-018-5331-y PMID: 29609567; PMCID: PMC5879615.
31. Soe K, Holland P, Mateus C. Association between maternal education and childhood mortalities in Myanmar. Asia Pac J Public Health. 2019;31(8):689–700. https://doi.org/10.1177/1010539519888299 Epub 2019 Nov 20. PMID: 31747773.
32. United Nation. World contraceptive use. 2011. Available at: http://www.un.org/esa/population/publications/contraceptive2011/any.pdf
33. Tin NK, Williamson J, Sonneveldt E. Setting the stage for strengthen annual monitoring of family planning program performance at the state/national level in Myanmar. 2019;3:154. https://doi.org/10.12688/gatesopenres.13012.2.
34. Ministry of health. Health in Myanmar, 2013. Naypyidaw: Ministry of Health; 2014.
35. Ministry of Immigration and Population. Summary of the provisional result. 2014. Available at: http://unstats.un.org/unsd/demographic/sources/census/2010_PHC/Myanmar/MMR-2015-05.pdf.
36. United Nation. Trends in contraception use worldwide 2015 (ST/ESA/SER.A/349). Available at: https://www.un.org/development/desa/pd/sites/www.un.org.development.desa.pd/files/undesa_pd_report_2015_trends_contraceptive_use.pdf. Accessed 20 Nov 2020.
37. Philippine Statistics Authority (PSA) and ICF. Philippines national demographic and health survey 2017: key indicators. Quezon City and Rockville: PSA and ICF; 2018. Available at: https://pdf.usaid.gov/pdf_docs/PBAAJ317.pdf
38. Nagai M, Bellizzi S, Murray J, Kitong J, Cabral EI, Sobel HL. Opportunities lost: Barriers to increasing the use of effective contraception in the Philippines. PLoS One. 2019;14(7):e0218187. https://doi.org/10.1371/journal.pone.0218187 PMID: 31344054; PMCID: PMC6657820.
39. Aung T, Hom NM, Sudhinaraset M. Increasing family planning in Myanmar: the role of the private sector and social franchise programs. BMC Womens Health. 2017;17(1):46. https://doi.org/10.1186/s12905-017-0400-4 PMID: 28668083; PMCID: PMC5493840.
40. Aung T, Thet MM, Sudhinaraset M, Diamond-Smith N. Impact of a social franchise intervention program on the adoption of long and short acting family planning methods in hard to reach communities in Myanmar. J Public Health (Oxf). 2019;41(1):192–200. https://doi.org/10.1093/pubmed/fdy005 PMID: 29538698; PMCID: PMC6459358.
41. Najafi-Sharjabad F, Zainiyah Syed Yahya S, Abdul Rahman H, Hanafiah Juni M, Abdul Manaf R. Barriers of modern contraceptive practices among Asian women: a mini literature review. Global J Health Sci. 2013;5(5):181–92. https://doi.org/10.5539/gjhs.v5n5p181 PMID: 23985120; PMCID: PMC4776867.
42. Miradora KG. Determinants of modern contraceptive use in the Philippines. Int J Pol Stu. 2017;8(1) Available at: researchgate.net/profile/Katrina_Miradora/publication/320444306_Determinants_of_Modern_Contraceptive_Use_in_the_Philippines/links/59e5d10d0f7e9b0e1ab25219/Determinants-of-Modern-Contraceptive-Use-in-the-Philippines.pdf.
43. Mello MM, Powlowski M, Nañagas JM, Bossert T. The role of law in public health: the case of family planning in the Philippines. Soc Sci Med. 2006; 63(2):384–96. https://doi.org/10.1016/j.socscimed.2006.01.010 Epub 2006 Feb 20. PMID: 16488063.
44. Gupta N, Katende C, Bessinger RE. Associations of mass media exposure with family planning attitudes and practices in Uganda. Stud Fam Plan. 2003;34(1):19–31. https://doi.org/10.1111/j.1728-4465.2003.00019.x.
45. Jacobs J, et al. Mass media exposure and modern contraceptive use among married west African adolescents. Eur J Contracept Reprod Health Care. 2017;22(6):439–49. https://doi.org/10.1080/13625187.2017.1409889.
46. Tiruneh FN, et al. Factors associated with contraceptive use and intention to use contraceptives among married women in Ethiopia. Women Health. 2016;56(1):1–22. https://doi.org/10.1080/03630242.2015.1074640.
47. Seidu AA, Hagan JE, Agbemavi W, Ahinkorah BO, Nartey EB, Budu E, et al. Not just numbers: Beyond counting caesarean deliveries to understanding their determinants in Ghana using a population based cross-sectional study. BMC Pregnancy Childbirth. 2020;20(1):1–10.
48. Nair S, Dixit A, Ghule M, Battala M, Gajanan V, Dasgupta A, Begum S, Averbach S, Donta B, Silverman J, Saggurti N. Health care providers' perspectives on delivering gender equity focused family planning program for young married couples in a cluster randomized controlled trial in rural Maharashtra, India. Gates Open Res. 2019;3.
49. Jensen R, Oster E. The power of TV: Cable television and women's status in India. Q J Econ. 2009;124(3):1057–94.
50. Mądra-Sawicka M, Nord JH, Paliszkiewicz J, Lee TR. Digital Media: Empowerment and Equality. Inform. 2020;11(4):225.

51. Leong C, Pan SL, Bahri S, Fauzi A. Social media empowerment in social movements: power activation and power accrual in digital activism. Eur J Inform Systems. 2019;28(2):173–204.
52. Servaes J, Malikhao P. Advocacy strategies for health communication. Public Relat Rev. 2010;36(1):42–9.
53. Aung MS, Soe PP, Moh MM. Predictors of modern contraceptive use and fertility preferences among men in Myanmar: further analysis of the 2015-16 demographic and health survey. Int J Community Med Public Health. 2019; 6(10):4209.
54. MacQuarrie KLD, Edmeades J, Steinhaus M, Head SK. Men and contraception: trends in attitudes and use, DHS analytical studies no.49. Rockville: ICF; 2015. Available at: https://www.popline.org/node/641293. Accessed on 10 May 2019
55. United States Agency for International Development. Essential considerations for engaging men and boys for improved family planning outcomes. Washington, D.C: Office of Population and Reproductive Health, Bureau for Global Health; 2018. Available at: https://www.usaid.gov/.../files/documents/1864/Engaging-men-boys-family-planning-508.pdf. Accessed on 10 May 2019
56. Tang K, Zhao Y, Li B, Zhang S, Lee SH. Health inequity on access to services in the ethic minorityregions of Northestern Myanmar: a cross-sectional study. BMJ. 2017;7:e017770.
57. Malik S, Courtney K. Higher education and women's empowerment in Pakistan. Gend Educ. 2011;23(1):29–45.
58. Claringbold L, Sanci L, Temple-Smith M. Factors influencing young women's contraceptive choices. Aust J Gen Pract. 2019;48(6):389.
59. Hornik R, McAnany E. Theories and evidence: mass media effects and fertility change. Commun Theory. 2001;11(4):454–71.
60. Wulifan JK, Brenner S, Jahn A, De Allegri M. A scoping review on determinants of unmet need for family planning among women of reproductive age in low and middle income countries. BMC women's health. 2015;16(1):1–5.
61. Chapagain M. Conjugal power relations and couples' participation in reproductive health decision-making: exploring the links in Nepal. Gend Techn Dev. 2006;10(2):159–89.
62. Landau SC, Tapias MP, McGhee BT. Birth control within reach: a national survey on women's attitudes toward and interest in pharmacy access to hormonal contraception. Contraception. 2006;74(6):463–70.
63. Wong LP. An exploration of knowledge, attitudes and behaviours of young multiethnic Muslim-majority society in Malaysia in relation to reproductive and premarital sexual practices. BMC Public Health. 2012;12(1):865 https://doi.org/10.1186/1471-2458-12-865.

# 3

# Dual contraceptive utilization and determinant factors among HIV positive women in Ethiopia

Alemu Degu Ayele[1*], Bekalu Getnet Kassa[1], Fentahun Yenealem Beyene[2], Dagne Addisu Sewyew[1] and Gedefaye Nibret Mihretie[1]

**Abstract**

**Background:** Dual contraceptive is the use of a barrier like condom along with any modern contraceptive methods which has double significance for the prevention STI including HIV and unintended pregnancy. The prevalence and determinants of dual contraceptive utilization described by different studies were highly inconsistent in Ethiopia. Therefore, this systematic review and meta-analysis aimed to estimate the pooled prevalence and determinants of dual contraceptive utilization among HIV positive women in Ethiopia.

**Methods:** International database mainly Pub Med, Google scholar, HINARI, EMBASE, Cochrane Library, AJOL was applied to identify original studies. STATA software version 14 was applied to analyze the pooled prevalence of dual contraceptive. $I^2$ test statistics was computed to check the presence of heterogeneity across the studies and eggers test was used to identify publication bias. The pooled prevalence of dual contraceptive utilization was estimated by using a random effects model. The associations between determinants and dual contraceptive utilization were evaluated by using both random and fixed effect models.

**Result:** A total 9 studies with 9168 HIV positive women were enrolled in this study. The pooled prevalence of dual contraceptive utilization among HIV positive women in Ethiopia was 26.14% (95% CI 21.20–31.08). Disclosure of HIV status (OR = 4.18,95%CI:2.26–7.72), partner involvement in post-test counselling (OR = 2.31,95%CI:1.63–3.25), open discussion about dual contraceptive with partner (OR = 4.27 95% CI:1.69–10.77), provision of counselling on dual contraceptives by health care provider (OR = 4.47,95% CI:3.81–5.24) and CD4 count > 350 cells/ $mm^3$ (OR = 3.87, 95%CI:3.53–4.23) were among the significant factors associated with dual contraceptive utilization.

(Continued on next page)

* Correspondence: degualemu53@gmail.com
[1]Department of Midwifery, College of Health Sciences, Debre Tabor University, Debre Tabor, Ethiopia

(Continued from previous page)

**Conclusion:** The overall prevalence of dual contraceptive utilization among HIV positive women was significantly low. Disclosure of HIV status, partner involvement in post-test counselling, open discussion about dual contraceptive with partner, counselling on dual contraceptive by health care provider and CD4 count > 350 cells/ $mm^3$ were positively affect dual contraceptive utilization. This study implies the need to develop plans and policies to improve partner involvement posttest counseling, integrate the counseling and provision of dual contraceptive at ART clinic at each level of health system.

**Keywords:** Dual contraceptive, Utilization, Determinants, Systematic review, Meta-analysis, Ethiopia

## Background

Human immune deficiency virus is the most common public health issue and continues to have disastrous multidimensional impacts on individuals, females, nations and the international community at large [1]. UNAIDS 2019 report, indicated that in the globe 37.9 million peoples were living with HIV, 1.7 million people became newly infected with HIV and around 770,000 people died from AIDS-related illnesses. In addition, an estimated number of 600 young women aged from 15 to 24 become infected by HIV. Among these new infections four out of five were from the sub-Saharan Africa [2]. This showed that the burden is highest in Sub Saharan Africa countries where, 60% of people reported to live with HIV/AIDS and more than half of them were females [3]. Likewise, Ethiopia is among the countries mostly affected by the HIV epidemic. According to the Ethiopian Demographic Health Survey (EDHS) 2016 report, the national adult HIV prevalence was 0.9% with women disproportionately infected, 1.2% compared to 0.6% in men [4].

Worldwide, due to poor contraceptive utilization and unsafe sex practices, greater than 2 million HIV positive women become pregnant every year, out of these, 600, 000 die due to pregnancy related complications [5]. Besides, unintended pregnancies responsible for 21.3% of new born HIV infections, 90% were from Sub Saharan African countries [6]. Ethiopia is among the sub-Saharan countries which is seriously affected by the epidemic with an estimated number of 24,000 HIV-positive pregnant women and 3800 new HIV infections among children in the 2016 [7].

HIV positive women can use most of the available contraceptive methods to limit and/or space their fertility including, hormonals, intra uterine device and sterilization. However, these methods do not protect against the transmission of both STIs/HIV between partners. At the same time, the efficacy of estrogen based hormonal contraceptive is also affected by drug to drug interaction with some Antiretroviral (ARV) drugs [8–10]. Due to these and other reasons HIV positive women needs barrier methods like condom in addition to the method the used to prevent unintended pregnancy.

Utilization of dual contraceptive is the use of two different methods, a barrier like condom along with any modern contraceptive methods which has double significance for those HIV positive women by preventing transmissions of STI including HIV and unintended pregnancy [11, 12].

In Ethiopia context different primary studies were conducted to estimate the prevalence of dual contraceptive utilization among HIV positive women [13–30] (Tewabe T, Abdanur A, Jenbere D, Ayehu M, Talema G: Contraceptive use and associated factors among sexually active HIV positive women attending ART clinic in FHRH in Bahir Dar, north west, Ethiopia. Facility based cross-sectional study. 2018. BMC Contraceptive and Reproductive Medicine Research Square Preprint current status, under review). These detached studies showed that prevalence of dual contraceptive utilization among HIV positive women in Ethiopia ranges from13.2% in University of Gondor Hospital Northwest Ethiopia [14] to 59.5 in West zone health facilities, Oromia Ethiopia [21]. From the reports of these studies there was a great variation and inconsistency related to prevalence of dual contraceptive utilization among HIV positive women throughout the country.

Women age, disclosure of HIV status to partner, partner involvement in post-test counselling, open discussion with partner on dual contraceptive use, provision of counseling on dual contraceptive by health care providers, having HIV negative partner and CD4 count were most frequently (twice and/or more) reported determinants of dual contraceptive utilization among HIV positive women in Ethiopia [13, 14, 18, 21, 24, 25, 28–30].

The reasons for the above variation in the prevalence and determinants of dual contraceptive utilization among Ethiopian HIV positive women's have not yet been investigated. Hence, it is important to have summarized evidence on the prevalence rate and determinant factors of dual contraceptive utilization among HIV positive women, as this helps the concerned bodies to identify existing gaps and propose supplementary strategies to increase the availability, accessibility and utilization of dual contraceptive in Ethiopia. Therefore, the aim of this study was to summarize the evidence of dual contraceptive utilization and determinant factors among HIV positive women in Ethiopia.

## Methods

### Study design and protocol

This study was a systemic review and meta-analysis of both published and unpublished relevant articles. The result of this meta-analysis was reported via systematic review and meta-analyses reporting PRISMA guidelines [31]. Protocol registration is not applicable in this systematic review and meta-analysis.

### Eligibility criteria

#### *Inclusion criteria*

**Study area** Only studies conducted in Ethiopia were included.

**Publication condition and period** Both published and unpublished articles from August 01 /2010 to August 01/ 2020 were considered.

**Study design** Cross-sectional studies which contain original data reporting the prevalence or/and determinants of dual contraceptive utilization was considered.

**Population** Studies on HIV positive women were considered.

#### *Exclusion criteria*

Studies without full content, anonymous reports, editorials, and qualitative studies were excluded. In addition, we exclude articles which were not fully accessed after we make contact with the primary author two times through email.

### Searching strategy and data source/data base

Major international databases such as PubMed, HINARI, EMBASE, Cochrane Library, Google Scholar, and African Journals Online databases were used to search relevant published studies. Google hand searching was also performed for unpublished studies.

The PECO (Population, Exposure, Comparison and Outcomes) search format has used this review to search pertinent studies.

#### *Population*

HIV positive women.

#### *Exposure*

Determinants of dual contraceptive utilization (socio-demographics such as age, educational status,) reproductive related factors (number of children, desire of future fertility, partner involvement in post -test counselling), health care and disease related factor (having HIV negative partner, disclosure of HIV status to partner, counseled about FP by health care provider, open discussion on dual contraceptive with partner).

#### *Comparison*

The reported reference groups for each determinant factor in each respective study such as, dual contraceptive utilization among HIV positive women who have open discussion with partner versus those who haven't open discussion, and dual contraceptive utilization among HIV positive women whose husband has involved in the post-test counselling versus their counterparts.

#### *Outcome*

Dual contraceptive utilization among HIV positive women.

Studies were searched exhaustively by 3 authors (AD, BG and FY) from international databases by using comprehensive searching strategies. Initially, pretested search strategies were developed to retrieve all pertinent studies. First, articles were searched by examining the full titles ("Dual contraceptive utilization and determinant factors among HIV positive women in Ethiopia") and then keywords ("dual contraceptive", "family planning"," "prevalence", magnitude, "determinants", "predictors", "associated factors", HIV positive", "reproductive age", "group," "women", and "Ethiopia"). These keywords were used independently and in combination using Boolean operators "OR" or "AND". Besides to this, studies were also searched from the reference lists of all included studies to find any other missed studies by our searching strategies. Furthermore, to find pertinent unpublished studies, Ethiopian universities digital libraries were searched (Addis Ababa University, University of Gondar and Haramiya University). The searching periods were from September 15, 2020 to October 15, 2020. Finally, all studies identified by our search strategy were imported and managed using Endnote X7 reference manager software (Additional file 1).

#### *Identification and study selection*

In the screening phase, three independent authors (AD, BG, FY) assessed the articles independently for inclusion and exclusion through a title, abstract and full review by using the search strategy. Any divergences and disagreement between three reviewers were managed by a discussion and consensus based on established criteria and if necessary, with the fourth and fifth authors (DA and GN). In the second phase of screening, those potentially eligible studies were undergoing full-text review to determine if they satisfy the predetermined inclusion criteria and assessed for duplicated records. When duplicate data were encountered, only the full-text article published was retained.

### Quality assessment

The scientific strength and quality of each incorporated original cross-sectional study was assessed by using the Newcastle-Ottawa Scale quality assessment tool adapted for cross-sectional study quality assessments [32]. The tool has three core components; the principal component of the tool graded from five stars and mainly emphasized on the methodological quality of each primary study. The second component of the tool graded from two stars and mainly concerns about the comparability of each study and the last component of the tool graded from three stars and used to assess the outcomes and statistical analysis of each original study. The quality of each original study was assessed by three authors independently using this tool. Disagreements between the three authors were resolved by the last two authors. Finally, the quality of the studies was weighed up based on these components. Overall, the quality of the eligible studies was moderate (Additional file 2).

#### *Data extraction*

All necessary data were extracted from 19 primary studies by three reviewers (AD, BG & FY) individually using pre tested standardized data extraction form. This form includes primary author, year of publication, study setting, sample size, study design, response rate, statistically significant factors, adjusted Odds ratio (AOR), 95% confidence interval, and covariance is considered. Uncertainties during the extraction process were resolved by logical consensus between the three authors and the final consensus was approved by the last two authors (DA and GN). In the case of incomplete data, we excluded the study or the parameter that was not available.

For the second objectives (determinants), the information extraction format was prepared for each specific determinant, i.e., women age, HIV status disclosure to partner, partner involvement in post-test counseling, open discussion with partner on dual contraceptive use, provision of counseling on dual contraceptive by health care providers, having HIV negative partner and CD4 count. In this study, variables were selected if at least two or more studies reported them as a significant factor.

### Outcome of interest

The primary outcome of this systematic and meta-analysis was the prevalence of dual contraceptive utilization among HIV positive Ethiopian women. The second objective of the review was to find out the determinants of dual contraceptive utilization.

### Publication bias and heterogeneity

To minimize the risk of bias comprehensive searches (electronic/database search and manual search) were used. Cooperative work of the authors was also critical in reducing bias, in selection of articles based on the clear objectives and eligibility criteria, deciding the quality of the article, in regularly evaluating the review process, and in extracting and compiling the data.

We examine publication bias with visual inspection of the funnel plot graph qualitatively. Besides, Egger's correlation tests at a 5% significant level were done to assess the presence of publication bias [33, 34]. Furthermore, to reduce the random variations among the point estimates of the primary study, subgroup analysis was done based on the study region, publication year and sample size. Heterogeneity across studies was evaluated using invers variance ($I^2$) statistics with its corresponding *p*-value using random effect model.

### Statistical analysis

To provide a comparable classification of the outcome and determinants of interest a Meta-analysis was performed for selected articles. The associated factors of dual contraceptive utilization were examined based on eligibility criteria. We had considered at least two studies were reported about one associated factors of dual contraceptive in common with their measure of effect and 95% confidence interval (CI). The significant association between factors affecting dual contraceptive utilization was estimated by calculating the effect size and 95% confidence interval (CI). Random effects model based on DerSimonian-Laird method was considered to assess for variations between the studies as well as within the studies. Data abstraction and analysis were done by using Microsoft Excel and STATA software version 14 respectively. The results were presented using texts, tables and forest plots with measures of effect and 95% confidence interval. Statistical heterogeneity was tested via the $I^2$ statistics at a $p$ value $\leq 0.05$ [35].

## Results

### Description of studies

Our literature search identified 669 primary studies by using medical electronic databases and other relevant sources searching mechanisms. Among the identified studies, 206 articles were removed after reviewing their titles due to duplication whereas 463 articles were allowed for further screening. Out of these 413 articles were removed due to irrelevance after being screened based on titles and abstracts. Then after the remaining 50 articles were assessed for eligibility and 31 of them were excluded due to inappropriate use of statistical analysis, irrelevant target population, inconsistent study

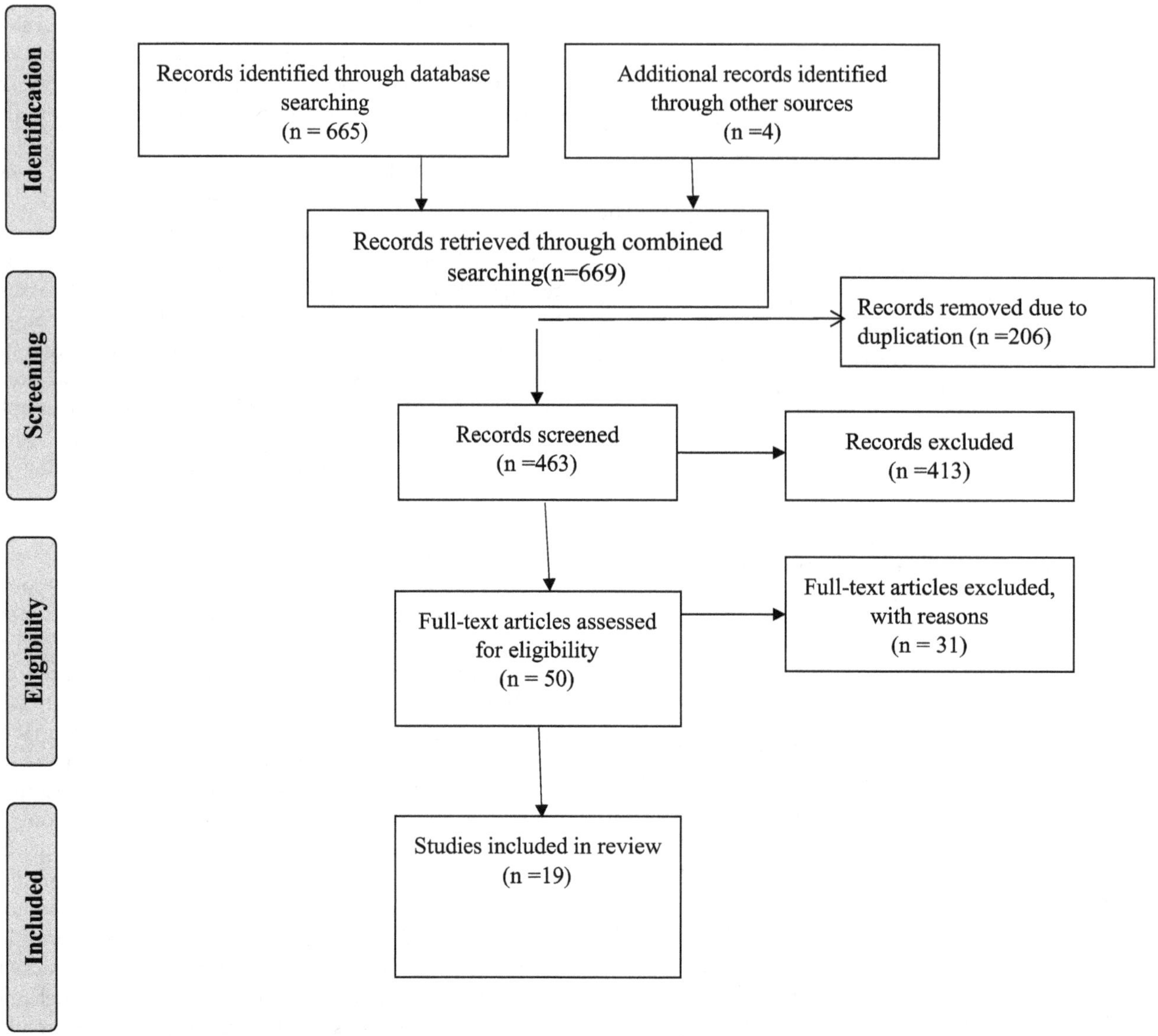


**Fig. 1** Flow chart describing the selection of studies for the systematic review and meta-analysis of prevalence and determinants of modern contraceptive utilization among HIV positive women's in Ethiopia, 2020

report, outcome of interest not reported, unavailability of full text and inconsistency with the predetermined inclusion criteria for the review. Finally, 19 articles were included in the systematic review and meta-analysis (Fig. 1).

### Characteristics of the included studies

All the 19 studies eligible for the current systematic review and meta-analysis were cross-sectional by study design, reported with English and conducted from 2013 to 220. The sample size ranges from 243 in Gebretsadik Shawo Hospital, found in South Nation Nationalities and peoples representatives (SNNPR), South West Ethiopia [30] to 1418 in Addis Ababa [17]. In this systematic review and meta-analysis, a total of 9168 HIV positive women were enrolled to estimate the pooled prevalence of dual contraceptive use. Regarding to geographical distribution of studies, six studies were from Oromia [18–23], five studies were from Amhara [13–16] (Tewabe T, Abdanur A, Jenbere D, Ayehu M, Talema G: Contraceptive use and associated factors among sexually active HIV positive women attending ART clinic in FHRH in Bahir Dar, north west, Ethiopia. Facility based cross-sectional study. 2018. BMC Contraceptive and Reproductive Medicine Research Square Preprint current status, under review), four studies from Tigray [24–27], two from SNNP [29, 30], one study from Addis Ababa [17] and one from Benishangul Gumuze [28]. The highest and lowest prevalence of dual contraceptive utilization were 59.5 and 13.2% respectively. In addition,

**Table 1** Characteristics of included primary studies showing dual contraceptive utilization and determinants among HIV positive women in Ethiopia, systematic review and meta-analysis, 2020

| Authors | Year of publication | Region | Study design | Sample size | Response rate (%) | Prevalence (95%CI) | Quality |
|---|---|---|---|---|---|---|---|
| Abay et al. [13] | 2020 | Amhara | C/S | 563 | 98 | 28.8 (26.83,30.77) | Low risk |
| Reta et al. [14] | 2019 | Amhara | C/S | 619 | 98.25 | 13.2 (11.72,14.68) | Low risk |
| Kebede et al. [15] | 2015 | Amhara | C/S | 420 | 99.04 | 26.7 (24.77,28.63) | Low risk |
| Egzeabher et al. [16] | 2015 | Amhara | C/S | 335 | 98.5 | 19 (17.29,20.71) | Low risk |
| Tewabe et al. | 2018 | Amhara | C/S | 308 | 100 | 26 (24.09,27.91) | Low risk |
| Asfaw et al. [17] | 2014 | AA | C/S | 1418 | 100 | 18 (16.32,19.68) | Low risk |
| Demissie et al. [18] | 2015 | Oromia | C/S | 357 | 100 | 32 (29.96,34.04) | Low risk |
| Sufa et al. [19] | 2013 | Oromia | C/S | 461 | 98.9 | 22.4 (20.58,24.22) | Low risk |
| Polis et al. [20] | 2014 | Oromia | C/S | 395 | 93.2 | 17 (15.36,18.64) | Low risk |
| Dereje et al. [21] | 2019 | Oromia | C/S | 323 | 94.1 | 59.5 (57.36,61.64) | Low risk |
| Feyissa et al. [22] | 2020 | Oromia | C/S | 360 | 100 | 17 (15.36,18.64) | Low risk |
| Tesfaye et al. [23] | 2014 | Oromia | C/S | 403 | 99.5 | 31.9 (29.86,33.94) | Low risk |
| Gebrehiwot et al [24] | 2017 | Tigray | C/S | 331 | 97.9 | 15.7 (14.11,17.29) | Low risk |
| Kalayu [25] | 2019 | Tigray | C/S | 632 | 100 | 45.2 (43.03,47.37) | Low risk |
| Melaku et al. [26] | 2014 | Tigray | C/S | 964 | 100 | 14 (12.48,15.52) | Low risk |
| Berhane.et al. [27] | 2013 | Tigray | C/S | 364 | 99.2 | 21.6 (19.80,23.40) | Low risk |
| Assefa et al. [28] | 2014 | Benishangul | C/S | 404 | 100 | 40.9 (38.75,43.06) | Low risk |
| Markos et al. [29] | 2019 | SNNP | C/S | 269 | 95.9 | 28.3 (26.34,30.26) | Low risk |
| Meseret et al. [30] | 2015 | SNNP | C/S | 243 | 98.78 | 19.8 (18.06,21.54) | Low risk |

*AA* Addis Ababa, *SNNP* Southern Nations Nationalities Peoples, *C/S* Cross-sectional

the response rate of the primary studies incorporated in the current study range from 93.2 to 100%. Among the 19 included studies 17 of them were published articles in reputable journal while two of them [25] (Tewabe T, Abdanur A, Jenbere D, Ayehu M, Talema G: Contraceptive use and associated factors among sexually active HIV positive women attending ART clinic in FHRH in Bahir Dar, north west, Ethiopia. Facility based cross-sectional study. 2018. BMC Contraceptive and Reproductive Medicine Research Square Preprint current status, under review) were repository articles (Table 1). Lastly, the primary studies included in the present systematic review and meta-analysis had a quality score of 6–9 out of 10 points (Additional file 2).

#### Dual contraceptive utilization

The overall pooled prevalence of dual contraceptive utilization among HIV positive women in Ethiopia was 26.14% (95% CI 21.20–31.08) (Fig. 2).

#### Heterogeneity and publication bias

According to the finding of this study there was a markedly high heterogeneity across the studies as evidenced by $I^2$ statistics ($I^2$ = 99.3%, $P \leq 0.001$). Due to this random effect model meta-analysis was applicable to determine the pooled prevalence of dual contraceptive utilization among HIV positive women in Ethiopia.

Publication biases among the included studies were examined by using both funnel plots and egger's regression test. The results of funnel plots showed an asymmetric shape, which indicates the presence of publication bias among those included studies (Fig. 3a). Objective assessments of publication bias by egger's regression test also showed the presence of publication bias across studies (*p*-value < 0.001). The Duval and Tweedie nonparametric trim and fill analysis were done to correct publication bias among the studies. Accordingly, publication bias was corrected when six missed studies were filled in the funnel plot by trim and fill analysis After six studies were filled, a total of 25 studies were included and computed via the trim and fill analysis to produce the pooled prevalence of 19.519% (95% CI, 13.744–25.294) by applying random effect model (Fig. 3b).

#### Sensitivity analysis

In the current meta-analysis, in order to determine the potential source of heterogeneity seen in the pooled prevalence of dual contraceptive utilization, the investigators performed a leave-one-out sensitivity analysis. The result of the sensitivity analysis indicated that the finding was not relay on a particular study. The pooled prevalence of dual contraceptive utilization was varied and ranges from 24.28% (20.37–28.18%) to 26.86% (21.79–31.92%) after deletion of six studies (Table 2).

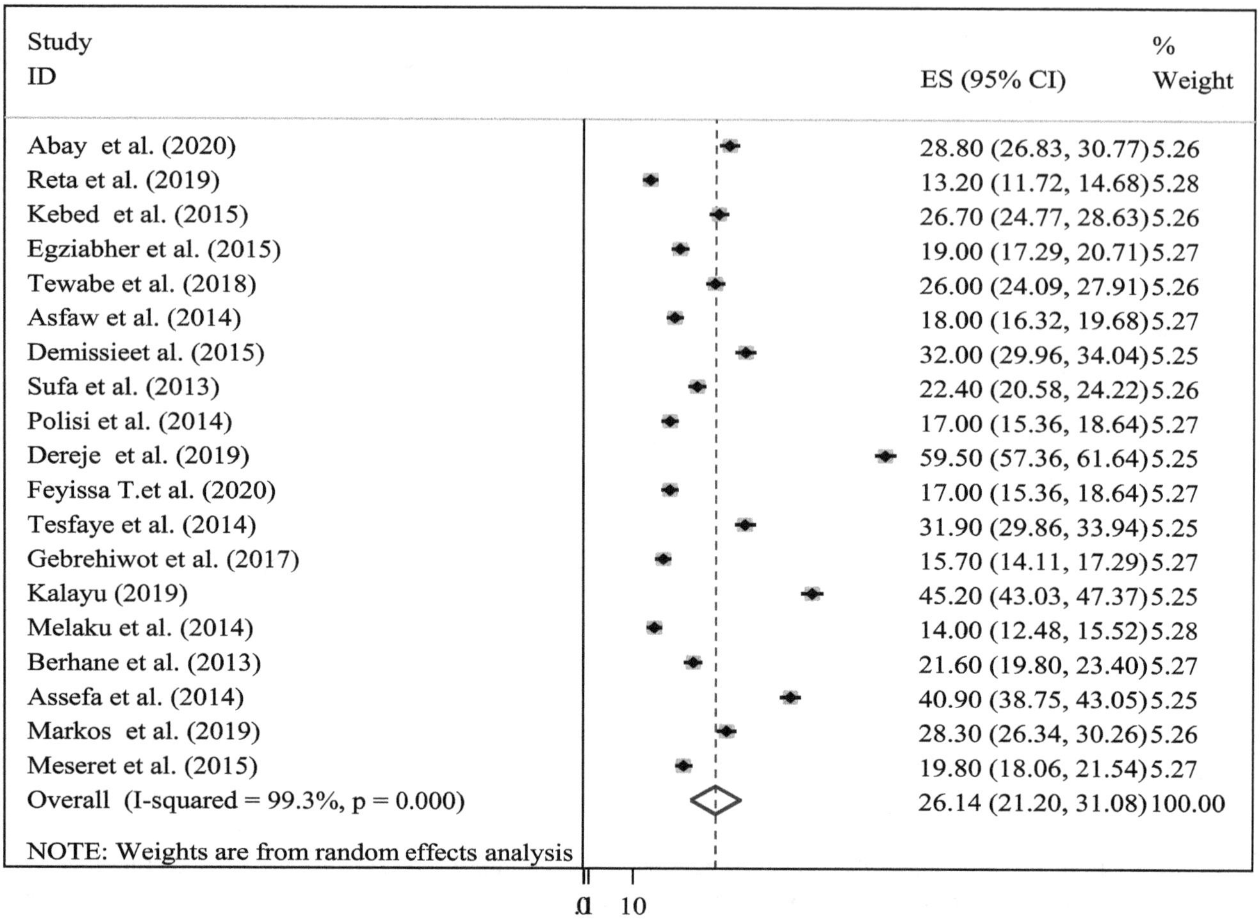


**Fig. 2** Forest plot of the pooled prevalence of dual contraceptive use among HIV positive women in Ethiopia, 2020

#### Subgroup analysis

We performed a subgroup analysis based on the region where the primary studies were done. As a result, the largest prevalence was observed in Oromia with a prevalence of 29.96% (95%CI, 17.98–41.93) and lowest in Amhara with prevalence of 22.72% (95%CI, 16.66–28.78). In addition, subgroup analysis was also checked by publication year and those studies published from 2019 to 2020 has the highest prevalence, 31.99(18.31–45.67) while, studies published from 2016 to 2018 has the lowest pooled prevalence 20.84(10.74–30.93). Lastly, we also executed subgroup analysis using sample size (< 400 and > 400) of the primary studies. The outcome of this subgroup analysis revealed that studies done with sample size of greater than 400 26.77% (95% CI, 19.60–33.94) were slightly higher in utilization of dual contraceptive compared to those studies done with sample size of greater than 400, 25.58(18.38–32.77) (Table 3).

#### Determinants of dual contraceptive utilization

The finding of this systematic review and meta-analysis revealed that dual contraceptive utilization among HIV positive women in Ethiopia were significantly associated with disclosure of HIV status to partner, partner involvement in post-test counselling, open discussion about dual contraceptive with partner, provision of counseling on dual contraceptive by health care providers, CD4 count >350cells/dl whereas having HIV negative partner is mentioned as a determinant factor for dual contraceptive use.

According to this study two primary articles identified that partner involvement in post-test counselling was significantly associated with dual contraceptive utilization [14, 28]. Those women whose partner was involved in the post-test counseling were 2.31 times (OR = 2.31,95%CI: 1.63, 3.25) more likely to use dual contraceptive than those women whose husband was not participated in the post-test counselling. Heterogeneity test indicated $I^2$ = 39.8%, hence random effect model was applicable for analysis (Fig. 4).

Based on the finding of the current study four primary studies showed that disclosure of HIV status to partner were significantly associated with dual contraceptive utilization [13, 21, 24, 28]. The odds of utilizing dual contraceptive methods were four times

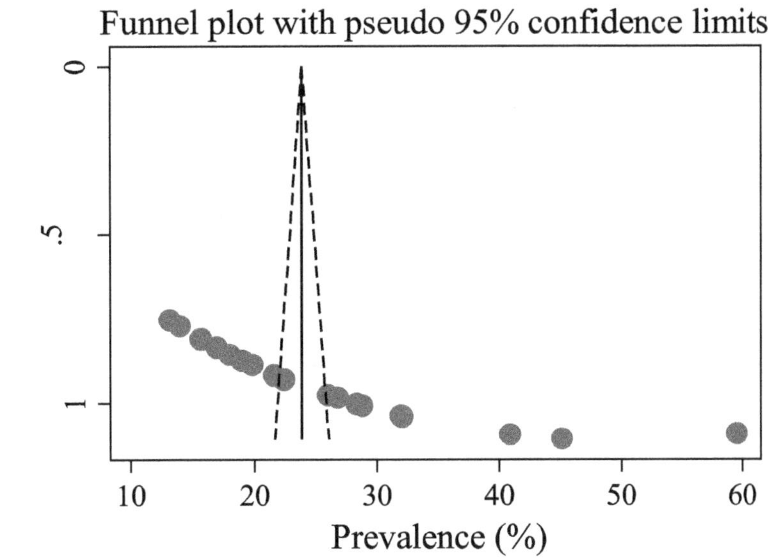


a

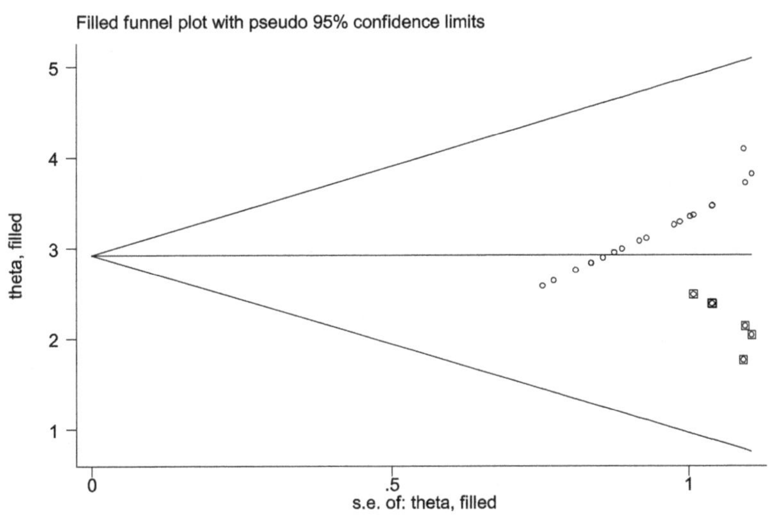


(b)

**Fig. 3** **a** Funnel plot to test publication bias of 19 studies. **b** Result of trim and fill analysis for adjusting publication bias of the 25 studies

(OR = 4.18,95%CI:2.26–7.72) higher among those who disclose their HIV status to their husband as compared to their counterparts. Since the heterogeneity test showed $I^2 = 51.7\%$ we used random effect model for analysis (Fig. 5).

Moreover, six primary studies also reported that open discussion on the issue dual contraceptive with partner was strongly associated with dual contraceptive use [14, 21, 24, 25, 28, 30]. HIV positive women who has open discussion on the issue of dual contraceptive use with their partner were 4.27 times (OR = 4.27, 95% CI:1.69–10.77) higher the odds of utilizing dual contraceptive as compared to those women who has no open discussion. Marked heterogeneity was observed across the studies (I -squared = 96.3%). As a result, random effect model analysis was used to assess the association between two variables (Fig. 6).

The result of this systematic review and meta-analysis concluded that getting counseling about dual contraceptive use by health care provider was another

**Table 2** Sensitivity analysis of the prevalence of dual contraceptive utilization among HIV positive women in Ethiopia 2020

| Study omitted | Prevalence (%) | 95%CI |
|---|---|---|
| Abay et al. (2020) [13] | 25.99 | 20.82–31.16 |
| Reta et al. (2019) [14] | 26.86 | 21.79–31.95 |
| Kebede et al. (2015) [15] | 26.11 | 20.92–31.30 |
| Egzeabher et al. (2015) [16] | 26.54 | 21.34–31.74 |
| Tewabe et al. (2018) | 26.15 | 20.95–31.35 |
| Asfaw et al. (2014) [17] | 26.59 | 21.40–31.78 |
| Demissie et al. (2015) [18] | 25.81 | 20.69–30.93 |
| Sufa et al. (2013) [19] | 26.35 | 21.13–31.56 |
| Polis et al. (2014) [20] | 26.65 | 21.47–31.82 |
| Dereje (2019) [21] | 24.28 | 20.37–28.18 |
| Feyissa et al. (2020) [22] | 26.65 | 21.47–31.82 |
| Tesfaye et al. (2014) [23] | 25.82 | 20.69–30.94 |
| Gebrehiwot et al. (2017) [24] | 26.72 | 21.57–31.87 |
| Kalayu (2019) [25] | 25.08 | 20.31–29.85 |
| Melaku et al. (2014) [26] | 26.81 | 21.72–31.91 |
| Berhane et al. (2013) [27] | 26.39 | 21.17–31.60 |
| Assefa et al. (2014) [28] | 25.32 | 20.40–30.23 |
| Markos et al. (2019) [29] | 26.02 | 20.84–31.19 |
| Meseret et al. (2015) [30] | 26.49 | 21.28–31.70 |

significant predictor of dual contraceptive use as mentioned by five primary studies [14, 21, 24, 28, 29]. The likely hood of using dual contraceptive methods in HIV positive women who has got counseling on dual method use by health care provider was 4.47 times (OR = 4.47,95% CI:3.81–5.24) higher than their counterparts. The heterogeneity test showed an I value of 0.0%, hence, we used fixed effect model for analysis (Fig. 7).

Finally, the association between dual contraceptive utilization and CD4 count was evaluated by using 2 studies [28, 30]. Dual contraceptive utilization was significantly associated with CD4 count, mentioned in two primary studies. HIV positive women who has CD4 count of > 350 cells/ $mm^3$ were almost four times (OR = 3.87,95%CI: 3.53–4.23) higher the odds of utilizing dual contraceptive methods as compared to women who has CD4 count of < 250. The investigators used a fixed effect model for the analysis because the $I^2$value was 0.0% (Fig. 8).

## Discussion

The hall mark of utilizing dual contraceptive methods includes the prevention of both unintended pregnancy and HIV transmission. It also has an added benefit in reducing the number of unsafe abortion and getting HIV free generation and as large improving the health status of the community. Hence, the current systematic review and meta-analysis is aimed to estimate the pooled prevalence of dual contraceptive utilization and its determinants among HIV positive women in Ethiopia. According to this meta-analysis, the pooled prevalence of dual contraceptive utilization among HIV positive women in Ethiopia was 26.14% (95% CI:21.20–31.08). This indicates that almost one from four women has been utilize dual contraceptive methods. The finding of this study was in lined with a multinational study done on African women (23.5%) [36], Sub-Saharan Africa (31%) [37], India (29.9%) [38], Malawi (26.5%) [39]. On the other hand, the finding of this study is lower than a survey conducted in USA (39%) [12]. This might be due to socio-demographic differences. Furthermore, the finding is lower than a survey done in Cameron (33.3%) [40], South Africa (33%) [41], Kenya (38.5%) [42]. This discrepancy might be due to the differences in women's negotiation ability to use condom as additional contraceptives due to socio cultural impact, respondents' level

**Table 3** Subgroup analysis of dual contraceptive utilization among HIV positive women in Ethiopia

| Variables | Characteristics | Included studies | Number of study participants | Prevalence (95% CI) | $I^2$(%), *P-value* |
|---|---|---|---|---|---|
| Region | Amhara | 5 | 2245 | 22.72 (16.66–28.78) | 98.3, < 0.001 |
| | Oromia | 6 | 2299 | 29.96 (17.98–41.93) | 99.6, < 0.001 |
| | A. A | 1 | 1418 | 18.00 (16.32–19.63) | – |
| | Tigray | 4 | 2291 | 24.11 (11.79–36.42) | 99.5, < 0.001 |
| | Benishangul | 1 | 403 | 40.90 (38.75–43.05) | – |
| | SNNP | 2 | 512 | 24.04 (15.71–32.37) | 97.5, < 0.001 |
| Sample size | ≤400 | 10 | 3285 | 25.58 (18.38–32.77) | 99.4, < 0.001 |
| | > 400 | 9 | ,5883 | 26.77 (19.60–33.94) | 99.3, < 0.001 |
| Year of publication | 2013–2015 | 11 | 5763 | 23.91 (19.43–28.40) | 98.5, < 0.001 |
| | 2016–2018 | 2 | 639 | 20.84 (10.74–30.93) | 98.5, < 0.001 |
| | 2019–2020 | 6 | 2766 | 31.99 (18.31–45.67) | 99.7, < 0.001 |
| Overall | | 19 | 9168 | 26.14 (21.20–31.08) | 99.3, < 0.001 |

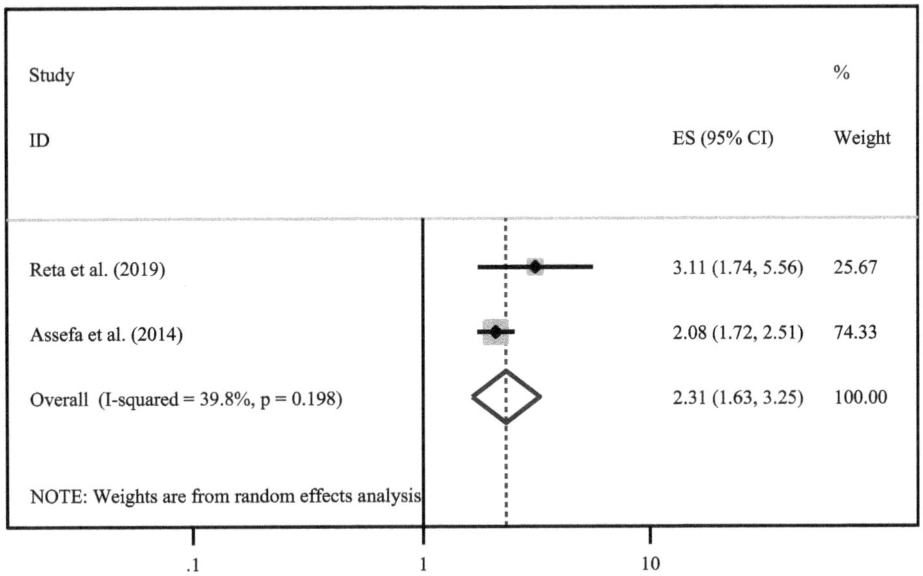


**Fig. 4** Association between partner involvment in post-test counseling with dual contraceptive utilization

of knowledge about unique benefit of using dual contraceptive methods other than preventing unintended pregnancy, availability of dual contraceptives and level of partner involvement between Ethiopia and across the respective countries.

However, the current pooled prevalence is higher than a survey performed in Zambia (17.7%) [43], Togo16.9% [44] South Malawi (18.9%) [45]. The possible explanation might be partly as a result of difference in socio-cultural parameters, study setting, time gaps of the primary studies conducted in the comparable countries. Nowadays the government of Ethiopia is highly committed in expanding of family planning programs including condom distribution that might be positively affect dual contraceptive.

In the present study we found significant dual contraceptive utilization among HIV positive women whose partner was involved in post-test counselling. Women whose partners were involved in post-test counselling were more likely to utilize dual contraceptives as

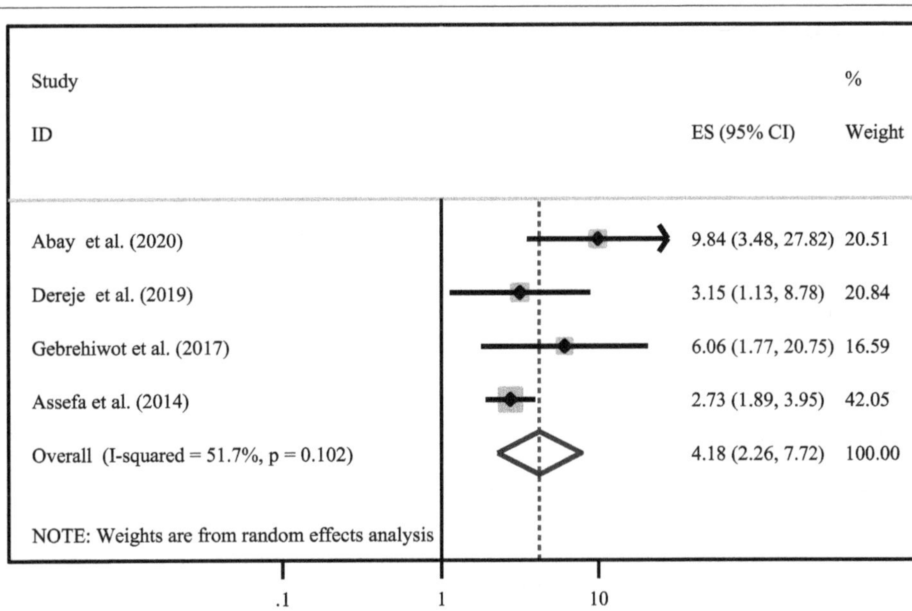


**Fig. 5** Association between disclosure HIV status to partner with dual contraceptive utilization. Moreover, six primary studies also reported that open discussion on the issue dual contraceptive

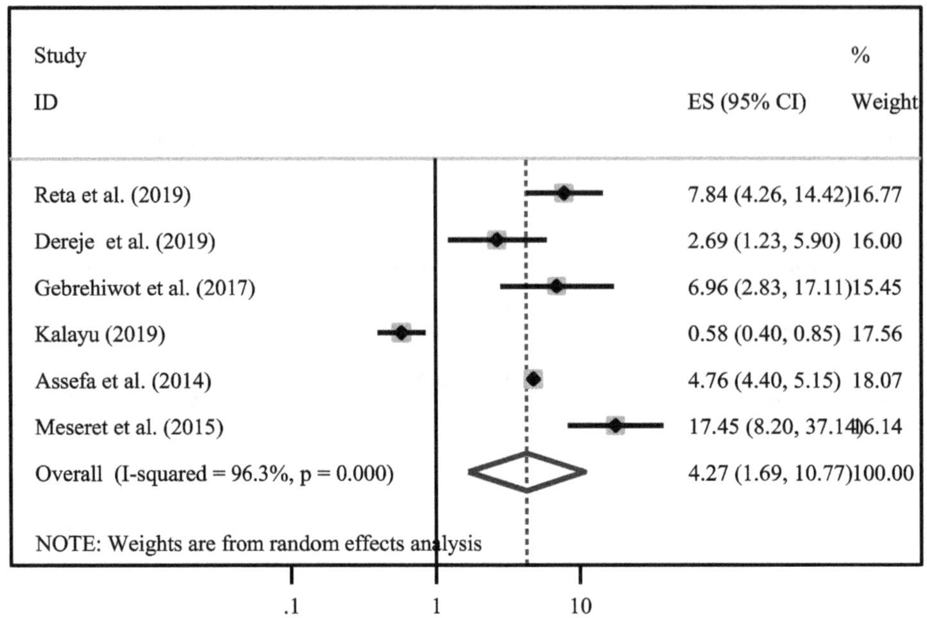


**Fig. 6** Association between open discussion about dual contraceptive with partner and utilization of it

compared to their counterparts. The finding is in agreement with study done in India [38]. This may be the reflection of involving partner in testing and counselling process help both of them to have open discussion in selecting the preferred contraceptive they utilize. The other reason might be now a day in Ethiopia, male partner involvement in the prevention of mother to child transmission of HIV/AIDS and related reproductive health services become highly advocated and exercised to scale up dual contraceptive utilization which eventually reduce the burden of both unintended pregnancy and HIV/AIDS.

In addition, women who have open discussion with partner regarding to dual contraceptive utilization increase the odds of utilizing dual contraceptives as compared to women who have not open discussed with their partner. This is in agreement with study conducted in India [46], south Africa [47], Tanzania [48], Northern Uganda [49]. Open discussion with partner may

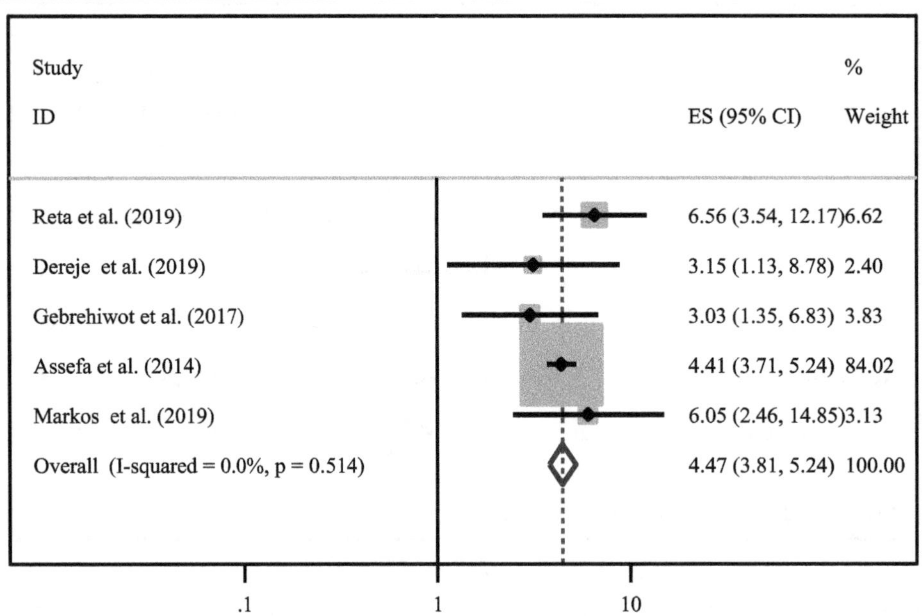


**Fig. 7** Association between provision of counseling on dual contraceptive by health care providers and utilization of it

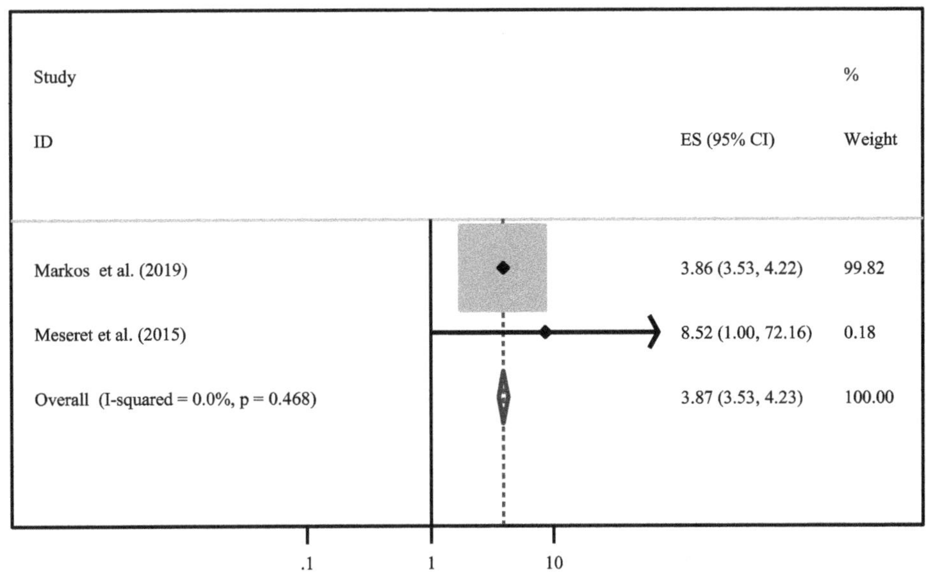


**Fig. 8** Association between CD4 count with dual contraceptive utilization

empower women to make informed decision on fertility and contraceptive options, inspire to disclose their HIV status and general speaking it play an important role to manage life very simply. In addition, open discussion may increase women's freedom to negotiate male partner in decision of limiting or spacing number of births and safer sex practice. Furthermore, in the majority of our community male partner plays a great role in decision making role either to support or prohibit the use of dual contraceptive thus open discussion is crucial to minimize/eliminate challenges encounter in using condom consistently and correctly in each sexual activity.

According to the finding of current meta-analysis, disclosing of HIV status to male partner is another crucial to scale up utilization of dual contraceptives. This is consistent with a study conducted in Kenya [42], Uganda [50], Lusaka Zambia [51]. This might be due to the fact that stigma/discrimination and misconception-related HIV/AIDS was reduced due to community awareness and higher partner care which leads HIV positive women to disclose their status to their partner. Moreover, HIV status disclosure is imperative to get support and facilitates open discussion with male partner in regard to safer sex practice. Disclosing HIV status also help the women to have common understanding regarding to the importance of dual contraceptives utilization and help to reach an agreement to utilize it.

Moreover, provision of counseling on dual contraceptive utilization by health care providers were significantly associated with utilization of them. Our finding is consistent with a study finding from Kenya [42], Tanzania [48], Zambia [43], Northern Uganda [49]. This might be due to provision of counseling empowers and allows women to make informed decision which may increase the uptake of dual methods. Counseling also offers information regarding to the importance of safer sex, build self-efficacy, and negotiation skills on consistent and correct use of condoms. On the other hand, counseling and providing of reproductive health interventions may have a positive influence on minimizing unmet need for dual contraceptive utilization.

Once more, the current meta-analysis finding showed that women who had CD4 count > 350 cells/ $mm^3$ were more likely to use dual methods than women with CD4 count < 250 cells/ $mm^3$. This was supported by study done in Zambia [43]. On the contrary this finding was inconsistent from study finding from India [38]. Perhaps this might be those women who have higher number of CD4 count may either have children or no farther intention for future fertility which might increase the use of dual methods.

### Limitation

This systematic review and meta-analysis have some limitations. All of the studies included in this systematic review and meta-analysis were cross-sectional in nature; as a result, the outcome variable might be affected by other confounding variables. Beside to this, some of the studies enrolled in the in this systematic review and meta-analysis had small sample size, which may affect the actual magnitude of utilization at the country level. Furthermore, all regions in Ethiopia were not represented in this systematic review and meta-analysis due to limited number of studies in the country (only five regions and one administrative town were represented in this study). As a result, the finding of this systematic review and meta-analysis may not exactly indicate the national prevalence of dual contraceptive utilization.

## Conclusion

The overall prevalence of dual contraceptive utilization among HIV positive women was significantly low in Ethiopia. Male partner involvement in post-test counselling, disclosure of HIV status to partner, open discussion about dual contraceptive with partner, provision of counselling on dual contraceptive and CD4 counts were found to be predictors of dual contraceptive. This study implies the need to develop plans and policies to improve male partner involvement during post-test counseling and provision of counseling on dual contraceptive at each level of health system. Besides to this, improving disclosure of HIV status to male partner and open discussion about dual contraceptive with partner were recommended.

#### Abbreviations

AIDIS: Acquired Immune Deficiency Syndromes; HIV: Human Immune Virus; FP: Family Planning; WHO: World Health Organization

#### Acknowledgements

Not applicable.

#### Authors' contributions

AD, BG, and FY inception and designed the review. AD, BG, and FY developed the search strings and select studies. DA and GN evaluated the quality of the articles. AD, DA and FY performed analysis and interpretation. AD and DA prepared the draft of the manuscript. All authors read and approved the final paper.

#### Author details

[1]Department of Midwifery, College of Health Sciences, Debre Tabor University, Debre Tabor, Ethiopia. [2]Department of Midwifery, College of Medicine and Health Sciences, Bahir Dar University, Bahir Dar, Ethiopia.

#### References

1. UNAIDS WHO. Global summary of AIDS epidemic report. Geneva: WHO; 2007. p. 23–5.
2. UNAIDS, Global HIV & AIDS statistics — 2019 fact sheet, 2019, https://www.unaids.org/en/resources/fact-sheet.
3. UNAIDS, AIDS. Epidemic update in united nation joint programme on HIV/AIDS. Geneva: WHO/UNAIDS; 2011.
4. Central Statistical Agency (CSA) [Ethiopia] and ICF. Ethiopia demographic and health survey 2016: HIV report. Addis Ababa and Rockville: CSA and ICF; 2018.
5. Collins L, Doupe A.Preventing HIV and unintended pregnancies: strategic framework 2011–2015; 2011.
6. Joint United Nations Programme on HIV/AIDS (UNAIDs). The gap report: Children and pregnant womenliving with HIV. 2015.
7. UNAIDS AIDS info, HIV and AIDS estimates. Country factsheets, Ethiopia. 2016. Available at https://www.unaids.org/sites/default/files/media_asset/2016-AIDS-data_en.pdf.
8. Agboghoroma CO. Contraception in the context of HIV/AIDS. Afr J Reprod Health. 2011;15(3):15–23.
9. Trussell J. Choosing a contraceptive: efficacy, safety, and personal considerations. In: Hatcher RA, Trussell J, Nelson AL, Cates Jr W, Stewart FH, Kowal D, editors. Contraceptive technology. 19th ed. New York: Ardent Media; 2008.
10. Cates W Jr, Steiner MJ. Dual protection against unintended pregnancy and sexually transmitted infections: what is the best contraceptive approach? Sex Transm Dis. 2002;29(3):168–74. https://doi.org/10.1097/00007435-200203000-00007.
11. Dual protection against unwanted pregnancy and HIV / STDs. Sex Health Exch. 1998;(3):8.
12. Wilson TE, Koenig LJ, Walter E, Fernandez I, Ethier K, Perinatal Guidelines Evaluation P. Dual contraceptive method use for pregnancy and disease prevention among HIV-infected and HIV-uninfected women: the importance of an event-level focus for promoting safer sexual behaviors. Sex Transm Dis. 2003;30(11):809–12. https://doi.org/10.1097/01.OLQ.0000086617.41012.14.
13. Abay F, Yeshita HY, Mekonnen FA, Sisay M. Dual contraception method utilization and associated factors among sexually active women on antiretroviral therapy in Gondar city, northwest, Ethiopia: a cross sectional study. BMC Womens Health. 2020;20(1):26. https://doi.org/10.1186/s12905-020-0890-3.
14. Reta M, et al. Prevalence of dual contraceptive use and associated factors among HIV positive women at University of Gondar Hospital, Northwest Ethiopia. BMC Res Notes. 2019;12. https://doi.org/10.1186/s13104-019-4053-2.
15. Kebede HG, Nahusenay H, Birhane Y, Tesfaye DJ. Assessment of contraceptive use and associated factors among HIV positive women in Bahir-Dar town, Northwest Ethiopia. Open Access Libr J. 2015;2:e1942. https://doi.org/10.4236/oalib.1101942.
16. Egzeabher SG, Bishaw MA, Tegegne TK, Boneya DJ. Modern family planning utilization and associated factors among HIV positive reproductive age women in Debre Markos Referral Hospital Northwest Ethiopia, 2014 G.C. Open J Epidemiol. 2015;5(01):32–40. https://doi.org/10.4236/ojepi.2015.51005.
17. Asfaw HM, Gashe FE. Contraceptive use and method preference among HIV positive women in Addis Ababa, Ethiopia: a cross sectional survey. BMC Public Health. 2014;14:566.
18. Demissie D, Girma T, Abdissa G. Dual contraceptive utilization and associated factors among people living with HIV attending ART clinic in Fitche Hospital, Ethiopia. J Health Med Nurs. 2015;2015:20.
19. Sufa A, Abera M, Admasu B. Utilization of family planning methods and associated factors among women living with HIV attending ART clinics in Nekemte Public Health Facilities, East Wollega Zone, Ethiopia. Sci Technol Arts Res. 2013;2(4):71.
20. Polisi A, et al. Modern contraceptive utilization among female ART attendees in health facilities of Gimbie town, West Ethiopia. Reprod Health. 2014;11(1):30.
21. Demissie DB, Gudisa T. Dual contraceptive use and associated factors among women living with HIV attending art clinics in West Zone Health Facilities Oromia, Ethiopia. EC Gynaecol. 2019;8(4):143–55.
22. Feyissa TR, et al. Contraceptive use among sexually active women living with HIV in western Ethiopia. PLoS One. 2020;15(8):e0237212.
23. Feyissa TR, Melka AS. Demand for modern family planning among married women living with HIV in western Ethiopia. PLoS One. 2014;9(11):e113008.
24. Gebrehiwot, et al. Utilization of dual contraception method among reproductive age women on antiretroviral therapy in selected public hospitals of Northern Ethiopia. BMC Reprod Health. 2017;14:125. https://doi.org/10.1186/s12978-017-0390-6.
25. Halefom Kalayu Redae. Dual contraceptive use and associated factors among HIV positive women on art follow up in Mekelle Town Tigray, Ethiopia. Proceedings of the 9th Multi-Disciplinary Seminar, Research and Knowledge Management Office, St. Mary's University, August 2017. Available at http://repository.smuc.edu.et/bitstream/123456789/3984/1/Halefom%20Kalayu%20Redae.pdf.
26. Melaku YA, Zeleke EG. Contraceptive utilization and associated factors among HIV positive women on chronic follow up care in Tigray region, northern Ethiopia: a cross sectional study. PLoS One. 2014;9(4):e94682.
27. Berhane Y, Berhe H, Abera GB, Berhe H. Utilization of modern contraceptives among HIV positive reproductive age women in Tigray, Ethiopia: a cross sectional study. ISRN AIDS. 2013;2013:1–8. https://doi.org/10.1155/2013/319724

28. Alemayehu A, Akililu J. Determinants of dual contraceptive use among HIV positive women in reproductive age group, Benishangul Gumuz region, northwest Ethiopia; 2018.
29. Markos SJ, Tilahun BH. Proportion of dual protection use at a time to prevent unwanted pregnancy and HIV/AIDS/sexually transmitted infections and its predictors among human immunodeficiency virus (HIV) positive women attending anti retro viral therapy (ART) Clinic Hosanna Hospital, Southern Ethiopia; institution based cross sectional study. JOJ Pub Health. 2019;4(5):555649. https://doi.org/10.19080/JOJPH.2019.04.555649.
30. Erashi MWM, Tesso FY, Beyene TT. Dual-contraceptive method utilization and associated factors among HIV positive women attending art clinic in Gebretsadik Shawo Hospital, SNNPR, south West Ethiopia. J Women's Health Care. 2015;4(06):267. https://doi.org/10.4172/2167-0420.1000267.
31. Moher D, Liberati A, Tetzlaff J, Altman DG. Preferred reporting items for systematic reviews and meta-analyses: the PRISMA statement. Ann Intern Med. 2009;151(4):264–9. https://doi.org/10.7326/0003-4819-151-4-2009081 80-00135.
32. Zeng X, Zhang Y, Kwong JS, et al. The methodological quality assessment tools for preclinical and clinical studies, systematic review and meta-analysis, and clinical practice guideline: a systematic review. J Evid Based Med. 2015; 8(1):2–10. https://doi.org/10.1111/jebm.12141.
33. Sterne JA, Egger M. Funnel plots for detecting bias in meta-analysis: guidelines on choice of axis. J Clin Epidemiol. 2001;54(10):1046–55. https://doi.org/10.1016/S0895-4356(01)00377-8.
34. Egger M, Smith GD, Schneider M, Minder C. Bias in meta-analysis detected by a simple, graphical test. BMJ. 1997;315(7109):629–34. https://doi.org/1 0.1136/bmj.315.7109.629.
35. Higgins JP, Thompson SG, Deeks JJ, Altman DG. Measuring inconsistency in metaanalyses. BMJ. 2003;327(7414):557–60. https://doi.org/10.1136/bmj.327.7414.557.
36. Heffron, et al. A prospective study of contraceptive use among African women in HIV-1 serodiscordant partnerships. Sex Transm Dis. 2010;37:10.
37. Antelman G, Medley A, Mbatia R, Pals S, Arthur G, Haberlen S, et al. Pregnancy desire and dual method contraceptive use among people living with HIV attending clinical care in Kenya, Namibia and Tanzania. J Fam Plann Reprod Health Care. 2015;41(1):e1. https://doi.org/10.1136/jfprhc-2 013-100784.
38. Chakrapani V, Trace K, Murali S, PeterA N, Deborah H, Robert D. Prevalence of and barriers to dual-contraceptive methods use among married men and women living with HIV in India. Infect Dis Obstet Gynecol. 2011;2011:376432 Hindawi Publishing Corporation.
39. Gausi GB, et al. HIV Sero-discordance and dual contraceptive method use among HIV-infected men and women in Lilongwe, Malawi. Sex Transm Dis. 2018;45(11):747–53. https://doi.org/10.1097/OLQ.0000000000000868.
40. Tsafack M, Essiben F, Momo RJ, Moyo GPK, Mpoah YM, Mbu RE. Dual contraception use and associated factors among HIV positive women follow-up at Treatment Center Unit of Yaounde Central Hospital, Cameroon. Open Access Libr J. 2020;7:e6225. https://doi.org/10.4236/oalib.1106225.
41. Kaida A, Laher F, Strathdee SA, Money D, Janssen PA, Hogg RS, et al. Contraceptive use and method preference among women in Soweto, South Africa: the influence of expanding access to HIV care and treatment services. PLoS One. 2010;5(11):e13868. https://doi.org/10.1371/journal.pone.0013868.
42. Mideva M, et al. Factors associated with uptake of dual contraception among HIV-infected women in Bungoma County, Kenya: a crosssectional study. Pan Afr Med J. 2017;28(Supp 1):2. https://doi.org/10.11604/pamj.supp.2017.28.1.9289.
43. Chibwesha CJ, et al. Modern contraceptive and dual method use among HIV-infected women in Lusaka, Zambia. Infect Dis Obstet Gynecol. 2011; 2011:261453–8. https://doi.org/10.1155/2011/261453 Hindawi Publishing Corporation.
44. Yaya I, Patassi AA, Landoh DE, Bignandi EM, Kolani K, Namoro ADD, et al. Modern contraceptive use among HIVinfected women attending HIV care centres in Togo: a cross-sectional study. BMJ Open. 2018;8(4):e019006. https://doi.org/10.1136/bmjopen-2017-019006.
45. Kopp DM, et al. Dual method use among postpartum HIV-infected and HIV-uninfected Malawian women: a prospective cohort study. Infect Dis Obstet Gynecol. 2017;2017:1475813–9. https://doi.org/10.1155/2017/1475813
46. Dugg P, Chhabra P, Sharma AK. Contraceptive use and unmet need for family planning among HIV-positive women: a hospital-based study. Indian J Public Health. 2020;64(1):32.
47. Chtherine M, et al. Predictors of dual method use for pregnancy and HIV prevention among adolescent south African women. Contraception. 2007; 75(5):383–9.
48. Damian DJ, George JM, Martin E, Temba B, Msuya SE. Prevalence and factors influencing modern contraceptive use among HIV-positive women in Kilimanjaro region, northern Tanzania. Contracept Reprod Med. 2018;3(1): 7.
49. Barbara N, et al. Family planning among people living with HIV in post-conflict Northern Uganda: a mixed methods study. BMC Confl Health. 2011; 5:18 http://www.conflictandhealth.com/content/5/1/18.
50. Wanyenze RK, Tumwesigye NM, Kindyomunda R, et al. Uptake of family planning methods and unplanned pregnancies among HIV-infected individuals: a cross-sectional survey among clients at HIV clinics in Uganda. J Int AIDS Soc. 2011;14(1):35.
51. Hancock NL, Chibwesha CJ, Bosomprah S, et al. Contraceptive use among HIV-infected women and men receiving antiretroviral therapy in Lusaka, Zambia: a cross-sectional survey. BMC Public Health. 2016;16(1):392.

4

# Utilization and predictors of long acting reversible contraceptive methods among reproductive age women in Hawassa city, South Ethiopia

Aklilu Tilahun[1], Amanuel Yoseph[2*] and Mesay Hailu Dangisso[2]

## Abstract

**Background:** Long acting reversible contraceptive methods are highly effective, safe and provide uninterrupted protection to women for 3 to 12 years, yet are little used in the Ethiopia. Assessment of the utilization and predictors of long acting reversible contraceptive methods assist health planners to prioritize promotion strategies, and is a fundamental step for intervention. Therefore, this study aimed to assess the utilization and predictors of long acting reversible contraceptives among reproductive age women in Hawassa city, South Ethiopia; 2019.

**Methods:** A community-based cross-sectional study was conducted using a mixed method among the sample of 660 reproductive age women in Hawassa city, South Ethiopia from January 1–30, 2019. We have used a systematic and purposive sampling technique to select the study participants. A structured interview-administrated questionnaire and focus group discussion were used to collect the data. The data were entered using Epi data version 3.1 and analyzed using SPSS version 20. Chi-square ($X^2$) test was used to determine the overall association between explanatory and outcome variables. The variables were entered into the multivariable model using the backward stepwise regression approach. Bi-variable and multivariable logistic regression analyses were conducted. The qualitative data were analyzed using a manual thematic analysis technique.

**Results:** The overall utilization of long acting reversible contraceptive methods was 22% (95% CI = 19.50–25.50%). Among this, 17.5 and 4.5% of women utilized the implants and IUCD, respectively. Good knowledge (AOR = 4.0; 95% CI = 1.66–9.60; $P = 0.001$) and positive attitude (AOR = 7.9; 95% CI = 3.84–16.10; $P = 0.001$) of women about LARC methods were positively associated with utilization of LARC methods. The odds of utilizing LARC methods increased 8.2 times for women who have no desire to have a child (AOR = 8.2, 95% CI = 3.13–21.30) as compared to those who have the desire to have a child. The discussion of women about LARC methods with providers (AOR = 4.1; 95% CI = 1.24–5.24) and husbands (AOR = 2.7; 95% CI =1.02–7.20) were positively associated with utilization of LARC methods. These findings were supported by the individual, institutional and socio-cultural qualitative findings.
(Continued on next page)

* Correspondence: amanuelyoseph45@gmail.com
[2]School of Public Health, College of Medicine and Health Sciences, Hawassa University, Hawassa, Ethiopia

(Continued from previous page)

**Conclusions:** The utilization of LARC methods far below the national target (22 V 40%) in the study area. Good knowledge and positive attitude about LARC methods, no desire to have a child, discussion with husbands and providers were major predictors of the LARC methods utilization. Increasing knowledge and positive attitude of the women about LARC methods using various methods of health education should be considered.

**Keywords:** Reproductive age women, Long acting reversible contraceptive methods, Utilization, Hawassa city and Ethiopia

## Background

Contraceptive methods are classified as modern and traditional methods. Modern methods include female sterilization, male sterilization, the intrauterine contraceptive device (IUCD), implants, injectable, the pill, male condoms, female condoms, emergency contraception, standard day's method (SDM), and lactation amenorrhea method (LAM). Methods such as rhythm, withdrawal, and folk method are grouped as traditional [1].

Hormonal contraceptive implants are a reversible long acting contraceptive which release a progestin hormone in the body. It can give a continuous protection for 3 to 5 years. The IUCD is also a reversible long acting contraceptive which is a small device placed in the uterus to prevent pregnancy [2].

Contraceptive use was estimated to prevent 218 millions of unintended pregnancies in developing countries. It also prevented 55 millions of unplanned births, 138 millions of abortions (of which 40 million are unsafe) and 25 million miscarriages. Moreover, it prevents 118, 000 maternal deaths and the loss of 240,000 healthy years from women's lives each year [3].

Globally, the prevalence of unintended pregnancies and unsafe abortion is high. Its implication in terms of public health is alarming. According to WHO report, it was estimated that 282 and 40 million women had unintended pregnancies and unsafe abortion, 30 million women were suffering from the most severe form of unsafe abortion complication and 5–10 million annual deaths were among 15–49 years in 2016 [4].

The economic cost of unintended pregnancies and unsafe abortion are substantial which leads to total loss of 10% disability-adjusted life years [5]. It also resulted in increases in fertility by 15% [3]. Consequently, unintended pregnancies and unsafe abortion might end up with 10% losses in productivity [4, 5].

Low utilization of the modern contraceptive methods is a great challenge in most low resource settings, no exception in Ethiopia. Among the six top underutilized countries (India, Nigeria, Pakistan, Afghanistan and the DRC) in which almost half of worldwide maternal mortality happens, an estimated maternal mortality ratio of Ethiopia is 420 per 100, 000 live births [1, 2].

The huge number of maternal death, specifically in low and middle income countries has been because of low level of LARC methods utilization. The low level utilization of LARC methods compounded by the extremely low ANC, skilled delivery and PNC utilization which are the major predictors for the high maternal deaths during the last two decades [6].

In addition, different predictors have been found to be associated with the utilization of LARC methods and can be grouped as socio-demographic, behavioral, institutional and service related factors [7].

In spite of the presence of many modern contraceptive methods options such as pills, injectable, implants, IUCD and sterilization, low utilization of LARC methods are a wide-spread problem in Ethiopia [2].

The Ethiopian Federal Ministry of Health developed health sector transformation plan and promised to achieve 40% utilization of the LARC methods by 2020 [8]. However, a study conducted in Adigrat town of Tigray region, Ethiopia shows that utilization of LARC methods is 28.7% [9]. Injectable and pills are the commonest and widely utilized contraceptive methods throughout country (Ethiopia) [2].

Modern contraceptive methods service utilization has been among the most relevant interventions strategy to reduce maternal morbidity and mortality [10]. Due to this evidence, Ethiopia has given a special consideration to it in the last three decades [8]. Moreover, modern contraceptive methods especially focus on LARC methods, which are among the six priority areas in the reproductive health strategy of the country to enhance maternal health [11].

In spite of the fact that modern contraceptive methods service utilization is very important for further improvement of maternal health, limited information exists on the utilization and predictors of LARC methods among reproductive age women in Hawasa city, South Ethiopia. In addition, information about LARC methods is also important because it is one of the targets for Ethiopian GTP 2 in 2012/2020 and the preparation for the third Growth and Transformation Plan in Ethiopia are fast approaching. Moreover, assessing the current level of utilization and identifying the predictors of LARC methods is important to guide public health planners, policymakers and implementers to plan and design appropriate intervention strategies in order to enhance LARC methods utilization. Therefore, the main aim of this study was to assess utilization and predicators of LARC methods among reproductive age women in Hawassa city, South Ethiopia, 2019.

## Methods

### Study area

The study was carried out in Hawassa city, South Ethiopia. The Hawassa city is located 275 km from Addis Ababa, the capital of Ethiopia. According to the central statistical agency report of Ethiopia, the total population of the city was estimated to be 359,358 (49% males and 51% females). The city has consisted of 8 sub-cities and 32 Kebeles (smallest administrative unit of Ethiopia). The health service coverage of the city was 94%. There is only one-government referral hospital, one general hospital, one primary hospital, 10 health centers and 32 health post. The city also consists of 12 private hospitals, 30 private clinics and 45 pharmacies. According to the health department report, the distribution of underutilization of LARC methods affects almost all Kebeles of the city. Trade is the main source of income in the Hawassa city; inhabitants of the rural sub-cities mainly produce enset (*Enset ventricosum*), cereals, cash crops (khat, coffee) and livestock (Hawassa City Administration: Annual health sector reports on health and other health related issues, unpublished).

### Study design and population

A community-based cross-sectional study was carried out using quantitative and qualitative methods in Hawassa city from January 1–30; 2019. The source and study population were all women in reproductive age group who were non-pregnant and all systematically selected women in reproductive age group who were non-pregnant and resided in the Hawassa city for 6 months, respectively. Pregnant women were excluded from the study.

### Sample size determination

For the first objective, the sample size was calculated by using a single population proportion formula in consideration of the following assumptions. The utilization/proportion (p) of long acting reversible contraceptive methods from the previous study done in Adigrat town, Northern Ethiopia was 28.7% [9], 95% confidence level, 5% margin of error. As a two-stage sampling technique was used to select the study participants, a design effect of 2 was considered and a 10% non-response rate was added to the calculated sample size. Therefore, the final sample size was 692. Similarly, the sample size (n) for the second objective was calculated by using the EPI-info TM 7 statistical package with the inputs of: 95% confidence level, 80% power, 1:1 ratio between exposed and unexposed and adjusted odds ratio (AOR) of 2.53. Thus, the final sample size was 392. A sample size of 692 obtained from the first specific objective was used because it was the largest sample size estimated and would be sufficient for the study.

### Sampling technique

A two-stage stratified sampling technique (i.e. considering each Kebele as stratum) was used to select a representative sample size. In the first stage, we have used simple random sampling technique to select a representative Kebeles from the Hawassa city. In the second stage, we used a systematic random sampling technique to select the study households. In Hawassa city, there are 32 Kebeles and from all 32 Kebeles, nine Kebeles were selected by using a simple random sampling technique. Households with reproductive age group women who were non-pregnant were identified by the house-to-house census and a sampling frame was prepared. Finally, study participants were selected using a systematic sampling method. The first woman was identified by using simple random sampling and then after, at regular intervals, another woman was selected until needed sample size reached. If woman was absent from the household for 3 consecutive visits and there were no other options, the next nearest woman was included. One woman was included by using simple random sampling when two or more women existed in the selected households. To select discussant women a purposive sampling technique was used by considering variation in age, socio-economic and education status. All women included in the FGD were not participants of the quantitative study.

### Study variables

The outcome variable was utilization of long acting reversible contraceptive methods. The independent variables were socio-demographic variables such as age, religion, ethnicity, family size, wealth index, maternal/paternal education and occupation, marital status, number and sex of living children, and media availability; reproductive factors such as history of abortion, experience of child death, need of more children; factors related to communication such as communication with husband and health professionals; health service availability and other factors like perception, knowledge and attitude.

### Study tools and data collection techniques

Data collection was administered by 8 clinical nurses. Two BSc nurses intensively supervised the data collection process. Qualitative data collected using focus group discussion (FGD) until information saturation was reached. Each FGD consisted of 8 participants and were selected purposively from one to five networks of reproductive age group women. FGD guideline was used to explore ideas of reproductive age group. It was triangulated with the quantitative method. Two experienced health officers were assigned for note taking and tape recording while the public health expert with MPH facilitated the FGD. Quantitative data were collected at their households while FGD were conducted at proximal community gathering area.

#### Data quality control

Data were collected using structured and interviewer-administered questionnaire. Firstly, the questionnaire was prepared in English. Secondly, it was translated into Amharic language. Finally, it was retranslated back to English to keep its consistency. The comparison was done to assess the inconsistency and non-accuracy between the two versions of the questionnaire. It was pretested on 5% of sample and one FGD was conducted in Kebeles which were not included in the actual study area. Then, any inconsistency and non-accuracy was corrected accordingly. Training was given for data collectors and supervisors by the principal investigator for 2 days. The training was focused on the objective, methods and data collection process. In addition, regular checkup for completeness and consistency of the data were made on a daily basis.

#### Operational definitions

**Long acting reversible contraceptive methods** are a modern contraceptive method which includes implant and Intra Uterine Contraceptive Device (IUCD) and provides uninterrupted protection to women for 3 to 12 years.

**Short acting reversible contraceptive methods** are a modern contraceptive methods which are used in short time intervals from single use (e.g. the condom), daily intake (e.g. the pill) to up to 3 monthly application (e.g. injectable contraceptives).

**Knowledge** was measured using the 7 knowledge assessment questions. Knowledge questions were scored and pulled together and the mean score was computed to determine the overall knowledge of the participants. Based on that good level of knowledge assigned when the respondent answered the sum score of greater than or equal 75% of 7 knowledge assessment questions; moderate level of knowledge, when the respondent correctly answered between 50 and 74%; and low level of knowledge, when the respondent answered below 50% of 7 knowledge assessment questions.

**Attitude** was measured using the 8 attitude assessment questions. Accordingly, those who scored above mean, mean and below mean to the correct answers considered as positive and negative attitude, respectively.

#### Data analysis

The data were entered into Epi Data 3.1 and exported to the Statistical Package for Social Sciences (SPSS) version 20.0 for analysis. All required variables recoding and computations were done prior to the main analysis. Descriptive analyses were conducted to obtain descriptive measures for the socio-demographic characteristics and other variables. Tables and graphs were used for the data presentation. Chi-square($X^2$) test was used to determine the overall association between explanatory and outcome variables. Cross tabulations was used to test the assumption of $X^2$. A sensitivity analysis was conducted to investigate the effect of missing data by multiple imputations. Binary logistic regression was used to identify predictors of LARC methods utilization. The binary logistic regression analysis started with unadjusted analysis in which each potential predictor was assessed separately for its association with LARC methods utilization. Variables with $p$-values $< 0.25$ on the unadjusted analysis were entered into a multivariable logistic regression model to find out independent predictors of LARC methods utilization adjusting for other factors in the model. The variables were entered into the multivariable model using the backward stepwise regression approach. The main assumptions of logistic regression model (absence of outliers, multicollinearity and interaction among independent variables) were checked to be satisfied. Accordingly, none of the interaction terms was statistically significant indicating absence of a significant effect modification. Multicollinearity between the independent variables was also assessed using multiple linear regression. No evidence of multicollinearity was found as the variance inflation factor (VIF) for all variables was less than 10 and the tolerance statistic was greater than 0.1. The fitness of logistic regression model was also evaluated in model using the Hosmer-Lemeshow statistic and greater than 0.05. The presence and strength of association between LARC methods utilization and the predictors was assessed using adjusted odds ratios (AORs) with 95% CIs. Statistically significant association was declared when the 95% CI of the AOR did not include 1. Qualitative data were transcribed verbatim from the local languages into English language and presented in narratives using the respondents own words. The transcripts were read and checked two times by the professional transcribers for verification. The qualitative data were analyzed using a manual thematic analysis technique.

### Results

Socio-demographic characteristics of the study participants have been summarized in Table 1. From a total of 692, only 660 study participants answered questions, making a response rate of this study 95.3%. The mean

**Table 1** Socio-demographic characteristics of study participants in Hawassa city, South Ethiopia, 2019 ($N = 660$)

| Variable | Categories | number | Percent |
|---|---|---|---|
| Age | 15–19 | 116 | 17.6 |
| | 20–36 | 481 | 72.9 |
| | 37–49 | 63 | 9.5 |
| Marital status | Single | 216 | 32.2 |
| | Married | 433 | 65.6 |
| | Others | 11 | 2.2 |
| Religion | Protestant | 403 | 61.1 |
| | Orthodox | 195 | 29.5 |
| | Musilim | 41 | 6.2 |
| | Others | 21 | 3.2 |
| Ethnicity | Sidama | 387 | 58.6 |
| | Amhara | 109 | 16.5 |
| | Wolaita | 64 | 9.7 |
| | Others | 100 | 15.2 |
| Educational level | No formal education | 44 | 6.4 |
| | Primary level | 235 | 34.2 |
| | Secondary level | 219 | 31.9 |
| | Higher/university level | 162 | 24.5 |
| Occupation | Housewife | 293 | 44.4 |
| | Government employer | 66 | 10.0 |
| | Merchant | 57 | 8.6 |
| | Daily employer | 244 | 37.0 |

(± standard deviation [SD]) of the age of participants was 25 (± 7) years. Majority of respondents were within the range of 20–35 years. The median family size of each household was 4 persons. According to this study, majority 387/660 (58.6%) of the study participants were from Sidama ethnic group. Majority 403/660 (61.1%) and 433/660 (65.6%) of the study participants were followers of protestant Christianity and married, respectively.

Two hundred twenty-seven (34.4%) of study participants had no child, 176(26.7%) had 1–2 children, 198 (30.0%) had 3–5 children and 59(8.9%) had greater than 5 children (Fig. 1).

#### Average number of children that needed for one household from group discussants illustrated as follows

*"Large family size is not good. It is difficult to raise children and difficult to cover school expense. It is enough if you get four children on average. But no problems if you get more children as you have economy".* **(G-1 D4 woman aged 32 years)**

*"Having four children, totally six family members are enough. Family size determined by household economy. What is the importance of having a large family size? It has no advantage; rather it is determined by economic status".* **(G-2 D5 women aged 37 years)**

*"Four children two males and two females are enough. Having many children is not good because in order to raise properly and live quality life, having large number of children is not good".* **(G-2 D2 women aged 28 years).**

*"People want to have 6 to 7 children but it is restricted by economy. Due to economic problems, saving and also preventing giving birth within short period of time is mandatory".* **(G-3 D2 29 years-old woman)**

*'At this time, having large family size or having many children is not good. A maximum of 6 children are enough. This (having limited number of children) is because, in order to raise children properly, and of economic problems. Previously, our mother gave up 12 children and at that time cost of living was not that much expensive and children were grown easily. Mothers are also not affected if she does not give many children and can raise her children in quality of life'.* **(G-3 D4 34 years-old woman)**

*"Even I want to have up to 12 children. It is a gift of God and I don't want to close my womb by my mouth. If God give me, I want to give birth but by interval and by raising my children properly. You know injection can't prevent God's will because for example, one of my friends was using implant but she became pregnant. That means implant cannot prevent God's will. Having many children has its own advantages because while you give birth, you plan and adjust your budget for it since you are giving birth by spacing."* **(G-3 D1 25 years-old woman)**

*"As discussant 1 said, no one hates children to have. Our mother said that 'if you have many children, they will be grown differently and their fate also different'. For example if you have only two children, raising two of them may be simple. For example, we are 7 in number and each of us has different behavior and fate. If one becomes weak, the other becomes strong and if one has good husband and other may not have as a previous one does, so having many children provide many choices. But according to present situation and as science says, children should be grown to have quality life and you have to educate them properly and address them to be in a good position".* **(G-3 D4 34 years-old woman)**

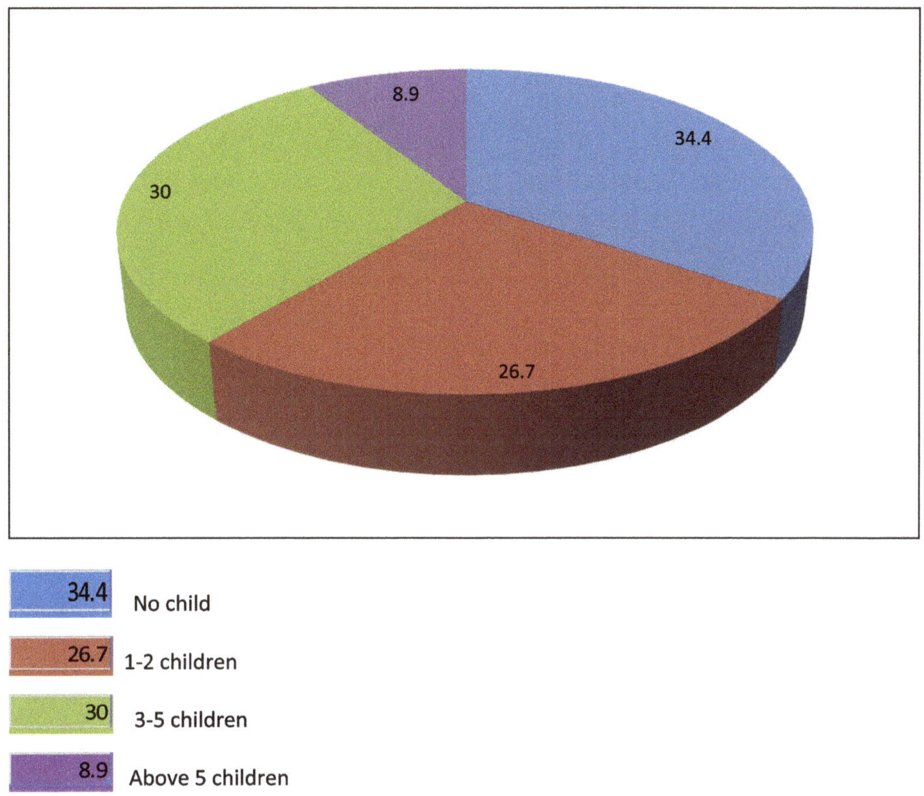


**Fig. 1** Number of children that reproductive age women have in Hawassa city, 2019

Only 242/660 (36.7%) of the study participants had good knowledge on long acting reversible contraceptive methods. Two hundred sixty-two (39.5%) of the study participants had positive attitude and the 399/660 (60.5%) had negative attitude on long acting reversible contraceptive methods (Table 2).

#### Utilization of long acting reversible contraceptive methods

The overall utilization of long acting reversible contraceptive methods was 22% (95% CI = 19.5–25.5%) in the study area. Majority, 428/660 (64.9%) of the study participants had ever used contraceptive methods during their lifetime. Five hundred thirty-seven (81.3%) of women had discussed with husband on contraceptive methods choice (Table 3).

**Table 2** Knowledge and attitude of the study participants towards long acting reversible contraceptive methods in Hawassa city, South Ethiopia 2019 ($N = 660$)

| Variables | Categories | Number | percent |
|---|---|---|---|
| Knowledge | Good knowledge | 242 | 36.6 |
| | Moderate knowledge | 141 | 21.4 |
| | Poor knowledge | 277 | 42.0 |
| Attitude | Positive attitude | 262 | 39.5 |
| | Negative attitude | 398 | 60.5 |

Currently, 357/660 (54.1%) of the study participants were using modern contraceptive methods. The implant was the leading long acting reversible contraceptive method 115/660 (17.4%), followed by IUCD 30/660 (4.5%) (Fig. 2).

#### Descriptive reasons for not utilizing long acting reversible contraceptive methods

The main descriptive reasons that study participants did not use contraceptive methods were, 188/660 (28.5%) fear of side effects, 62/660 (9.4%) choose not to accept method at this time, 30/660 (4.6%) desire more children (Fig. 3).

##### *Qualitative reasons for not utilizing long acting reversible contraceptive methods according to discussants expressed during group discussions are illustrated as follows*

> *"I am using injectable and one of my friends uses implant and it causes dizziness, weight loss or body decrement or thinness and when she went to a health facility, health professionals were not okay to remove it. So she went to a private facility and removed it by payment. Now she becomes healthy after*

**Table 3** Utilization of long acting reversible contraceptive methods among reproductive age women in Hawassa city, South Ethiopia, 2019 ($N = 660$)

| Variables | Categories | Number | Percent |
|---|---|---|---|
| Ever used contraceptive methods | Yes | 428 | 64.9 |
| | No | 232 | 35.1 |
| Currently use contraceptive methods | Yes | 357 | 54.1 |
| | No | 303 | 45.9 |
| Currently using | Long acting Reversible | 145 | 22.0 |
| | Short acting | 515 | 78.0 |
| Communication with husband | Yes | 537 | 81.3 |
| | No | 123 | 18.7 |

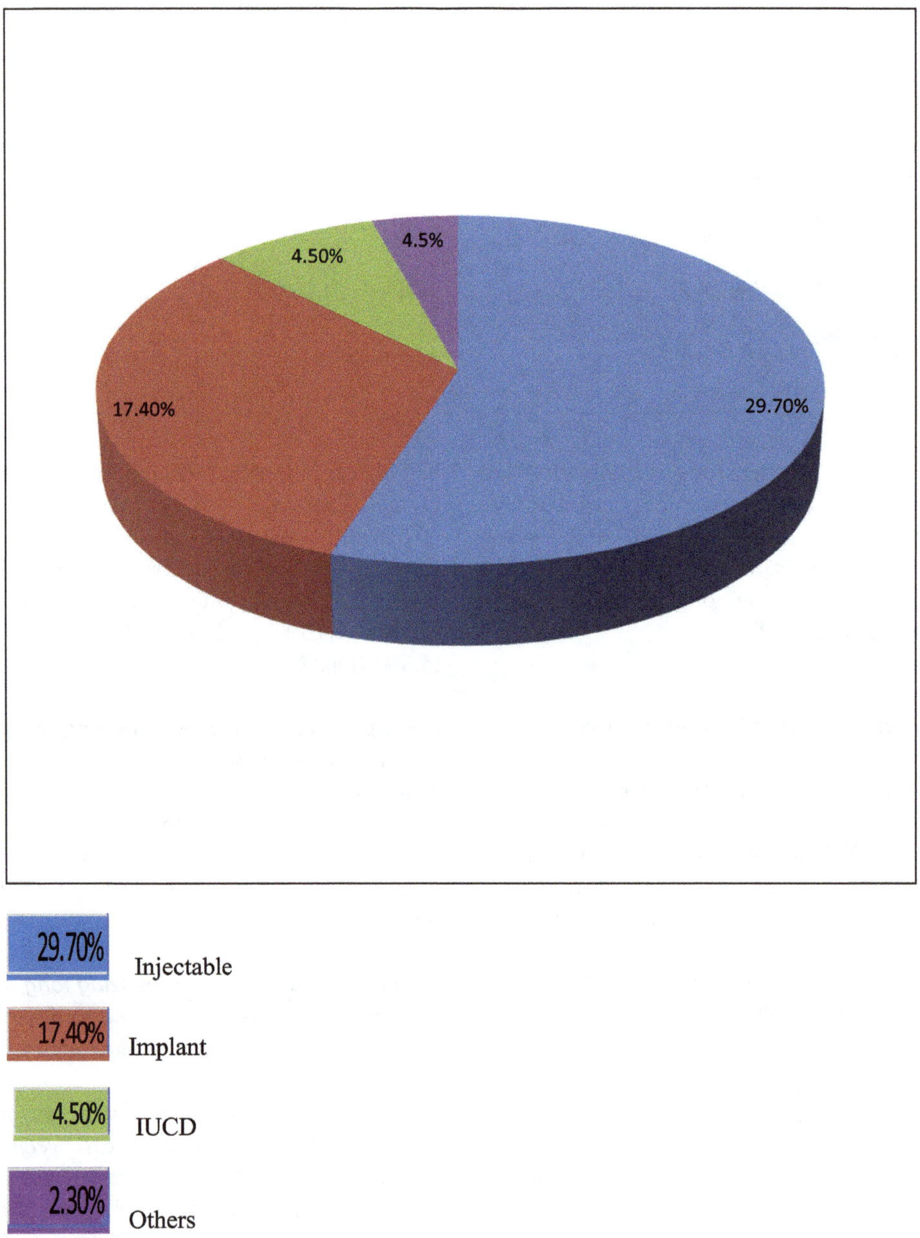


**Fig. 2** Current utilization of the modern contraceptive methods among reproductive age women in Hawassa city, 2019

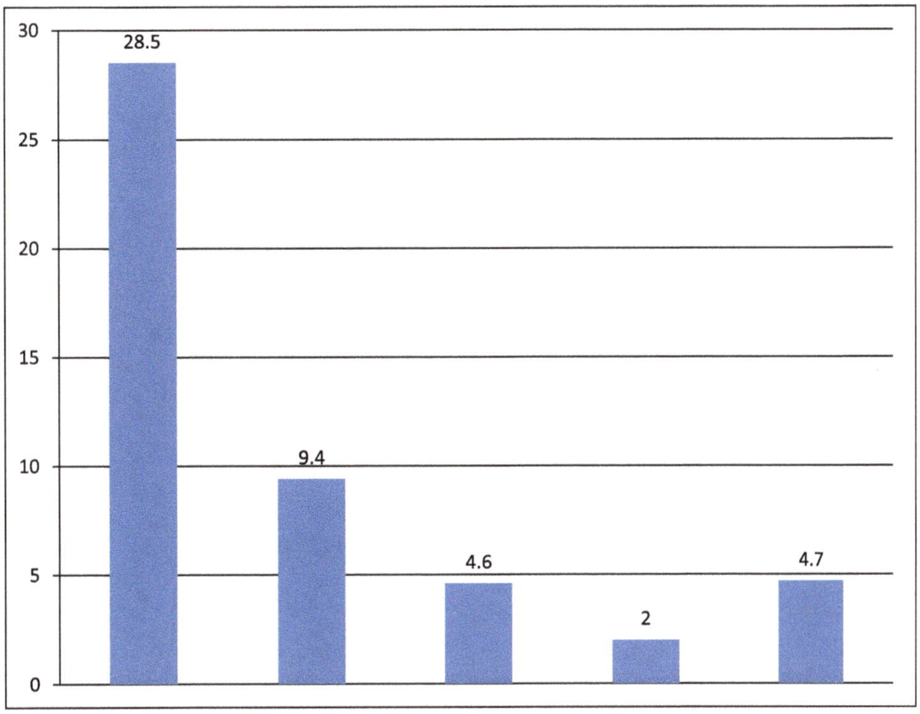


**Fig. 3** Descriptive reasons for non-utilization of the contraceptive methods among reproductive age group in Hawassa city, 2019

*removing it. So when I saw this, I don't want to use implant. Also people said that injectable causes hypertension since it prevents menstruation, pills cause softening of uterus and causes cancer so it is difficult".* (**G-1 D4 34 years-old woman**)

*"First, community members want to use it but after insertion some nurses were not okay to remove it if mother demanded to remove it. When I asked my friends "why they are not using long acting family planning" like five years implant, they said that "after insertion some health professionals refused to remove it", and I think they were not using long acting reversible contraceptive due to that reason".* (**G-3 D1 25 years-old woman**)

*"I have used implant and it has problem like wound, itching sensation and when I went to a health facility to remove it, they (health professionals) said that 'for short period of time it may cause symptoms just like that and it will be resolved after your body adapt it'. When we wanted to remove it, they (health professionals) were not okay and simply they said that 'if you have a problem, we will remove it'. Implant has so many problems like dizziness, itching sensation and irritability. What was a reason for this?"* (**G-3 D6 38 years-old woman**)

*"There were mothers who complained that "why does a pregnancy happen while we are using family planning methods?" Health professionals do not accepting mothers' request to remove if mother demanded to remove it. They were not okay to remove if time were not reached as they said. My brother's wife begun to have DM and HTN after using implant and when she went to remove implant, they were refused to remove and said that 'implant inserted for three years, so its time is not reached'. Finally, they (health professionals) were removed implant when her husband fighting with them (health professionals) and she remained with these diseases".* (**G-3 D7 25 Years-old Woman**)

### Predictors of long acting reversible contraceptive methods utilization

Results of the logistic regression analysis of LARC methods are shown in Table 4. Both bi-variable and multivariable analyses of predictors revealed that odds of LARC methods utilization were 4.0 times higher in women who have good knowledge as compared to those who have poor knowledge about LARC methods (AOR = 4.0; 95% CI = 1.66–9.60; $P = 0.004$). The odds of utilizing LARC methods increased 7.9 times for women who have a positive attitude (AOR = 7.9, 95% CI = 3.84–16.10) than women who have a negative attitude about LARC methods. The findings of FGD also support this. Focus group discussant said *"Some people believe that long*

**Table 4** Bivariable and multivariable logistic regression analysis of predictorsof LARC methods utilization among reproductive age group in Hawassa city, South Ethiopia, 2019 ($N = 660$)

| Variables | Bivariate analysis | | Multivariate analysis |
|---|---|---|---|
| | Level | CI (95%) | CI (95%) |
| Knowledge | Good | 19.00 (10.12–35.76)* | 3.99 (1.66–9.60)** |
| | Moderate | 3.80 (1.84–8.11)* | 1.34 (0.50–3.60) |
| | Poor | 1 | 1 |
| Attitude | Positive | 21.60 (12.56–37.22)* | 7.90 (3.80–16.10)** |
| | Negative | 1 | 1 |
| Source of information | Health professionals | 1 | 1 |
| | Mass media | 0.05 (0.02–0.15) | 0.60 (0.13–2.83) |
| | Others | 0.12 (0.04–0.33)* | 0.43 (0.11–1.70) |
| Educational level | No formal education | 1 | 1. |
| | Primary level | 1.87 (0.24–14.61) | 0.27 (0.09–8.65) |
| | Secondary | 0.98 (0.21–4.52) | 0.36 (0.03–4.72) |
| | Higher | 6.80 (1.60–29.15) * | 1.77 (0.13–23.31) |
| Discussion with husband | Yes | 4.60 (2.20–9.60)* | 2.70 (1.02–7.20)* |
| | No | 1 | |
| Ever use contraceptive | Yes | 8.26 (4.40–15.30)* | 2.30 (0.80–6.46) |
| | No | 1 | 1 |
| Number of children | 0 | 1 | 1 |
| | 1–2 | 5.90 (2.88–12.38)* | 0.56 (0.07–4.26) |
| | 3–5 | 10.60 (5.26–21.35)* | 0.86 (0.11–6.61) |
| | Above 5 | 25.70 (11.38–58.10)* | 2.28 (0.25–20.61) |
| No desire to have children | Yes | 2.53 (1.57–4.10) | 8.20 (3.13–21.33)** |
| | No | 1 | 1 |
| Discussion with providers | Yes | 4.90 (2.20–11.30)* | 4.10 (1.36–12.55)** |
| | No | 1 | 1 |

Note: 1 indicates the reference categories; a single asterisk (*) indicates a significant association ($p$-value < 0.05); double asterisk (**) indicates a highly significant association ($p$-value < 0.01)

*acting contraceptives (Implant and IUCD) cause infertility if women used it for a long period of time. Even previously they believe that contraceptives cause infertility, but now they have started to use it after having awareness. Some people, who have no awareness and knowledge, by considering as it causes infertility, remove LARC but those who have knowledge about LARC using it properly".* **(G-1 D1 27 years-old woman)** *"Community beliefs on LARC were, it causes infertility if they (women) stay for long period of time without giving birth. We know that within a community there are community members, who are not using family planning, and even they prefer to give birth until they have 6 to 7 children and some are using family planning accordingly, and their awareness is different".* **(G-1 D4 34 years-old woman)**.

In addition, discussion of women about LARC methods with health care provider (AOR = 4.1; 95% CI = 1.24–5.24) and husband (AOR = 2.7; 95% CI =1.02–7.20) were positively associated with utilization of LARC methods. Moreover, the odds of utilizing LARC methods increased 8 times for women who have no desire to have a child (AOR = 8.2, 95% CI = 3.13–21.30) as compared to those who have the desire to have a child.

## Discussion

A community-based cross-sectional study was conducted to assess utilization and predictors of LARC methods using mixed methods among reproductive age women in Hawassa city, South Ethiopia. The utilization of long acting reversible contraceptive methods among reproductive age women in Hawassa city was 22%. Good knowledge and positive attitude of women about LARC methods, no desire to have children, women discussion with health care providers and husbands had a significant association with utilization of the LARC methods.

In this study the utilization of the modern contraceptive and LARC methods among women of the reproductive age were 54.1 and 22%, respectively. Among this, majority of women (17.4%) utilized implant, followed by IUCD (4.5%). In contrary to the present finding, EDHS 2016 reported a lower utilization of modern contraceptives (36%) and implants (8%) [2]. This discrepancy might be due to the fact that EDHS survey included both rural and urban study participants. However, our study included study participants from urban area. In addition, a lower utilization of the modern contraceptive methods also reported from studies done in Arbaminch, Mekelle and Durame town, Ethiopia [12–14]. This difference might be due to the fact that difference in the sample size, study setting, and study period. However, the study conducted in Gedeo zone, south Ethiopia reported a higher utilization of modern contraceptive methods (74.8%), IUCD (6.6%) and implants (26.1%) than our study [15].

Multivariable analysis revealed that odds of LARC methods utilization were 4.0 times higher in women who have good knowledge as compared to those who have poor knowledge about LARC methods. This is consistent with the study findings from Arbaminch and Gedeo zone, Southern Ethiopia and Kicukiro town, Ruanda [15–17]. This might be attributed to the fact that women who have a good knowledge about LARC methods are more likely to outweigh the benefits and risks of using contraceptives. Moreover, it increases women's capacity to make decision to utilize it.

The odds of utilizing LARC methods increased 7.9 times for women who had a positive attitude than women who had a negative attitude about LARC methods. This finding is in agreement with the studies done in Gesuba town, Gedeo zone, Addis Ababa city, Ethiopia and Calabar Metropolis, Southern Nigeria [15, 16, 18, 19]. This might be because of women who have a positive attitude about LARC methods are confident and more likely to minimize rumors of LARC methods. In addition, it increases women's confidence to make decision about its utilization.

In addition, discussion of women about LARC methods with health care providers and husbands were positively associated with utilization of LARC methods. This finding is in agreement with studies conducted in North Shoa, Jigjiga Town, Ethiopia and Nepal [20–22]. This might be because women who had a discussion with health care providers and husbands were more likely to have information about LARC methods like duration of pregnancy prevention, effectiveness, method failure, and side effect. Also, these women were more confident to minimize rumors of LARC methods. Moreover, it increases women confidence to make decision about its utilization.

Moreover, the odds of utilizing LARC methods increased 8 times for women who had no desire to have a child as compared to those who had the desire to have a child. This finding agreed with studies conducted in North Shoa, West Harerge and Debre Markos town, North Ethiopia and Kucikiro district of Rwanda [17, 21, 23, 24].

### Limitation of the study

This study had a number of strengths. Among these, the community based nature and using both quantitative and qualitative methods provided representative and valuable information for all reproductive age group which is important to develop relevant policy strategy for efficient promotion of LARC methods utilization. Regardless of its strengths, our study has some basic limitations that might be considered while interpreting the findings. First, the cross-sectional nature of the study design does not exactly establish the cause and effect relationship. Secondly, the study might be prone to recall bias because of the information was collected by the study participants self-report.

## Conclusions

The utilization of LARC methods was far below the targeted health sector growth and transformation plan (22% v 40%) in the study area. The low utilization of LARC methods in the study area indicated that much work remains to be done to improve the health of women.

Good knowledge and positive attitude about LARC methods, women discussion with health care providers and husbands about LARC methods and no desire to have children were pertinent predictors of LARC methods utilization. Therefore, increasing knowledge and positive attitude of the women about LARC methods using various methods of health education should be considered. In addition, women's discussion with health care providers and husbands about LARC methods to have an explicit understanding is also important. Moreover, providing relevant information about LARC methods for women who have no desire to have a child is also of paramount importance. Finally, further research using analytical study design to identify predictors of LARC methods utilization is required.

#### Abbreviations

AOR: Adjusted odds ratio; ANC: Antenatal Care; CI: Confidence Interval; DRC: Democratic Republic Congo; FGD: Focus group discussion; GTP 2: Growth and transformation plan 2; IRB: Institutional Review Board; IUCD: Intra-uterine contraceptive device; LARC: Long acting reversible contraceptive methods; OR: Odds ratio; PNC: Postnatal Care; SD: Standard Deviation; SPSS: Statistical packages for social science; WHO: World Health Organization

#### Acknowledgements

First of all, authors thank Almighty God. They also would like to thank the Hawassa University, School of Public Health for approval of ethical clearance. Our deep gratitude goes to Hawassa city health department for their support. The authors are also very grateful for data collectors and study participants. Finally, our special thanks go to Frehiwot Teshome for her genuine support.

**Authors' contributions**

AT- Involved in initiation of the research question, prepared the research proposal, carried out the research, did the data entry and analysis. AY- did data analysis, wrote and revised manuscript. MHD- conducted edition, advising, prepared research tools with PI and revised the manuscript. All authors have read and approved the final manuscript.

**Author details**

[1]Adare General Hospital, Maternal and Child Health service case team, Hawassa, Ethiopia. [2]School of Public Health, College of Medicine and Health Sciences, Hawassa University, Hawassa, Ethiopia.

**References**

1. Elma *P. Laguna*, Maria Paz N. Marquez and Maria Midea M. Kabamalan of the UP Population Institute. 1 in 3 Pinays use traditional over modern contraceptives. August 8, 2017 13:45. Available from https://upd.edu.ph/1-in-3-pinays-use-traditional-over-modern-contraceptives/.
2. Central Stastical Agency (CSA). Ethiopian Demographic and Health Survey. Key indicators report ICF Rockville, Maryland, USA, 2016.
3. World Health Organization (WHO). Benefits of family planning and contraception fact sheet Available from https://apps.who.int/iris/bitstream/handle/10665/112319/WHO_RHR_14.07_eng.pdf?ua=1.
4. World Health Organization (WHO). Public health implication of unintended pregnancy and unsafe abortion. Geneva, Switherland: WHO; 2016.
5. World Bank. Global burden of diseases series 12 report. Comparative quantification of health risks in global and regional burden of disease attributable to selected major risk factors 2016.
6. World Health Organisation (WHO). Trends in maternal mortality and maternal health service utilization : 1990 to 2015. Geneva, Switzerland: World Health Organization; 2016.
7. World Health Organisation (WHO). Trends of contraceptive methods utilization and associated factors report. Geneva, Switherland: WHO; 2016.
8. The Federa Democratic Republic of Ethiopian Ministry of Health (FMOH). Health Sector Transportation Plan (2015/16–2019/20), Addis Ababa, Ethiopia.
9. Gebru AA, Fantahun A, Gebrekidan KG. Assessment of Factors Affecting Long acting reversible contraceptives utilization in Adigrat Town, Tigray, North-East Ethiopia. Am J Health Res. 2018;3:239–47.
10. World Health Organisation (WHO). Global causes of maternal death especial consideration of family planning: a WHO systematic analysis. Lancet Glob Health. 2016.
11. Federal Ministry of Health(FMOH). National reproductive health strategy to improve maternal and child health, Addis Ababa, Ethiopia. 2016-2020. 2015.
12. Alemayehu M, Belachew T, Tilahun T. Factors associated with utilization of long acting and permanent contraceptive methods among married women of reproductive age in Mekelle town, Tigray region, North Ethiopia. BMC Pregnancy Childbirth. 2016.
13. Tamrie YE, Gebre E, Argaw MD. Determinants of long acting reversible contraception method use among mothers in extended postpartum period, Durame Town, Southern Ethiopia: a cross sectional community based survey; 2015.
14. Getnet S, Amin M, Hailu D. Long acting contraceptive method utilization and associated factors among reproductive age women in Arba Minch Town, Ethiopia. Greener J Epidemiol Public Health. 2014;2:23–31.
15. Akine E. Contraceptive method mix utilization and its associated factors among married women in Gedeo zone, Southern Nations,Nationality and People Region-Ethiopia: a community based cross sectional study; 2015.
16. Belayneh F, Abreha S, Meskele M. Knowledge, attitude and factors associated with the use of long acting and permanent contraceptive methods among women of reproductive age in Gesuba Town, Southern Ethiopia. J Biol Agriculture Healthcare. 2015;5:16–7.
17. Bikorimana E. Barriers to the use of long acting contraceptive methods among married women of reproductive age in Kicukiro District, Rwanda. Int J Sci Res Publ. 2015;5(12):513–21.
18. Tizita Dadi. Assessment on utilization of long acting reversible contraceptive methods and its associated factors among reproductive aged women in selected health centers in Addis Ababa, 2015 Unpublished thesis.
19. Eko Jimmy E, Kalu O, Osuchukwu NC. Prevalence of contraceptive use among women of reproductive age in Calabar Metropolis, southern Nigeria. Int J Humanities Soc Sci Invention. 2015;2.
20. Abdisa B, Mideksa L. Factors associated with utilization of long acting and permanent contraceptive methods among women of reproductive age Group in Jigjiga Town. Int Hum Anat Physiol. 2017;7(2):6.
21. Mohammed A, Woldeyohannes D, Feleke A, Megabiaw B. Determinants of modern contraceptive utilization among married women of reproductive age group in North Shoa Zone, Amhara Region, Ethiopia. BMC Reproductive Health. 2014;11:13.
22. Penny Murphy, Woman's health stats and facts in Nepal. The American Congress of Obstetricians and Gynecologists, 2015 Available from https://ww1.prweb.com/prfiles/2018/05/01/15456577/MediaKit_Womens%20Health%20Source.pdf.
23. Jemal Alemu. Utilization of long acting reversible contraceptive and associated factors among women of family planning users in Chiro zonal hospital west Harerge, Eastern Ethiopia, Unpublished thesis, 2015.
24. Gudaynhe SW, Zegeye DT, Asmamaw T, Kibret GD. Factors affecting the use of long-acting reversible contraceptive methods among married women in Debre Markos Town, NorthWest Ethiopia 2013. Glob J Med Res. 2014;14(5).

5

# Spousal age difference and its effect on contraceptive use among sexually active couples in Ethiopia: Evidence from the 2016 Ethiopia demographic and health survey

Sena Belina Kitila[1*], Yonas Biratu Terfa[1], Adugna Olani Akuma[1], Ayantu Kebede Olika[2] and Alemi Kebede Olika[3]

**Abstract**

**Background:** Age difference among spouses can be considered as an indicator of the nature of the marital bond, and influences the couple's fertility expectations. The age difference is one of the features of the traditional African marriage system. However, the likelihood that women use of contraceptives and spousal age differences is not well studied. Thus, this study was to examine the spousal age difference on contraceptive use.

**Objective:** This study was aimed to examine spousal age differences and its effect on contraceptive use among sexually active couples in Ethiopia.

**Methods:** The related variables for this study were extracted from Ethiopian Demographic and Health Survey 2016 data. IBM SPSS statistics version 20 software was used for analysis. Logistic regression was conducted to see the association between spousal age difference and contraceptive use. All analyses were adjusted for sample weights.

**Results:** Out of the 7268 selected women for contraceptive usage questions, one fourth (25.3%) of them were between ages 25 and 29 and in almost all 7061 (98.4%) of them there was spousal age differences, 1555 (21.4%) of them were from poor socioeconomic group. Nearly all 7184 (98.8%) of them knew contraceptive method. However, among those sexually active in the last 4 weeks only two in five (41.2%) were using a contraceptive method. Spousal age difference was found to be significant factor and women older than their spouses were (AOR: 1.771, 95%CI: 1.276, 2.459) more likely and women having spouse's age difference greater than 10 years were 1.2% (AOR: .988, 95%CI: .848, 1.150) less likely to use contraception compared to those age difference is ten or less than years respectively.

Also, women who were living in urban areas (AOR: 1.482, 95%CI: 1.161 to 1.890), current working status (AOR: 1.170; 95%CI: 1.033 to 1.325), from richest economic category (AOR: 2.560; 95%CI: 2.000 to 3.278) husband's education, couples' fertility preference (AOR: 1.233; 95%CI: 1.070 to 1.420) were contraception use predictors. Similarly, being

(Continued on next page)

* Correspondence: senabalina26@gmail.com
[1]Faculty of Health Sciences, School of Nursing and Midwifery, Jimma University Institute of Health Science, Addis Abeba, Ethiopia

(Continued from previous page)
Muslim by religion (AOR: .579 95%CI: 0.496 to 0.675) and husband based decision for their health care use were (AOR: .847, CI: .729 to .985) less likely to use contraception.

**Conclusion and recommendation:** This study found association between spousal age differences and contraceptive use. Similarly, women's age, age difference, place of residence, religion, current working status, socioeconomic, husband's education, living children and current pregnancy, the couples' fertility preference and who decides on health care use were found to be predictors of contraceptive use. Strengthening strategies for improving women's educational status, socio-economic and demographic that will help to limit the age differences and improve contraceptive use. Further study, including qualitative is recommended to dig out the why components and better understand this finding.

**Keywords:** Spousal, Age difference, Contraceptive, Couples, Ethiopia

## Introduction

The age difference among spouses can be considered as an indicator of the charactertics of the marital bond, and influences the couple's fertility expectations. At the individual level, a large age difference makes the distance between the spouses, since age is vital for forming a relationship of subordination, and it generates a generational and cultural gap between spouses those are at different phases in their life cycle and who had different experiences and understanding of pre-marital life [1].

A big age difference between couples is one of the features of the traditional African marriage system [1] and this age difference between spouses influence marital stability, marital satisfaction, family size preference and contraceptive use [2].

Also the likelihood that women use contraceptives may be reduced when they are significantly younger than their husband, because such age differences are often accompanied by incongruences in social position, resources and life experiences, which may make marital relationships integrally unequal [3].

The study conducted in India to assess the influence of the age gap between couples on contraception and fertility indicated that age at marriage for husband and wife, the age gap between spouses, desire for additional child, household structure, residence, education, religion, caste, standard of living and mass media exposure affect the use of contraception and fertility behavior [4].

The secondary analysis of the Tanzania Demographic Health Survey (TDHS), 2010 indicated that women empowerment, male-female age difference, child desire, partners education and advice given at health care facilities on family planning were predictors of modern contraceptive use [5].

The analysis of 2008/09 Kenya Demographic and Health Survey (DHS) to look at the effect of age difference on contraception use indicated that the spousal age difference has no association with contraception use [6].

The analysis of 2014 Kenya Demographic and Health Survey (DHS) to look at the determinants of modern contraceptive use found that region of residence, marital status, religion, wealth, interaction with a health care provider, fertility preference, number of sexual partners and access to media were all significantly associated with modern contraceptive use [7].

The cross sectional study conducted in Urban Kenya to see the Couple Characteristics and Contraceptive use showed spouses' education, religion and income were correlated with contraceptive use [8].

The analysis of 2008 Nigeria Demographic and Health Survey (DHS) to assess the age difference between partners and contraceptive use indicated that there was no association between age differences between partners' and women's contraceptive use but household wealth and regional differences were predictors [3].

The cross sectional study conducted in Jimma zone to assess spousal discordance on fertility preference and its effect on contraceptive practice indicated that wife's age, husband's desire for more children, husband's favorable attitude towards family planning and husband's preparedness to accept his wife's use of contraceptives without his consent are significant contributors for contraceptive use [9]. Due to the nature of human sexual reproduction, men more attracted to women who appear to be healthy and fertile. Thus age is an important visible cue of a woman's fertility, given that women have a limited reproductive window. This helps to explain why younger men's age preferences are not as pronounced as those of older men. That is, preferring younger and younger partners are more likely to result in successful reproduction [10].

All women who want to prevent pregnancy are able to obtain and use modern contraceptives, that they are given their choice otherwise impair their health and limit their prospects for productive participation in society. Yet, unplanned pregnancies among women happen despite the best of contraceptive intentions [11–13], (https://www.worldometers.info/world-population/population-by-country/). Hence, this study was aimed to examine the spousal age difference and its effect on contraceptive use among married couples at county level.

## Methodology

### Study setting

Ethiopia is, the largest nation in the Horn of Africa, and country bounded by Eritrea from the north, Sudan and South Sudan from the West, Kenya from the South, and Somalia and Djibouti from the East. The capital city of the country is Addis Ababa. Ethiopia is the second most populous country in Africa and 12th in the world with an estimated population of 112.73 million. The male to female ratio is almost 1:1 (https://www.worldometers.info/world-population/population-by-country/). Women of childbearing age account for about 57% of the female population and 30% of the total population. Hence, the contraceptive prevalence rate (CPR) for currently married women age 15–49 was 36% and unmet need for family planning among currently married women is 22% [14].

### Sampling

The data for this study was obtained from the 2016 Ethiopian Demographic and Health Survey (EDHS). The sampling frame for the study was a complete list of 84, 915 enumeration areas (EAs) created for the 2007 population and housing census [PHC]. EDHS typically adopt a two-stage sample design. Each region was stratified into urban and rural areas, which yielded 21 sampling strata. Samples of Enumeration areas [EAs] were selected independently in each stratum in two stages. The first stage involves randomly selecting clusters, EAs. Two hundred two, 202 urban and 443 rural clusters were selected. At the second stage a systematic sample of households is drawn from a listing of households in each of the sampled clusters-28 households per each cluster were selected.

#### *Data collection*

Women between 15 and 49 years who were either permanent residents of the selected households or visitors who stayed in the household the night before the survey were eligible to be interviewed and one woman per household was selected. The EDHS data collection tools were divided into five sets: The Household Questionnaire, the Woman's Questionnaire, the Man's Questionnaire, the Biomarker Questionnaire, and the Health Facility Questionnaire. Data on contraceptive use was collected using The Woman's Questionnaire.

Interviewers selected for the survey used tablet computers to record responses during the interviews. The tablets were equipped with Bluetooth technology to enable remote electronic transfer of files. Transfer of assignment sheets from team supervisor to interviewers and transfer of completed questionnaires from interviewers to the supervisor were performed electronically through the CSPro software [15].

### Variables

**Dependent variables:** contraceptive use (Yes/No).

**Independent variables**: Age category, age difference (Age difference = Husband's Age minus Wife's Age), place of residence, religion, region, sex of household head, wealth status, women's level of education, husband/ partner's education level, respondent's current working condition, knowledge of any method, recent sexual activity, fertility preference of the husband and fertility preference of the women were taken as independent variables.

### Data processing and analysis

Relevant variables for this study were extracted from Ethiopian Demographic and Health Survey [EDHS] 2016 data. We used IBM SPSS statistics version 20 software for analysis. The data were described using frequency and percentage. Bivariate logistic regression was conducted to examine the crude association between spousal age difference and contraceptive use. Finally, multiple logistic regressions were conducted to identify independent predictors of contraceptive use. Variables with $p$ value less than 0.05 were considered as significantly associated with contraceptive use. All analyses were adjusted for clusters and sample weights.

## Results

### Description of study participants

This section describes the distribution of women ($N$ = 7268) by their selected background characteristics using the EDHS data set. The highest proportion 1841 (25.3%) of women were within age groups of 25 and 29 years. Almost two fifth 2897 (39.9%) of the women were from the Oromia regional state. Most of the women 6237(85.8%), were residents of rural areas. Three thousand and sixty-four (42.2%) were Orthodox by religion followed by Muslim 2442 (33.6%). Almost all 6969(95.9%) of the households were headed by males. Only 454 (6.2%) and 247 (3.4%) of the husbands and wives had attained their higher education respectively. Nearly one fifth 1555 (21.4%) of them were from poor socioeconomic group (Table 1).

### Experience of contraceptive use

Regarding knowledge of contraceptive method almost all 7189 (98.9%) of them knew the contraceptive methods. On the other hand, only three in five 4438 (61.1%) of them had history of contraceptive use to delay or avoid getting pregnant. As to the sexual practice in the last 4 weeks almost nine in ten (87.2%) were active. However, only two in five 2608 (41.2%) were using contraceptive

**Table 1** Distribution of women by their selected background characteristics, 2016 EDHS

| Variable | Category | Frequency($n$ = 7268) | Percent |
|---|---|---|---|
| Age | 15–19 | 419 | 5.8 |
| | 20–24 | 1272 | 17.5 |
| | 25–29 | 1841 | 25.3 |
| | 30–34 | 1468 | 20.2 |
| | 35–39 | 1169 | 16.1 |
| | 40–44 | 681 | 9.4 |
| | 45–49 | 417 | 5.7 |
| Region | Oromia | 2897 | 39.9 |
| | Amhara | 1879 | 25.9 |
| | SNNPR | 1526 | 21.0 |
| | Tigray | 408 | 5.6 |
| | Addis Adaba | 214 | 2.9 |
| | Somali | 163 | 2.2 |
| | Others [a] | 181 | 2.5 |
| Residence | Urban | 1031 | 14.2 |
| | Rural | 6237 | 85.8 |
| Religion | Orthodox | 3064 | 42.2 |
| | Muslim | 2442 | 33.6 |
| | Protestant | 1612 | 22.2 |
| | Other[b] | 150 | 2 |
| Sex of household head | Male | 6969 | 95.9 |
| | Female | 299 | 4.1 |
| Husband/partner's education level | No education | 3229 | 44.4 |
| | Primary | 2908 | 40.0 |
| | Secondary | 639 | 8.8 |
| | Higher | 454 | 6.2 |
| | Don't know | 38 | .5 |
| Highest educational level women | No education | 4465 | 61.4 |
| | Primary | 2131 | 29.3 |
| | Secondary | 425 | 5.8 |
| | Higher | 247 | 3.4 |
| Respondent currently working | No | 5076 | 69.8 |
| | Yes | 2192 | 30.2 |
| Wealth Index | Poorest | 1280 | 17.6 |
| | Poorer | 1555 | 21.4 |
| | Middle | 1514 | 20.8 |
| | Richer | 1504 | 20.7 |
| | Richest | 1414 | 19.5 |

Others [a] Afar, Benishangul, Gambela, Harari and Dire Dawa
Other[b] Catholic, Traditional, Other

method currently. Also 1692(45.4%) do not intend to use the contraceptive. The majority 4619 (63.6%) and 4142 (57.0%) of the husbands and wives have fertility preference respectively. More than one fifth 1640 (22.6%) them have six and above children (Table 2).

**Decision making and Age difference**

Decision on contraceptive use was made a jointly 2108 (75.6%), likewise there was joint decision on health care aspects among 5163(71.0%). However, in matters concerning household expenditure, one in five 318 (22.9%)

**Table 2** Distribution of women by their experience of contraceptive use, 2016 EDHS

| Variable | Category | Frequency($n$ = 7268) | Percent |
|---|---|---|---|
| Knowledge of any method | Knows no method | 79 | 1.1 |
| | Knows methods | 7189 | 98.9 |
| Ever used contraceptive | No (Not used outside and in calendar) | 2830 | 38.9 |
| | Yes (used outside and in calendar) | 4438 | 61.1 |
| Recent sexual activity | Active in last 4 weeks | 6335 | 87.2 |
| | Not active in last 4 weeks | 932 | 12.8 |
| Current use of contraceptive($n$ = 6335) | Not using | 3728 | 58.8 |
| | Using | 2608 | 41.2 |
| Intention to use ($n$ = 3728) | Use later | 1942 | 52.1 |
| | Unsure about use | 94 | 2.5 |
| | Does not intend | 1692 | 45.4 |
| Fertility preference of the Husband | Have another | 4619 | 63.6 |
| | Undecided | 222 | 3.1 |
| | No more | 2265 | 31.2 |
| | Others [a] | 162 | 2.3 |
| Fertility preference of the women | Have another | 4142 | 57.0 |
| | Undecided | 386 | 5.3 |
| | No more | 2622 | 36.1 |
| | Others [a] | 118 | 1.7 |
| Living children and current pregnancy | No child | 456 | 6.3 |
| | One Child | 1105 | 15.2 |
| | Two Children | 1135 | 15.6 |
| | Three Children | 1107 | 15.2 |
| | Four Children | 994 | 13.7 |
| | Five Children | 831 | 11.4 |
| | Six and above Children | 1640 | 22.6 |

[a] Sterilized (respondent or partner and Declared infecund

respondents were reported independent decision making. The age difference is calculated by using husband's age minus wife's age and further categorized negative (Age of wife is greater), equal greater than 10 years and less than 10 years to see the implication of age deference indeed, age-gap by more than 10 years perceive substantially more social disapproval regarding their relationship than do couples with only a minimal or no age gap. More than three fourth (78.6%) of husbands' were in age difference less than 10 year compared to their wife. (Table 3).

### Association between spouses age difference and contraceptive use

Women age, age difference, place of residence, religion, current working status, socioeconomic, husband's education, women's education, living children and current pregnancy, the couples' fertility preference and who decides on health care use were candidate variables for multiple logistic regression. And in the final model women age, age difference, place of residence, religion, current working status, socioeconomic, husband's education, living children and current pregnancy, the couples' fertility preference and who decides on health care use were remained statistically significant determinants of contraceptive use.

A spousal age difference was found to be a significant factor affecting the use of contraceptives. Women, older than their spouses were 1.77 times [AOR = 1.771, CI (1.276, 2.459) more likely to use contraceptives compared to those women, their husband age is greater than their age by ten or less years. Also, women having older spouse's age differences greater than 10 years were by 1.2% [AOR = .988, CI, .848, 1.150] less likely to use contraception compared with those women and husband age differences is ten or less than years. Also women who were living in urban area were 1.482 times (AOR = 1.482, CI, 1.161 to 1.890) more likely to use contraception compared to a woman living in rural area.

The probability of contraception use was 1.170 times (AOR: 1.170; 95%CI: 1.033 to 1.325) more likely among women who were currently working compared to

**Table 3** Distribution of women by their age difference and decision making, 2016 EDHS

| Variable | Category | Frequency | Percent |
|---|---|---|---|
| Decision maker for using contraception ($n = 2788$) | Mainly respondent | 523 | 18.8 |
| | Mainly husband, partner | 154 | 5.5 |
| | Joint decision | 2108 | 75.6 |
| | Other | 3 | .1 |
| Person who usually decides on respondent's health care | Respondent alone | 760 | 10.5 |
| | Respondent and husband/partner | 5163 | 71.0 |
| | Husband/partner alone | 1322 | 18.2 |
| | Other | 22 | .3 |
| Who decides how to spend respondent's earnings($n = 1388$) | Respondent alone | 318 | 22.9 |
| | Respondent and husband/partner | 949 | 68.4 |
| | Husband/partner alone | 121 | 8.7 |
| Age of the husbands' to women's | Negative (Age of wife is greater) | 208 | 2.9 |
| | Age of husband is equal to that of wife | 158 | 2.2 |
| | Age of husband is greater by ≤10 years | 5710 | 78.6 |
| | Age of husband is greater by >10 years | 1192 | 16.4 |

women who were not working at the time of the survey. Being women from the richest household economic category were 2.560 times more likely to use contraception compared with women from the poorest households (AOR: 2.560; 95%CI: 2.000 to 3.278).

Similarly, the partner's education level was found to be an important determinant of contraceptive use and husband with primary and higher education were 1.042 and 1.282 times more likely to use contraceptives, respectively, than women with no formal education. In addition, those whose husbands had no more fertility preference were 1.233 times (AOR: 1.233; 95%CI: 1.070 to 1.420) more likely to use contraceptives compared with those who have no fertility preference.

Moreover, contraceptive use was 15.1% less likely among women decision make for their health care use was their husband alone compared to women who made the decision by themselves (AOR: .847, CI: .729 to .985) (Table 4).

## Discussion

This analysis shows that just nearly nine in ten (87.2%) of the women were sexually active during the last 4 weeks of the survey period. However, only two in five (41.2%) were reported the contraceptive use during the study. This implies that three fifth of them were not using the contraceptives, although, almost all (98.8%) of them knew the contraceptive methods. This indicated that besides the knowledge factor, as a number of socioeconomic, demographic and cultural factors contribute to the contraceptive use [4].

This study further revealed the relationship between the spouses' age difference and contraceptive use. And the age difference of the spouses was found to be a significant factor affecting the use of contraceptives, women whose husbands' age was greater than their age was less likely to use a contraceptive compared with those who were older than their husbands.

Also, in the social and psychological literatures, age-gap carries some meaning for partners in any relationship and differences beyond 10 years appear to be regarded as non-normative, this leads to marital satisfaction declines. Substantially leads to more social disapproval regarding their relationship than does couples with only a minimal or no age gap [10, 16]. The finding was also in line with the study conducted in India, where the age difference between spouses influence marital stability, marital satisfaction, family size preference and contraceptive use [2]. This may be due to when the husbands are older than their wives; there is possible disparity in social position, resources and life experiences. Thus, women with older husbands, therefore tend to have lesser autonomy in the socioeconomic sphere like education, economic activity, access to resources, and in interpersonal and family relationships, such as freedom of speech, freedom to travel, decision-making power regarding childbearing and contraceptive use [1, 3, 17].

Similarly, women age, participant's residence, religion, current working status, socioeconomic, husband's education, living children and current pregnancy, the couples' fertility preference and who decides on health care use were found to be important contributing factors for contraceptive use [4].

This finding is consistent with the analysis from 2010 Tanzania Demographic Health Survey (TDHS), 2014

**Table 4** Bivariate and multivariate logistic regression model showing predictors of spouses' age difference and contraceptive use, 2016 EDHS

| Variable and its category | | COR [95% CI] | AOR [95% CI] |
|---|---|---|---|
| Women age classification | 15–19 | .713(.564, 900) | .892 (.665, 1.197) |
| | 20–24 | .890 (.764, 1.037) | .941 (.784, 1.128) |
| | 25–29 | 1 | |
| | 30–34 | .825 (.711, 956) | .886 (.746, 1.052) |
| | 35–39 | .773 (.659, 907) | .882 (.723, 1.077) |
| | 40–44 | .805 (.666, 974) | .877 (.687, 1.120) |
| | 45–49 | .348 (.266, 454) | .455 (.326, 636)* |
| Age difference | Negative (Age of wife is greater) | 1.506 (1.131, 2.006) | 1.771 (1.276, 2.459)* |
| | Equal to that of wife | .960 (.677, 1.361) | .790 (.542, 1.153) |
| | Age of husband greater by ≤10 years | 1 | |
| | Age of husband greater by 10 years | .963 (.839, 1.106) | .988 (.848, 1.150) |
| Type of place of residence | Urban | 2.612 (2.258, 3.022) | 1.482 (1.161, 1.890)* |
| | Rural | 1 | 1 |
| Religion | Orthodox | 1 | |
| | Protestant | .818 (.719, 930) | .966 (.808, 1.155) |
| | Muslim | .359 (.317, 405) | .579 (.496, 675) * |
| | Other | .618 (.419, .912) | .944 (.611, 1.459) |
| Current working status | Not working | 1 | |
| | Working | 1.506 (1.352, 1.677) | 1.170 (1.033, 1.325) * |
| Wealth Index | Poorest | 1 | 1 |
| | Poorer | 1.967 (1.640, 2.358) | 1.796 (1.479, 2.180) * |
| | Middle | 2.662 (2.224, 3.186) | 2.314 (1.906, 2.809) * |
| | Richer | 2.854 (2.385, 3.415) | 2.454 (2.015, 2.988) * |
| | Richest | 4.668 (3.891, 5.601) | 2.560 (2.000, 3.278) * |
| Husband/partner's education level | No education | 1 | |
| | Primary | 1.321 (1.183, 1.475) | 1.158 (1.013, 1.323) * |
| | Secondary | 1.684 (1.404, 2.021) | 1.040 (.823, 1.316) |
| | Higher | 3.120 (2.505, 3.885) | 1.282 (.941, 1.746) |
| | Don't know | 1.043 (.524, 2.079) | .828 (.397, 1.723) |
| Highest educational level women | No education | 1 | |
| | Primary | 1.474 (1.318, 1.649) | 1.042 (.904, 1.202) |
| | Secondary | 2.524 (2.033, 3.134) | 1.142 (.859, 1.518) |
| | Higher | 3.439 (2.579, 4.585) | 1.175 (.786, 1.756) |
| Living children and current pregnancy | No child | 2.013 (1.611, 2.516) | 1.674 (1.193, 2.349) * |
| | One Child | 2.155 (1.815, 2.560) | 2.148 (1.636, 2.820) * |
| | Two Children | 2.795 (2.358, 3.313) | 2.669 (2.093, 3.404) * |
| | Three Children | 1.978 (1.666, 2.348) | 1.844 (1.478, 2.302) * |
| | Four Children | 1.793 (1.501, 2.141) | 1.681 (1.362, 2.076) * |
| | Five Children | 1.318 (1.088, 1.598) | 1.331 (1.073,1.650) * |
| | Six and above Children | 1 | |
| Fertility preference of the women | Have another | 1 | 1 |
| | Undecided | .604 (.469, 778) | .813 (.614, 1.077) |
| | No more | 1.123 (1.010, 1.248) | 1.603 (1.391, 1.849) * |

**Table 4** Bivariate and multivariate logistic regression model showing predictors of spouses' age difference and contraceptive use, 2016 EDHS *(Continued)*

| Variable and its category | | COR [95% CI] | AOR [95% CI] |
|---|---|---|---|
| | Others | .386 (.235, 634) | .118 (.039,.353) * |
| Fertility preference of the Husband | Have another | 1 | 1 |
| | Undecided | .957 (.710, 1.289) | 1.229 (.870, 1.736) |
| | No more | 1.084 (.972, 1.209) | 1.233 (1.070, 1.420) * |
| | Sterilized | .342 (.176, 666) | .231 (.088,.603) * |
| | Declared infecund | .299 (.163, 547) | .430 (.220, 841) * |
| Who decides on health care | Respondent alone | 1.021 (.863,1.208) | .900 (.745, 1.087) |
| | Respondent and husband/partner | 1 | |
| | Husband/partner alone | .647 (.564,.742) | 847 (.729,.985) * |
| | Other | 5.988 (2.019, 17.765) | 15.235 (4.456, 52.085)* |

*Significant $p \leq 0.05$

Kenya Demographic and Health Survey (DHS), the cross sectional study conducted in Urban Kenya, Turkey where women empowerment, male-female age difference, partners education and advice given at health care facilities on family planning, region of residence, marital status, religion, wealth, interaction with a health care provider, fertility preference, number of sexual partners and access to media were found to be predictors of modern contraceptive use [6, 8, 9, 17].

Also consistent with the study conducted in India, where the age gap between couples contraception use and fertility influenced by age at marriage for husband and wife, the age gap between spouses, desire for additional child, household structure, residence, education, religion, standard of living and mass media exposure [4]. This could be due to the reason that the more the husband is educated, the more access to media, have stable household structure, health seeking behavior and he would be aware of the benefits of contraceptive, less desire for more child as development itself is the best contraceptive so that he encouraged his wife to use contraceptive.

The age difference between spouses may be one of the sign for woman' s autonomy, rural women usually have less access than urban women to contraception, information about contraceptive methods and access to health care that leads to less use of the contraceptive, there are also differences in contraceptive use by education, as the level of education is likely to affect their knowledge of contraceptive methods, its side effects, perceptions about contraception and factors like socioeconomic, demographic and cultural connotations these reasons might be among the contributing factors to contraceptive use.

However, this finding was unlike the analysis of 2008/09 Kenya Demographic and Health Survey (DHS) and 2008 Nigeria Demographic and Health Survey (DHS) where the spousal age difference has no association with contraception use but household wealth and regional differences were predictors [3, 6].

## Conclusion

This study found an association between spousal age differences and women's contraceptive use. Similarly, women age, age difference, participant's residence, religion, current working status, socioeconomic, husband's education, living children and current pregnancy, the couples' fertility preference and who decides on health care use were found to be predictors of contraceptive use. Strengthening strategies for improving women's educational status, socio-economic and demographic that will help to limit the age differences and improve contraceptive use. Further study, including the use of qualitative study is recommended to dig out the why components and better understand this finding.

### Abbreviations

EDHS: Ethiopian Demographic and Health Survey; SPSS: Statistical Package for the Social Sciences; AOR: Adjusted Odd ratio; CI: Confidence Interval; TDHS: Tanzania Demographic Health Survey; DHS: Demographic and Health Survey; EAs: Enumeration areas; PHC: Population and housing census

### Acknowledgements

We would like to thank the Demographic and Health Surveys (DHS) Program for availing the data and Professor Susan Anand for proofreading.

### Authors' contributions

Conceptualization: Sena Belina. Formal analysis: Sena Belina. Methodology: Sena Belina, Yonas Biratu, Ayantu Kebede, Alemi Kebede, Adugna Olani. Writing original draft: Sena Belina. Writing review and editing: Sena Belina, Yonas Biratu, Ayantu Kebede, Alemi Kebede, Adugna Olani. The author(s) read and approved the final manuscript.

### Author details

[1]Faculty of Health Sciences, School of Nursing and Midwifery, Jimma University Institute of Health Science, Addis Abeba, Ethiopia. [2]Department of Epidemiology, Faculty of Public Health, Jimma University Institute of Health, Addis Abeba, Ethiopia. [3]Population and Family Health Department, Faculty of Public Health, Jimma University Institute of Health Science, Addis Abeba, Ethiopia.

## References

1. Magali Barbieri, Véronique Hertrich and Madeleine Grieve. Age Difference between Spouses and Contraceptive Practice in Sub-Saharan Africa. 2019;60(5): 617–54. https://www.jstor.org/stable/4148187.
2. Age K. Levels , trends and patterns of age difference among the couples in India. 257629. Retrival date ,Agust 2020 https://iussp.org/sites/default/files/event_call_for_papers/Levels%20and%20trends%20of%20age%20difference%20among%20couples%20in%20India_IUSSP2013.pdf.
3. Ibisomi L. Is Age Difference Between Partners Associated with Contraceptive Use Among Married Couples in Nigeria ? International Perspectives on Sexual and Reproductive Health, 2014, 40(1):39–45. https://doi.org/10.1363/4003914.
4. Das KC, Gautam V, Das K, Tripathy PK. Influence of Age gap between couples on contraception and fertility. J Fam Welf. 2011;57(2):30–8.
5. Kidayi PL, Msuya S, Todd J, Mtuya CC, Mtuy T, Mahande MJ. Determinants of Modern Contraceptive Use among Women of Reproductive Age in Tanzania: Evidence from Tanzania Demographic and Health Survey Data. 2015;(July):43–52.
6. Odaa Beatrice Akotli. (2010). The Effect of Age Difference on Contraception Use Among Married Women in Kenya. Reg. Number Q56/64022/2010.
7. Ochako R, Temmerman M, Mbondo M, Askew I. Determinants of modern contraceptive use among sexually active men in Kenya; 2017. p. 1–15.
8. Irani, et al. Couple characteristics and contraceptive use among women and their Partners in Urban Kenya. Int Perspect Sex Reprod Health. 2014;40(1): 11–20. https://doi.org/10.1363/4001114.
9. Tilahun T, Coene G, Temmerman M, Degomme O. Spousal discordance on fertility preference and its effect on contraceptive practice among married couples in Jimma zone, Ethiopia; 2014. p. 1–10.
10. Lehmiller J, Agnew C. May–December paradoxes: an exploration of Age-gap relationships in Western society; 2011.
11. Biddlecom A, Riley T, Darroch JE, Sully E, Kantorová V. Future Scenarios of Adolescent Contraceptive Use, Cost and Impact in Developing Regions, New York: Guttmacher Institute. 2018. https://www.guttmacher.org/report/adolescent-contraceptive-use-in-developing-regions.
12. Fact sheet on teenage pregnancy in Ethiopia. https://www.rutgers.international/sites/rutgersorg/files/PDF/RHRNHLPF_A4leaflet_Ethiopia.pdf.
13. Chandra-mouli V, Parameshwar PS, Parry M, Lane C, Hainsworth G, Wong S, et al. A never-before opportunity to strengthen investment and action on adolescent contraception , and what we must do to make full use of it. Reproductive Health. 2017;14:85. https://doi.org/10.1186/s12978-017-0347-9.
14. Federal democratic Republic of Ethiopia. Ministry of health. National Reproductive health Strategy 2016–2020, Addis Ababa, Ethiopia. October 2016.
15. Central Statistical Agency (CSA) [Ethiopia] and ICF. 2016. Ethiopia Demographic and Health Survey 2016. Addis Ababa, Ethiopia, and Rockville, Maryland: CSA and ICF.
16. Lee, McKinnish. The marital satisfaction of differently aged couples. J Popul Econ. 2018 April;31(2):337–62. https://doi.org/10.1007/s00148-017-0658-8.
17. Barbieri M, Barbieri M, Barbieri M. Age difference between spouses and contraceptive practice in sub-Saharan Africa; 2005.

6

# The relationship of maternal anxiety, positive and negative affect schedule and fatigue with neonatal psychological health upon childbirth

Sara Dokuhaki[1], Fateme Dokuhaki[2] and Marzieh Akbarzadeh[3*]

**Abstract**

**Background:** Exposure of mothers to negative moods and stress before childbirth leads to negative consequences for the infants. Given the importance of psychological health, this study aimed to examine the effect of these factors on the infants' psychological health.

**Method:** This cross-sectional study was conducted in Shiraz hospitals on 110 pregnant women selected with multistage random sampling. Research tools included The McGill Pain Questionnaire (MPQ) to measure fatigue with three criteria; The Positive and Negative Emotion Schedule (PANAS); and The Spielberger State-Trait Anxiety Inventory (STAI) were used to measure maternal mood and anxiety level. Also, neonatal psychological health was assessed by a checklist. Neonatal psychological health's correlation with maternal anxiety, fatigue, and mental state was assessed. Data were analyzed by SPSS-19 software using Pearson correlation coefficient and statistical regression at the significance level of 0.05.

**Result:** Although there was no significant relationship between maternal anxiety score and neonatal psychological health after birth ($p = 0.231$; $r$=-0.343), the relationship was significant immediately after birth with positive ($P < 0.001$; $r = 0.343$) and negative affect scores ($P < 0.001$; $r$=-0.357).

**Conclusions:** There was a statistically significant relationship between the neonatal psychological health and maternal fatigue ($p \leq 0.001$; $r$ = -0.357) and PANAS ($p \leq 0.001$) of the mother; however, it had no significant relationship with maternal anxiety ($p = 0.231$; $r$=- 0.343). Therefore, nurses and midwives can reduce maternal anxiety and improve neonatal mental health by supporting mothers.

**Keywords:** Anxiety, Mood, Fatigue, Infant, Health

* Correspondence: marzieh.akhbar@gmail.com
[3]Maternal-fetal Medicine Research Center, Department of Midwifery, School of Nursing and Midwifery, Shiraz University of Medical Sciences, Shiraz, Iran

## Introduction

Anxiety, depression, stress and excitement of pregnancy period, especially upon childbirth, are usually overlooked in women [1]. Anxiety and stress have deleterious effects on the mother and infant [2]. Studies show that exposure of the mother to negative excitement and stress before childbirth increases the risk of behavioral and psychological problems in the infant's life after birth. Maternal psychological stress is basically known as a teratogen, a factor that can entail deleterious prenatal consequences [3, 4]. Higher pregnant mothers' anxiety scores are associated with the higher likelihood of cesarean childbirth and lower successful breastfeeding [5]. Anxiety gives rise to lower Apgar scores of infants upon birth and at minute 5; in this regard, Stuart et al. reported that low Apgar scores at minute 5 after birth were associated with a slight cognitive disorder in didactic performance [6].

In fact, the human embryo is extremely sensitive to maternal stress and affective moods. Post-natal stress can affect birth results and may cause neurobehavioral development in damaged infants. In a study, training on decreasing anxiety and increasing fetal affection toward pregnant mothers during the pregnancy increased neonatal psychological health upon birth [7, 8].

Neonatal exposure to maternal stress before birth was associated with low birth weight and smaller head perimeter. Improved maternal mood and calmness, and thus more neonatal improvement results in quicker attainment of motor development indicators [9, 10]. Similarly, physical indicators (weight, height, and head perimeter) were significantly greater than those of infants whose mothers have not received the necessary training during pregnancy [11, 12], which is due reduced anxiety, improved mood, and more kindness toward the fetus.

Several studies also showed that maternal stress reduced neonatal cognitive functions and brain volume, leading to learning and memory problems. Similarly, some reports on maternal anxiety or childbirth anxiety pointed out the emotional problems, hyperactivity, attention deficiency, and Tourette syndrome among such children.

Pregnancy stress appears to be one of the determinant factors of delayed growth and mental progress in 8-month infants and might be a risk factor for subsequent developmental problems.

On the other hand, in addition to anxiety and stress, mothers experience fatigue during pregnancy and after birth [13, 14]. In fact, during pregnancy, fatigue mostly comes with depression, anxiety, fear, and long duration of work; therefore, it can bring about similar effects, i.e. stress-derived fatigue and pregnant women usually report fatigue (87.2 to 96.5) [15]. Also, prenatal fatigue comes with postnatal depression, anxiety, premature childbirth, and cesarean section. In other words, maternal fatigue and anxiety have similar effects on the women's and consequently, infants' health; and psychological health problems during childhood will be a major challenge for their general health in the future [16].

That is often the main reason for impaired learning and social disorder that can also continue with greater severity at older ages; as the studies of neural sciences, biology, genetics, and social sciences within the past two decades have shown that the first 1000 days of life (childbirth period and first two years of life) is the golden age of brain development and psychological health of the infant [17–19]. Most of the studies revealed the relationship between deleterious effects of stress, fatigue, and mother's mood on neonatal physical health, growth, and development. The detrimental effects on neonatal psychological health indicators have not been addressed sufficiently [20–23], which are dealt with in the present study.

## Materials and methods

This descriptive study (correlation type) was conducted on 110 pregnant women aged 18–40 years old, who have referred to the hospital for labor. The inclusion criteria were gravida one, singleton and term pregnancy, and natural childbirth. Thus, mothers lacking severe and chronic diseases and willing to take part in the study were enrolled. The exclusion criteria were suffering from any physical or mental problems. The mothers were selected from the maternity ward of Hazrat Zeinab (P.B.U.H), Shoushtari, and Hafez hospitals affiliated with Shiraz University of Medical Sciences using random multistage sampling. The degree of anxiety was measured using STAI. Also, positive and negative emotion scores and pregnant mothers' fatigue were measured through standard questions. Neonatal psychological health was determined after birth using questionnaires related to the neonatal psychological health upon birth. Data were analyzed with SPSS software using the Pearson correlation coefficient and statistical regression at the significance level of 0.05.

The research tools used in this study were as follows:

1. Spielberger State-Trait Anxiety Inventory (STAI): It is used for assessing maternal anxiety level. It has 40 items, 20 of which are about positional anxiety and 20 are about character anxiety, and are scored based on a 3-point Likert scale. A total score of 0–19 indicates no anxiety; 20–40 indicates slight anxiety; 41–60 indicates average anxiety; and 61–80 indicates severe anxiety. Aqamohammadi et al. (2007) used STAI on 150 patients under surgery and reported a reliability of 97 %. The validity and reliability of the questionnaire have been reported

by Aqamohammadi et al., which was the basis of the present study [24].

2. The McGill Pain Questionnaire (MPQ): It is used to measure measuring the affective status and fatigue with three mental, cognitive, psychological criteria .
3. The Positive And Negative Affect Schedule (PANAS) is used for assessing the participants' mood at a specific time (like the time of conducting the test). It is made up of 20 words, each of which denotes different feelings and emotions, which are scored based on a 3-point Likert scale from very low or not at all to very high. The positive and negative PANAS are obtained from the sum of the scores of ten positive and ten negative words, respectively. Positive and negative words are retrieved in a scattered manner. In this study, the Cronbach alpha and test-retest correlation for the positive section of PANAS were 0.88 and 0.85, respectively. These were 0.87 and 0.89 for the negative part of PANAS, respectively.
4. Neonatal psychological health assessment checklist upon childbirth is developed based on the neonatal psychological health indicators derived from psychological health and development of psychology and pregnancy books. Upon childbirth, the neonatal psychological health indicators cannot be separated from its physical health, so an attempt was made to measure the main indicators of psychological health using these questions.

The checklist upon childbirth has 9 questions, scores 0, 1 or 2.; Finally, the scores of the 9 questions are summed up; the overall score of the checklists ranges from 0 to 18. Higher scores indicate higher neonatal psychological health. Cronbach alpha and split-half scores for this checklist were 0.89 and 0.72, respectively. The content validity of the checklist was calculated through scoring and assessing by 6 pediatricians. Given the obtained validity and reliability derived from the study conducted by Shayeqhian et al., we used this questionnaire in this study [25].

## Results

The mean age of the participants in this study was 26.42 ± 5.60 years; their mean anxiety level was 29.99 ± 14.05, their mean fatigue was 38.37 ± 16.11, their positive emotion was 37.22 ± 7.33, and mean neonatal psychological health upon birth was 16.68 ± 1.35 (Table 1). The Kolmogorov Smirnov test was used to assess data normality which indicated normal distribution of all data. Therefore, the Pearson correlation coefficient was used for obtaining the linear relationship, which showed no statistical relationship between maternal anxiety score and neonatal psychological health after birth. Moreover, there was a statistically significant relationship between neonatal psychological health score immediately after birth and a positive emotion score ($P < 0.001$; $r = 0.516$) and maternal fatigue score ($p < 0.001$; $r$=-0.357) (Table 2).

## Discussion

The present study found no significant relationship between maternal anxiety and neonatal psychological health after birth ($r$=-0.115; $p = 0.231$), or neonatal psychological health scores including Apgar score, and birth weight. Keenan et al. also reported that birth weight and Apgar score were not related to maternal anxiety and depression [26].

However, Hassanjanzadeh et al. emphasized the relationship of neonatal outcomes with pregnancy stress and depression and anxiety during pregnancy [27]. In their study, the results of correlation of depression, stress, and anxiety variables with birth weight, length and perimeter of the head, and Apgar score of infants showed significant differences ($P < 0.05$). Multiple regression analysis showed that interpersonal relationship was correlated with birth weight prediction (B=-0.324), anxiety with height prediction (B=-0.197); stress with head perimeter prediction (B=-0.350); and depression with Apgar score prediction (B=-0.323; $p < 0.001$).

Although this study found an obvious relationship between neonatal psychological health and other emotional maternal indicators such as maternal mood and fatigue upon childbirth, measurement should be carried out on a periodical basis and during pregnancy, not only upon childbirth since maternal anxiety diagram within

**Table 1** Neonatal Mental Health Assessment by Maternal Anxiety Level

| Maternal Anxiety Score | N | Mean ± SD Neonatal Mental Health | 95 % Confidence Interval for Mean | | Minimum | Maximum |
|---|---|---|---|---|---|---|
| | | | Lower bound | Upper bound | | |
| **Normal** | 33 | 16.87 ± 1.24 | 16.43 | 17.31 | 14 | 18 |
| **Mild** | 50 | 16.68 ± 1.46 | 16.26 | 17.09 | 13 | 18 |
| **Medium** | 27 | 16.44 ± 1.28 | 15.93 | 16.95 | 14 | 18 |
| **Severe** | 0 | - | - | - | - | - |
| **Total** | 110 | 16.68 ± 1.35 | 16.42 | 16.93 | 13 | 18 |

**Table 2** Pearson Correlation with Neonatal Mental Health at Birth

| Items | Mean ± SD | Min | Max | Pearson correlation coefficient with mental health | *P* value |
|---|---|---|---|---|---|
| **Anxiety score** | 29.99 ± 14.05 | 6 | 60 | _ 0.115 | 0.231 |
| **Positive PANAS score** | 37.22 ± 7.87 | 15 | 50 | 0.343 | < 0.001 |
| **Negative PANAS score** | 18.55 ± 7.33 | 10 | 38 | _ 0.574 | < 0.001 |
| **Total PANAS score** | 18.67 ± 13.38 | _ 16 | 40 | 0.516 | < 0.001 |
| **Fatigue** | 38.37 ± 16.11 | 0.00 | 71.67 | _ 0.357 | < 0.001 |
| **Neonatal Mental Health** | 16.68 ± 1.35 | 13 | 18 | 1 | - |

pregnancy is U-shape, while in this study the anxiety experienced by the mothers during the early postpartum months was not taken into account. Similarly, in the study carried out by Zijlmans et al., it was indicated that pregnancy anxiety and increased cortisol levels in pregnant mothers were associated with respiratory diseases and children's digestion problems until the age of 3 [28]. These findings showed that the possible effects of anxiety and negative mood of mothers extend beyond the first year of life and into the childhood.

Fan et al. reported a direct relationship between maternal mood and neonatal health and indicated that maternal anxiety had deleterious effects on the infants including their birth weight. Their results showed that the long-term effect of maternal mood during pregnancy leads to cardiovascular responses among infants [29]. In a study carried out by Chien et al., increased fatigue elevated the rate of cesarean Sec. [14]. Also, in our study, the extent of mothers' fatigue was considered as one of the factors affecting neonatal psychological health.

Staneva et al. in their study entitled "the effect of mothers' depression, anxiety and perceived stress during the pregnancy period on the premature accouchement" concluded that depression, anxiety, and stress of pregnant women had a significant relationship with detrimental consequents and premature accouchement in infants [30]. Distress and undesired mood effects within the mother's pregnancy are routinely characterized with premature childbirth but without medical etiology. Overall, we could find no similar studies investigating the relationship of the neonatal psychological status with reduction of maternal fatigue and anxiety, and improvement of mood during the first 24 h after vaginal childbirth. However, several studies have been conducted on post-cesarean and vaginal delivery pain, fatigue, and maternal mood [30–34]. The present study had some limitations. Participants were selected from only two childbirth centers. This group of participants may not be representative of the target population. The sample size was small, and we did not control some confounding variables such as delivery time and the psychological status during pregnancy. Therefore, studies with larger sample sizes and longer duration are recommended.

## Conclusions

There was a significant relationship between the neonatal psychological health and the scores of mothers' PANAS mood and fatigue; however, no significant relationship was found with maternal anxiety. Therefore, healthcare personnel like physicians, midwives, nurses, and psychologists who work in the field of pregnancy caregiving should support pregnant mothers during accouchement and childbirth. Also, supporting mothers can result in improvement of maternal outcomes and neonatal psychological health.


#### Acknowledgements

The authors would like to thank Shiraz University of Medical Sciences, Shiraz, Iran; Center for Development of Clinical Research of Nemazee Hospital. Dr. Nasrin Shokrpour is sincerely thanked for editorial assistance.


#### Authors' contributions

SD and MA: Made substantial contributions to conception and design. FD: contributed to the analysis and data interpretation, data acquisition, drafting the manuscript, and revising it critically for important intellectual content. All authors read and approved the final manuscript.


#### Author details

[1]Community Based Psychiatric Care Research Center, Department of Midwifery, School of Nursing and Midwifery, Shiraz University of Medical Sciences, Shiraz, Iran. [2]Department of Psychology, Islamic Azad University of Marvdasht, Marvdasht, Iran. [3]Maternal-fetal Medicine Research Center, Department of Midwifery, School of Nursing and Midwifery, Shiraz University of Medical Sciences, Shiraz, Iran.


#### References


1. Rezaee R, Framarzi M. Predictors of mental health during pregnancy. Iran J Nurs Midwifery Res. 2014;19:45–50. .
2. Dunkel Schetter C, Tanner L. Anxiety, depression and stress in pregnancy: implications for mothers, children, research, and practice. Curr Opin Psychiatry. 2012;25:141–8. https://doi.org/10.1097/YCO.0b013e3283503680 .
3. Barker DJP. The developmental origins of chronic adult disease. Acta Paediatr. 2007;93:26–33. https://doi.org/10.1111/j.1651-2227.2004.tb00236.x.
4. Jacobson JL, Jacobson SW. Methodological considerations in behavioral toxicology in infants and children. Dev Psychol. 1996;32:390–403. https://doi.org/10.1037/0012-1649.32.3.390.
5. Adedinsewo DA, Fleming AS, Steiner M, Meaney MJ, Girard AW. Maternal Anxiety and Breastfeeding. Journal of Human Lactation. 2013;30:102–9. https://doi.org/10.1177/0890334413504244.
6. Stuart A, Otterblad Olausson P, Källen K. Apgar Scores at 5 Minutes After Birth in Relation to School Performance at 16 Years of Age. Obstetrics Gynecology. 2011;118:201–8. https://doi.org/10.1097/AOG.0b013e31822200eb.

7. dokuhaki S, Heidary M, Akbarzadeh M. Investigation of the effect of training attachment behaviors to pregnant mothers on some physical indicators of their infants from birth to three months based on the separation of male and female infants. Pediatrics Neonatology. 2018. https://doi.org/10.1016/j.pedneo.2018.08.002.
8. Akbarzadeh M, Dokuhaki A, Joker A, Pishva N, Zare N. Teaching attachment behaviors to pregnant women: a randomized controlled trial of effects on infant _mental health from birth to the age of three months. Ann Saudi Med. 2016;36:175–83. https://doi.org/10.5144/0256-4947.2016.175.
9. Weinstock M. Brain. The potential influence of maternal stress hormones on development and mental health of the offspring. Behavior Immunity. 2005; 19:296–308. https://doi.org/10.1016/j.bbi.2004.09.006.
10. Dokuhaki A, Akbarzadeh M, Pishava N, Zare N. A study of the effect of training pregnant women about attachment skills on infants' motor development indices at birth to four months. Fam Med Prim Care Rev. 2017:114 – 22.
11. Sandman CA, Davis EP, Buss C, Glynn LM. Exposure to prenatal psychobiological stress exerts programming influences on the mother and her fetus. Neuroendocrinology. 2012;95:8–21.
12. Huizink AC, Robles de Medina PG, Mulder EJ, Visser GH, Buitelaar JK. Stress during pregnancy is associated with developmental outcome in infancy. J Child Psychol Psychiatry. 2003;44:810–8. .
13. Fairbrother N, Hutton EK, Stoll K, Hall W, Kluka S. Psychometric evaluation of the Multidimensional Assessment of Fatigue scale for use with pregnant and postpartum women. Psychol Assess. 2008;20:150–8. https://doi.org/10.1037/1040-3590.20.2.150 .
14. Chien LY, Ko YL. Fatigue during pregnancy predicts caesarean deliveries. J Adv Nurs. 2004;45:487–94. .
15. Kamysheva E, Wertheim EH, Skouteris H, Paxton SJ, Milgrom J. Frequency, severity, and effect on life of physical symptoms experienced during pregnancy. J Midwifery Womens Health. 2009;54:43–9. https://doi.org/10.1016/j.jmwh.2008.08.003 .
16. Pugh LC, Milligan RA. Patterns of fatigue during childbearing. Appl Nurs Res. 1995;8:140–3. .
17. Ko YL, Wu YC, Chang PC. Physical and social predictors for pre-term births and low birth weight infants in Taiwan. J Nurs Res. 2002;10:83–9. .
18. Costello EJ, Egger H, Angold A. 10-year research update review: the epidemiology of child and adolescent psychiatric disorders: I. Methods and public health burden. J Am Acad Child Adolesc Psychiatry. 2005;44:972–86. https://doi.org/10.1097/01.chi.0000172552.41596.6f .
19. Costello EJ, Foley DL, Angold A. 10-year research update review: the epidemiology of child and adolescent psychiatric disorders: II. Developmental epidemiology. J Am Acad Child Adolesc Psychiatry. 2006;45: 8–25. https://doi.org/10.1097/01.chi.0000184929.41423.c0 .
20. Rutter M, Kim-Cohen J, Maughan B. Continuities and discontinuities in psychopathology between childhood and adult life. J Child Psychol Psychiatry. 2006;47:276–95. https://doi.org/10.1111/j.1469-7610.2006.01614.x .
21. Fox SE, Levitt P, Nelson CA 3rd. How the timing and quality of early experiences influence the development of brain architecture. Child Dev. 2010;81:28–40. https://doi.org/10.1111/j.1467-8624.2009.01380.x .
22. Crawford JR, Henry JD. The positive and negative affect schedule (PANAS): construct validity, measurement properties and normative data in a large non-clinical sample. Br J Clin Psychol. 2004;43:245–65. https://doi.org/10.1348/0144665031752934 .
23. Nejati H. Developmental psychology. Tehran: Mehshad Publications; 1992.
24. Aghamohammadiyan H, Roshan R, Zamani Z, Tabatabaey K. Developmental Psychology. Tehran: Misagh Publications; 1996.
25. Shayeghian Z, Tabatabaey S. Effect of Maternal Anxiety during Third Trimester on Pregnancy Outcomes and Infants' Mental Health. Hayat. 2008;14.
26. Keenan K, Sheffield R, Boeldt D. Are prenatal psychological or physical stressors associated with suboptimal outcomes in neonates born to adolescent mothers? Early Hum Dev. 2007;83:623–7. https://doi.org/10.1016/j.earlhumdev.2007.01.002 .
27. Hasanjanzadeh P, Faramarzi M. Relationship between Maternal General and Specific-Pregnancy Stress, Anxiety, and Depression Symptoms and Pregnancy Outcome. J Clin Diagn Res. 2017;11:VC04–7. https://doi.org/10.7860/JCDR/2017/24352.9616 .
28. Zijlmans MAC, Beijers R, Riksen-Walraven MJ, de Weerth C. Maternal late pregnancy anxiety and stress is associated with children's health: a longitudinal study. Stress. 2017;20:495–504. https://doi.org/10.1080/10253890.2017.1348497.
29. Fan F, Zou Y, Tian H, Zhang Y, Zhang J, Ma X, et al. Effects of maternal anxiety and depression during pregnancy in Chinese women on children's heart rate and blood pressure response to stress. J Hum Hypertens. 2016;30:171.
30. Staneva A, Bogossian F, Pritchard M, Wittkowski A. The effects of maternal depression, anxiety, and perceived stress during pregnancy on preterm birth: A systematic review. Women Birth. 2015;28:179–93. https://doi.org/10.1016/j.wombi.2015.02.003 .
31. Vaziri F, Shiravani M, Najib FS, Pourahmad S, Salehi A, Yazdanpanahi Z. Effect of Lavender Oil Aroma in the Early Hours of Postpartum Period on Maternal Pains, Fatigue, and Mood: A Randomized Clinical Trial. Int J Prev Med. 2017 May 4;8:29. doi: https://doi.org/10.4103/ijpvm.IJPVM_137_16. PMID: 28567231; PMCID: PMC5439291.
32. Hannah P, Adams D, Lee A, Glover V, Sandler M. Links between early post-partum mood and post-natal depression. Br J Psychiatry. 1992;160:777–80.
33. Adewuya AO. Early postpartum mood as a risk factor for postnatal depression in Nigerian women. Am J Psychiatry. 2006;163:1435–7.
34. Conrad P, Adams C. The effects of clinical aromatherapy for anxiety and depression in the high risk postpartum woman – A pilot study. Complement Ther Clin Pract. 2012;18:164–8.

# 7

# Improving public health service delivery response to address contraceptive needs of socio-economically disadvantaged HIV positive people in Maharashtra, India

Beena Joshi[1*], Bhushan Girase[1,2], Siddesh Shetty[1], Vinita Verma[3], Shrikala Acharya[4], Pramod Deoraj[5], Ragini Kulkarni[1] and Shahina Begum[1]

**Abstract**

**Background:** People living with HIV (PLHIV) receive free antiretroviral treatment (ART) in public health facilities of India. With improved life expectancy, unmet sexual and reproductive health needs of PLHIV have to be addressed through a converged programmatic response strategy. Evidence shows that socioeconomically disadvantaged women are most vulnerable to high reproductive morbidities, especially HIV positive women with an unmet need of contraception.

**Methods:** Programmatic convergence by linking ART and family planning services were strengthened at two public health facilities (district hospitals) generally accessed by disadvantaged socio-economic sections of the society. Barriers to linking services including stigma and discrimination were addressed through analysis of existing linkage situation, sensitization and training of healthcare providers and system-level interventions. This facilitated provider-initiated assessment of contraceptive needs of PLHIV, counseling about dual contraception using a couple approach, linkage to family planning centers and maintaining data about these indicators. Six hundred eligible PLHIV seeking care at ART centers were enrolled and followed up for a duration of 6 months. Acceptance of family planning services as a result of the intervention, use of dual contraception methods and their determinants were assessed.

**Results:** Eighty-seven percent HIV couples reached FP centers and 44.6% accepted dual methods at the end of the study period. Dual methods such as oral contraceptive pills (56.2%), IUCDs (19.4%), female sterilization (11.6%), injectable contraception (9.9%) and vasectomy (2.9%) in addition to condoms were the most commonly accepted methods. Condom use remained regular and consistently high throughout. The study witnessed seven unintended pregnancies, all among exclusive condom users. These women availed medical abortion services and accepted dual methods after counseling. Female index participants, concordant couples, counseling by doctors and women with CD4 count above 741 had higher odds of accepting dual contraception methods. Standard operating procedures (SOP) were developed in consultation with key stakeholders to address operational linkage of HIV and family programs.

(Continued on next page)

* Correspondence: bjoshithane@gmail.com
[1]Indian Council of Medical Research- National Institute for Research in Reproductive Health (NIRRH), Mumbai, Maharashtra, India

(Continued from previous page)
**Conclusion:** The study saw significant improvement in acceptance of dual contraception by PLHIV couples as a result of the intervention. Implementation of SOPs with supportive supervision can ensure efficient linkage of programs and provide holistic sexual and reproductive healthcare for PLHIV in India.

**Keywords:** Dual contraception, HIV-FP linkage, Women living with HIV, Unmet need for contraception, Unintended pregnancy, Prevention of parent to child transmission

## Background

Human Immunodeficiency Virus (HIV) infection remains a major global public health concern with 38 million infected individuals and 1.7 million new cases in the year 2019 [1]. An estimated 1.3 million pregnant women in the world lived with HIV, exposing them to the risk of maternal to child transmission [2]. The disease is successfully suppressed by the highly effective antiretroviral therapy and is recommended for all People Living with HIV (PLHIV) including pregnant and breastfeeding women. A four-pronged strategy for Prevention of Parent to Child Transmission (PPTCT) namely preventing HIV infection in women of childbearing age, preventing unintended pregnancies in HIV infected women, preventing transmission of HIV from infected mother to her infant by drug therapy and providing appropriate treatment, care and support to the needs of the mother, child and family are outlined by the World Health Organization (WHO) [3].

India has managed to reverse the HIV epidemic owing to its phased national programs. The Indian national program provides direct access to free diagnostics, free Anti-Retroviral Therapy (ART) therapy, PPTCT services, management of opportunistic infections including tuberculosis (TB) all through a single-window approach. Consequently, the country has contributed to global success by making significant national gains in reducing new HIV infections by more than 60% since the year 2000 and 71% reduction in Acquired Immunodeficiency Syndrome (AIDS) related deaths since the year 2005 [4]. At an adult HIV prevalence of 0.22%, India had an estimated 22,677 (10927–40,605) pregnant women living with HIV in the year 2017 [4]. India is signatory to the 90:90:90 United Nations (UN) strategy and aims to end HIV/AIDS by the year 2030. The country has prioritized elimination of mother to child transmission as one of its immediate objectives to achieve HIV elimination [5]. India has adopted the WHO four-pronged strategy for its federally implemented PPTCT program, but efforts have primarily focused on the third prong i.e. preventing transmission from mother to child using Option B plus prophylaxis. As a result, the opportunity of preventing unintended pregnancy itself is missed, increasing the investment burden of resources needed for third prong of the program [6]. Avoiding unintended pregnancies among the immuno-compromised PLHIV population presents a potential opportunity to safeguard their sexual and reproductive health (SRH) rights. Comprehensive access to contraception services facilitate PLHIV to plan their family desires, reduces transmission of sexually transmitted infections (STI) and helps getting screened for reproductive health morbidities. This benefits the larger population health outcomes. For women, contraception specifically offers control of reproduction cycle, helps delay first birth, improves spacing, reduces total number of children borne and prevents high-risk and unintended pregnancies thus also reducing the need for unsafe abortions. Preventing unintended pregnancy gains added significance as it can potentially reduce number of infants born with HIV or children getting orphaned as a result of losing their parent [7]. The current consensus suggests HIV infected women can use any of the available modern contraceptive methods [8]. Using condom alone prevents STIs and pregnancy but comes with a drawback of a high failure rate as a contraceptive and is not a woman-controlled method.

Global advocacy agenda has shifted to implementation of interventions addressing combined HIV and SRH needs most recently stated by the 2018 'Call to Action' for attaining universal health coverage [9]. Consistent and correct use of male or female condoms supplemented by other methods is endorsed for providing contraception services in context of HIV treatment programs [10]. This becomes crucial for India as it has an unmet need for family planning (FP) at 13% in the general population with a higher reported need of 17% in PLHIV group [11, 12]. Further, women's socioeconomic status could have an association with their serostatus, as HIV-positive women are significantly more likely to have low levels of education than their HIV-negative counterparts [13]. Association of socio-economic determinants like age, education, place of residence along with gender-based discrimination and domestic violence faced by Indian women make them vulnerable to both HIV and unintended pregnancies. The current HIV/AIDS service delivery in India typically focuses on condoms as the method for preventing spread of STIs and HIV but fails to acknowledge strengths of dual methods of contraception. FP service provided by the Indian PPTCT program is limited to providing general information regarding contraception as and when demanded by PLHIV. There is no active assessment of unmet contraception need or provider-initiated referral to FP centers. Management Information System (MIS) is without indicators for reporting and monitoring of these measures. Inequity in access to healthcare services further poses challenges as a result of HIV related stigma and discrimination or lack of proper knowledge among healthcare providers about services that can or cannot be provided to HIV positive people. Healthcare providers are expected to play an integral role in identifying and meeting sexual and reproductive health needs of this marginalized population. Non-HIV related service providers often are not sensitized to their needs, have misconceptions or sometimes fear about the iatrogenic spread of infection [14, 15]. Their personal belief sometimes leads to unfriendly attitudes resulting in delaying or refusal of treatment [16]. This results in poor health-seeking behavior and reduces access opportunities to the already disadvantaged sub-groups like low socio-economic sections of this vulnerable population.

This study aimed at upscaling a pretested intervention at district hospital settings to improve system level efficiency and effectiveness of linkage between HIV and family planning services with a focus on dual contraception to prevent unintended pregnancies among PLHIV. The objectives of this study included assessment of the current situation of linkage between HIV and family planning services, assessment of knowledge, attitude and practices of contraception among PLHIV, implementation of the pretested intervention linkage package with modifications based on situation analysis and assessment of post intervention acceptance of dual methods of contraception and its determinants among PLHIV.

## Methods

This implementation study was conducted between April 2016 to May 2018. The up-scaling of this implementation research was framed based on experience from a previous study undertaken by the authors that focused on linking HIV and family planning services and promoting use of dual contraception among PLHIV at two tertiary care centers in Mumbai, India between 2011 and 2013. The study conducted among 300 HIV positive women had demonstrated improved uptake of dual methods without reduction in consistent use of condoms. Fewer unintended pregnancies in the experiment group were also reported [17, 18]. The program implementation agency i.e. NACO recommended implementation of this study to be undertaken at district level settings. Two district hospitals namely Civil hospital, Parbhani and District hospital, Aundh, Pune from the state of Maharashtra in India were chosen as the sites for this study after fulfilling criteria such as patient load at ART center, availability of staff at facility and considering operational feasibility. Ethical approvals from requisite institutions and administrative approvals from the chosen hospitals were obtained before initiating the study. Privacy and confidentiality of participants was ensured throughout. An informed consent was obtained from PLHIV before enrollment to the study.

### Situation analysis of HIV-FP linkage

Healthcare providers and program managers were interviewed to assess the existing linkage status and estimate training needs to facilitate provision of linked services. A total of seven medical doctors, six counselors and two nursing staff from the study sites were selected as key informants based on convenience sampling strategy and were interviewed using a semi-structured interview schedule adapted from an internationally developed rapid assessment tool for SRH and HIV linkage [19]. Participatory observations, facility survey checklists and informal interaction with program managers were additionally used to assess physical infrastructure, referral linkage and availability of Information, Education and Counseling (IEC) materials and supplies at the study sites. Details and methods used to assess provider perspective is also published elsewhere [20].

### PLHIV enrollment and baseline assessment of knowledge, attitude and practices of contraception

HIV positive couples at ART centers of the two chosen district hospitals were screened for eligibility of acceptance of dual contraception methods. HIV concordant or discordant couples (women aged 18–40 years) not having undergone permanent sterilization and using only condoms as a contraceptive method, if did not wish pregnancy for a year and were willing to follow-up for 6 months were considered eligible for the study. An estimated sample size of 246 couples from each centre i.e. 492 couples from the two district hospitals was calculated based on average statistics of PLHIV attending HIV facilities and considering 20% increase in acceptance of dual methods [17]. Further assuming a loss to follow-up, the estimated sample size was increased to 600 couples. A total of 2663 PLHIV clients visited the chosen ART facilities during the study period. Based on the pre-defined inclusion and exclusion criteria for participation, a successive/consecutive sampling technique was used to enroll 259 index participants at Pune site and 311 participants at Parbhani facility, thus enrolling 570 eligible couples for the study after obtaining the written informed consent. Age criteria, permanent sterilization, marital status (separated/divorced/widow) or pregnancy at enrollment were the commonest causes for exclusion of cases. Among those enrolled, there were four deaths (three male and one female index participant) due to tuberculosis, one couple refused further participation, five couples separated during the study course, one woman underwent hysterectomy for dysfunctional uterine bleeding and two were lost to follow-up. Eventually, data of 556 eligible couples, 256 from Pune and 300 from Parbhani facility completing all follow-ups were considered for analysis. This number was over and above the expected sample size of 492 due to fewer losses to follow-up.

A pretested semi-structured interview schedule divided into two sections with the first section administered at enrollment to collect information on study participants and at followup. Data on socio-economic status, contraception use, sexual practice, fertility desires, reproductive health knowledge and psychological well-being of the individuals was obtained at enrollment.

#### Intervention package, implementation challenges and actions taken

The intervention focused on providing linked HIV and FP services and promoting dual contraception among enrolled couples at designated healthcare facilities of chosen district hospitals. The following health system interventions were strengthened to fill gaps identified by situation analysis and stakeholder engagement.

(a) Healthcare providers at both HIV and FP centers were trained to impart desired skills for service provisioning. Workshop using lectures, group discussions, role plays, brainstorming of case studies were used to impart knowledge and skills of counseling techniques and desired service provisioning. Midterm refresher training was conducted to sensitize providers. Orientation and planning meeting were held with key stakeholders to operationalize the linkage strategy.

(b) Information, Education and Counseling (IEC) strategies were developed to improve awareness on HIV, STI, FP and modern contraception. Posters and pamphlets of dual protection, prevention of unintended pregnancies (UIP), FP methods, information on medical eligibility criteria for contraceptive use, pregnancy checklist, etc. by adapting government guidelines for providers were developed in local language of the study sites.

(c) Provider-initiated assessment of unmet need for contraception were established at ART centers by training counsellors for assessment of eligibility for contraception use as per WHO eligibility criteria, identification and assessment of needs and determinants of unmet contraception, clinical assessment and importance of provider-initiated referrals.

(d) Eligible PLHIV were referred from ART center to FP center using referral slips as a substitute to existing oral referrals.

(e) A couple approach was used to counsel eligible PLHIV on dual methods of contraception along with correct and consistent use of condoms.

(f) Management Information Systems (MIS) was maintained at both sites to capture referrals from ART centers, FP services attendance of referred cases and acceptors of dual methods.

(g) Enrolled PLHIV were followed up bi-monthly during their routine medication visit to ART center.

(h) Convergence and cross talks were facilitated between HIV and FP center staff. These interactions helped chalk out constraints faced by providers in implementation and identify solutions for the same.

(i) Many challenges were faced during implementation of the intervention package. This included supply-side challenges such as apprehensive attitude of providers, undue referrals to tertiary facilities and stock-out of FP commodities and drugs. Attitudinal issues comprised discrimination of PLHIV by delaying consultations, counseling or advising unwarranted pathophysiological investigations with associated surgical procedures. Table 1 summarizes the actions taken against broad challenges faced in implementation of the intervention.

#### Assessment of uptake of dual methods post intervention

The couples after initial enrollment and counselling at ART center were referred to FP centers using referral slips and facility-level linkages. Provisioning of accepted dual methods was done at the FP center. Enrolled PLHIV couples were then followed up bimonthly for up to six consecutive months at ART centers for follow-up counseling, assessment of acceptance and uptake of dual contraception. Section two of the semi-structured interview schedule was designed to assess and keep track of the respondent's health status, sexual activity, change in fertility desire, menstruation if applicable, any pregnancy or abortion, reasons for non-use of contraception and challenges faced in accessing contraception services.

#### *Data analysis*

SPSS Version 19 (SPSS Statistics for Macintosh, Version 19.0 (Armonk, NY: IBM Corp) was used for data analysis. Open-ended answers were coded. Categorical variables are presented as numbers, percentages and means. Bivariate comparisons were analyzed using a chi-squared test for categorical variables. Logistic regression analysis was run to assess determinants associated with acceptance of dual contraception methods. The adjusted Odds

**Table 1** Challenges faced during implementation of the study and corresponding actions undertaken

| Activity | Challenges | Action Taken |
|---|---|---|
| **HIV-FP linked services** | **Discriminatory services and negative work attitude of providers** | ▪ Brainstorming and experience sharing with health providers regarding their apprehensions about providing services to people living with HIV (PLHIV)<br>▪ Refresher training to guide district-level health providers in assessing medical eligibility of PLHIVs for contraceptive use<br>▪ Advised health providers to follow universal safety measures while performing IUCD insertion, medical termination of pregnancy (MTP), Tubal Ligation (TL) and delivery of HIV positive women |
| **Supplies** | **Inopportune indenting and frequent stock-out** | ▪ Liaised with the district, regional and state officials of Family Welfare Bureau and State AIDS Control Society in issuing required FP commodities and STI kits<br>▪ Supplied Information Education Counselling (IEC) materials on FP and dual methods of contraception |
| **Management Information System** | **No/under-reporting of FP indicators** | ▪ Strengthened monitoring to maintain records of HIV-FP linked services at Obstetrics and Gynecology (OBGY) and Out-Patient Department (OPD)<br>▪ Conducted concurrent meetings with concerned health providers at ART, ICTC, and STI centers to report FP related indicators in monthly reporting formats |

Ratio (OR) and 95% Confidence Interval (CI) was calculated and is presented in the results section.

## Results

### Existing HIV-FP linkages status

The ART centers were providing testing, counseling, free antiretroviral drug distribution and support services as mandated. Though condom promotion was encompassed by free distribution, demonstration of its use was demand specific. Nearly half the provider respondents (58% at Pune and 44% at Parbani) were engaged in providing FP services and post-abortion counselling. Male clients were not allowed to enter obstetrics-gynecology out-patient department (OPD) and female clients seeking FP advice were neither provided condoms nor were counseled on its correct use. Nearly 80% respondents from FP centers revealed that no mechanism for follow-up of referral cases existed. Existing referrals were exclusively for sero-positive pregnant women unless a specific service was demanded.

The respondent workforce was academically qualified, experienced and trained during induction as mandated but desired refresher training. Half the key informants presumed condom use alone to be sufficient to prevent pregnancies. Nearly half (47%) providers perceived contraceptives to be harmful or contra-indicated for PLHIV. Most respondents were unaware of mother-to-child transmission rate at their respective facilities.

Indenting and supply of FP commodities was irregular, inopportune and dependent on demand at facilities. Oral Contraception (OC) pills despite being available at pharmacy of the district hospitals was not supplied at respective FP facility. Emergency contraceptives were unavailable at both hospitals. The district hospitals were well-equipped for IUCD and permanent sterilization. IEC material on FP services for PLHIV was limited to only condom promotion with complete lack of materials for dual methods of contraception.

The ART facilities maintained patient and program monitoring records periodically as mandated. Though patient card had provisions for recording contraception and obstetric history, these were not updated for FP indicators including number of condoms distributed at the facility. The reproductive health facilities at district hospitals maintained registers for OPD, IUCD, antenatal clinics and high risk pregnancy but did not list indicators pertaining to FP service such as method advised by provider, method accepted by client, reason for any method ineligibility, follow-up date and reason for discontinuation of a given method. Moreover, seropositive status of FP acceptors at FP facility was not recorded.

### PLHIV characteristics and health status at enrollment

At enrollment, the mean age of men and women participants was 36.16 (±6.3) and 30.15 (±5.3) years respectively. Women accounted for 43.3% (241/556) of all index participants accessing ART services. Nearly one-third (165/556) participants, predominantly from Parbhani district (158/165) resided in rural areas. Nearly 19 % (105/556) participants resided in urban slums and remaining 51.3% (286/556) were from urban localities. Based on the modified Kuppuswamy scale for socio-economic classification-2019 used in Indian context, more than 93% (518/556) couples belonged to either lower-middle or lower socio-economic categories [21]. Only 3.6% (20/556) females in the study cohort as compared to 38% (212/556) males were in skilled or semi-skilled occupations. Nearly 90% (501/556) females were unskilled workers as compared to 35.9% (200/556) unskilled male counterparts. Illiteracy was more common in females with 16% (89/556) illiterate women as compared to 12.4% (69/556) illiterate males in the cohort. Nearly 82% (456/556) PLHIV couples lived in nuclear families. A mean family size of 3.96 (±1.34) members and mean 1.64 (±1.06) children in the family were reported. A monthly median household income of Indian

Rupee (INR) 8000 (United States Dollar (USD) 117) [Interquartile Range (IQR) INR 5000–12,000 (USD 73–175)] was reported as per the 2018 currency exchange rate [22]. Median per capita income was INR 2500 (USD 37) [IQR INR 1549–4000 (USD 23–58)]. Table 2 enlists socio-demographic characteristics of all participants that completed the study from two chosen district hospitals of Maharashtra, India.

Almost 99% (549/556) index participants had disclosed HIV status to their spouse. The study comprised 55% (306/556) concordant and 42.4% (236/556) discordant couples. The remaining 2.5% (14/556) participants did not know HIV status of their spouse. Participants had HIV for a mean duration of 4.14 (±3.27) years. Of the total 556 couples who completed the study, 88.3% (492/556) women had children, with 9.9% (49/492) women having one or more HIV infected children. Thirteen percent (75/556) index participants had experienced symptoms of Reproductive Tract Infection/Sexually Transmitted Infection (RTI/STI) of which only one third i.e. 36% (27/75) had sought treatment. Obstetric history revealed that 28% (156/556) women had previously undergone Medical Termination of Pregnancy (MTP). The risk of fear of HIV to fetus and unwanted pregnancy accounted for being the commonest reason for women diagnosed with HIV undergoing an abortion.

Overall knowledge about safe sexual practice was limited to only use of condoms during sexual activity with 98.2% (547/556) participants aware of this practice. Nearly one-third i.e. 29.5% (164/556) were aware of avoiding risky sexual partners. Nineteen percent (106/556) participants were aware of avoiding multiple sexual partners. Awareness about use of methods of contraception was highest for male condoms at 98.2% (554/556), followed by female sterilization at 89% (495/556), IUCD at 61.7% (343/556), OC pills at 56.5% (314/556) and vasectomy at 51.9% (289/556). Only 2 % (11/556) participants were aware of female condoms as a method of contraception. Knowledge of dual protection was again restricted to only use of condoms. Nearly 73% (406/556) participants were aware of use of condoms to prevent pregnancy outcomes, HIV, and STIs. None of the participants had knowledge of using two methods i.e. a more effective method in addition to condoms for dual

**Table 2** Socio-demographic characteristics of PLHIV respondents

| **Variable** | | **Percentage (%) (*n* = 556)** | |
|---|---|---|---|
| **Age** | | Male | Female |
| | 19–25 | 3.4 | 24.3 |
| | 26–32 | 27.5 | 42.8 |
| | 33–40 | 49.3 | 30.8 |
| | 41–45 | 19.8 | 2.2 |
| **Educational status** | Illiterate | 12.4 | 16.0 |
| | Primary & Middle | 24.3 | 34.7 |
| | High school & intermediate | 48.4 | 41.9 |
| | Graduate | 8.8 | 4.9 |
| | Professional degree | 6.1 | 2.5 |
| **Occupation** | Skilled & semi-skilled | 37.9 | 3.6 |
| | Unskilled | 36.0 | 90.1 |
| | Professional or semi-professional | 2.7 | 1.4 |
| | Business, farmer, clerical | 22.8 | 4.7 |
| | Unemployed | 0.5 | 0.2 |
| **Place of residence** | Urban slum | 18.9 | |
| | Urban non-slum | 51.3 | |
| | Rural | 29.7 | |
| **Socio-economic classification of the family** | Modified Kuppuswamy classification, 2019 | | |
| | Upper | 0.0 | |
| | Upper-middle | 6.8 | |
| | Lower-middle | 46.9 | |
| | Upper-lower | 45.0 | |
| | Lower | 1.3 | |

protection. Nearly 90% (500/556) participants believed condoms provided 100% protection against pregnancy. Nearly 16 % (87/556) participants believed that contraception was harmful to PLHIV. Of these, 72.4% (63/87) perceived IUCDs to be harmful for reasons such as perforation and other associated side effects. OC pills were perceived to be harmful by 25.3% (22/87) participants for reasons like abdominal pain, irritation, weakness and need for daily medication intake. Decision making for use of contraception was dependent most commonly on the doctor in 42.7% (237/556) cases, followed by choice of the sexual partner in 39% (217/556) cases and other family members in case of 3.9% (22/556) participants. Awareness about drugs and other treatment provision availability for preventing parent to child transmission of HIV was observed in 58% (323/556) participants.

Contraception use history revealed 11.3% (63/556) participants to have used modern methods of contraception before knowing their HIV status. None of the participants had previously used dual methods of contraception. Eighty-eight percent (492/556) participants did not desire children. Completed family in 49.7% (245/492) cases, risk of HIV transmission to child among 38.8% (191/492) were the commonest reasons given for not desiring children. Government facilities were used by 52.8% (294/556) participants to access condoms. Remaining 47.2% (249/556) sought pharmacies (246/249) or other Non-Governmental Organizations (NGOs) to avail it. Counseling at ICTC centers involved demonstration of correct use of condoms in 64% (356/556) participants previously.

### Impact of intervention

The intervention package resulted in a significant improvement in participant's knowledge of contraceptives [from a baseline score of 3.84 to post-intervention score of 6.72] (highest score being 8) and safe sex practice [from a baseline score of 1.54 to 3.25 post-intervention] (highest score being 4). Awareness of using condoms in spite of both partners being HIV positive improved from 86.3% (480/556) to 100% by end of the study.

The intervention package resulted in 87% of participants reaching FP centers after being referred from ART center. Acceptance of dual contraception methods improved over time with 44.6% (248/556) participants accepting dual contraception methods by end of the study. The most preferred method in addition to condoms was OC pills followed by IUCDs, tubectomy, Injectable, and vasectomy. Noticeable turn-around time for acceptance of dual contraception methods was seen with 50% (124/248) acceptors accepting dual methods within first follow up after referral. Condom use among sexually active participants remained steadily high with 96.16% (526/547) participants regularly using condoms at end of the study period. Table 3 shows the type of dual contraception method in addition to condoms accepted and continued by participants until the end of the study period.

**Table 3** Type of dual contraceptive method accepted and continued during the study period

| Characteristic | Total (%) |
|---|---|
| **Method initially accepted along with condom (dual method)** | (*n* = 242) |
| Oral Contraceptive pills | 136 (56.2%) |
| IUCD | 47 (19.4%) |
| Injectable | 24 (9.9%) |
| Tubectomy | 28 (11.6%) |
| Vasectomy | 7 (2.9%) |
| **Method used at the end of the study period along with condom** | (*n* = 248) |
| Oral Contraceptive pills | 131 (52.8%) |
| IUCD | 55 (22.2%) |
| Injectable | 14 (5.6%) |
| Tubectomy | 39 (15.7%) |
| Vasectomy | 9 (3.6%) |
| **Regular condom use among sexually active participants over time** | (*n* = 541/547) |
| At Enrollment | 512/547 (93.6%) |
| 1st Follow Up | 526/547 (96.2%) |
| 2nd Follow Up | 524/547 (95.8%) |
| 3rd Follow Up | 526/547 (96.2%) |

Participants reported a change in fertility desire over course of the study period. Fifteen women reported pregnancy. Eight women had planned pregnancies. Seven unplanned pregnancies were reported. All seven unplanned pregnancies occurred among non-acceptors of dual methods i.e. only using condoms as the method of contraception. Six of these seven women underwent medical termination of pregnancy whereas one case reported a spontaneous abortion. These women were counseled post-abortion which resulted in four women accepting OC pills, one accepting an IUCD, one continuing with condoms, and one couple opting for vasectomy. Discontinuation was observed for OC pills (30 cases), three monthly Injectable (12 cases), and IUCDs (1 case) among dual methods. Switching of the dual method was also seen, commonly for OC pill acceptors (24 cases), injectable users (4 cases) and IUCD acceptors (3 cases). Table 4 shows acceptance, switching, and discontinuation of dual methods among participants in the study.

### Determinants of dual contraception acceptance

Logistic regression analysis was run to assess determinants of acceptance of dual methods by couples. Female index participants [OR 2 (99% CI: 1.42–2.81)], concordant couples [OR

**Table 4** Dual method acceptance, switching and discontinuation of methods among participants in the study

| Type of FP Methods | FP method accepted in addition to condom as the dual method by end of the study | Method switching during the Study | Discontinued at study completion |
|---|---|---|---|
| Oral Contraceptive pill | 131 | 24 | 30 |
| Intra Uterine Contraceptive Device | 55 | 3 | 1 |
| Tubal Ligation | 39 | – | – |
| Injectable | 14 | 4 | 12 |
| Non-Scalpel Vasectomy | 9 | – | – |
| Total (N) | 248 | 31 | 43 |

1.97 (99% CI: 1.4–2.77)], decision making enabled by counseling provided by doctor [OR 1.63 (95% CI: 1.04–2.53)], CD4 counts above 741 [OR 1.7 (95% CI: 1.07–2.71)] were cases more likely to accept dual methods of contraception in study group apart from the ones who preferred method other than condoms [OR 4.92 (99% CI: 3.26–7.44)]. Table 5 describes these findings of determinants of dual contraception acceptance.

As a study output, Standard Operating Procedures (SOP) for providing linked HIV and FP services were developed with a consensus of a team of experts representing program managers, international NGOs and academicians to synthesize technical guidance for use by the programs. SOPs provided a brief overview and stated convergence strategy details of operationalizing linkage between HIV/STI and FP facilities. Job descriptions were detailed out for various healthcare providers at both ART and FP centers. Training modules with various case studies, role models, and pre- and post-assessment forms were generated. The WHO eligibility criteria wheel was described in detail. The essential supply of drugs and commodities along with MIS was elaborated eloquently to strengthen monitoring of services.

## Discussion

Contraceptive use in India is skewed with majority women in reprodutive age group resorting to sterilization and only 10% using condoms. However, when it comes to PLHIV the skew is reversed such that almost all resort to using only condoms and other methods are rarely used. The unmet need of contraception among PLHIV is not distinctly different to that of the general population. A recent Indian study at ART center in an urban tertiary hospital reported an unmet family planning need at 17% among PLHIV women [11]. Reliance on less effective methods such as condom alone moreover predisposes PLHIV to the risk of unfavorable outcomes such as an unintended pregnancy.

This study implemented a strategy linking HIV and FP services to improve use of dual contraception methods among disadvantaged PLHIV group. The study cohort primarily composed of socio-economically deprived subsections of the PLHIV population. The majority in this cohort were in unskilled occupations and had low education and income levels. Nearly half the participants were from urban slums or rural regions. Association of such socio-economic determinants to non-adherence of

**Table 5** Determinants of dual contraception acceptance

| Background Variables | | Unadjusted Odds Ratio | Adjusted Odds Ratio |
|---|---|---|---|
| **Index client** | Male | 1 | 1 |
| | Female | 2** (1.42–2.81) | 1.66* (1.12–2.46) |
| **Education Status** | Literate | 1 | 1 |
| | Illiterate | 1.62 (0.96–2.72) | 1.44 (0.8–2.59) |
| **CD4 count above 80th Percentile** | No | 1 | 1 |
| | Yes | 1.26 (0.83–1.9) | 1.7* (1.07–2.71) |
| **Partner HIV Status** | Negative | 1 | 1 |
| | Positive | 1.97** (1.4–2.77) | 1.65* (1.13–2.43) |
| **Decision Making** | Self | 1 | 1 |
| | Husband/Family/Doctors/Others | 1.63* (1.04–2.53) | 1.26 (0.77–2.08) |
| **Method preference** | Condom Only | 1 | 1 |
| | Dual methods | 4.92** (3.26–7.44) | 4.56** (2.94–7.06) |

**$p < 0.001$, *$p < 0.05$

Variables like religion, place of residence, type of family, per capita income, ART status, perception of family planning method being harmful, sexual partner other than the spouse, currently sexually active, desiring another child in future, spouse desiring the same number of children, any illness in last one month showed insignificant results

ART treatment services in spite of universal coverage of services has been documented in varied settings suggesting the need for support measures beyond treatment services [23, 24]. In this study, we have demonstrated feasibility and effectiveness of linking HIV and FP programs by counseling and referral mechanisms to improve FP uptake by PLHIV. Majority (87%) of the enrolled couples in this study reached FP centers as a result of the intervention. With zero participants using dual methods at enrollment, this study showed significant improvement uptake of 44% acceptance by end of the six follow up months as a result of motivation and promotion of dual methods. Our previous study at two urban tertiary hospitals showed a 33% uptake of dual methods [17]. This present study additionally included couple counseling and linkage referral services in the intervention package compared to the previous study which provisioned contraception methods to only PLHIV women. Both our studies from varied settings in India have reported a higher acceptance and is higher than a similar study from Tanzania (Africa) showing an 18% improvement in acceptance of dual methods [25]. Our study findings also report improved acceptance of long-term contraceptives among dual method users, in line with similar evidence from Thailand. This may be attributed to contraceptive effectiveness and low associated risks [26]. Oral contraceptives, IUCDs and tubal ligation were found to be the most commonly accepted dual method in our study with good continuation rates. Our study contradicts dual hypothesis theory that suggests condom use reduces if a PLHIV uses more effective contraception [27]. After the intervention, condom use in our study improved and remained consistently high throughout the study. The seven unplanned pregnancies in our study were addressed early by counseling to ensure access to further medical care. Subsequently, almost all unplanned pregnancies underwent medical termination of pregnancy as per the desires of the women after taking an informed decision. This was followed by counseling and acceptance of post-abortion contraception by all women.

Studies conducted in African context have shown HIV–FP integration or linkage interventions to be successful in terms of health outcomes and cost-effectiveness, but evidence for India in this case remains limited. India has a relatively low HIV prevalence among the general population. A bidirectional linkage between HIV and FP services for India would be cumbersome and expensive given the large-scale resource investment needed for such a strategy and India's declining HIV prevalence. The current PPTCT program in India is limited by way of its pregnant woman centricity. Guidelines focus on provisioning of a therapeutic regimen to HIV infected pregnant women while less emphasis is laid on prevention of an unwanted pregnancy itself. The use of dual methods of contraception widely ensures better protection against unintended pregnancies, HIV and other sexually transmitted infections. PLHIV like other non-infected women may not be eager to practice contraception and base decisions on various contextual factors such as spouse, family, desires, etc. A systematic review evaluating studies focusing on integration programs across sub-Saharan Africa has observed the need for integration efforts especially in low contraceptive use prevalence to address community-wide and HIV specific barriers in using FP methods along with improvement of access to information, commodities, and services within routine care [28]. Our study has focused on improving such intangible intricacies within the healthcare system to ensure comprehensive FP services to PLHIV by linking mechanisms. Provider aspects such as easy hospital registration procedure, delivery of comprehensive counseling services, training, providing available clear guidelines on medical eligibility of contraception use, sensitization to prevent stigma and discrimination have been addressed in this study which needs to be factored in decision making for the diverse Indian public health system.

This study recognizes the unidirectional linkage mechanism to be a feasible strategy to improve health outcomes that can potentially contribute to the Indian national program realizing its aim of convergence and mainstreaming of HIV into general health services.

In Phase IV of the National AIDS Control Program (NACP), India is striving to achieve the target of zero new infections. To achieve this, many preventive strategies have been planned but emphasis on unintended pregnancy prevention is missing thus far. With emergence of newer challenges for universal coverage of curative programs, it is imperative to simultaneously focus on cost-effective preventive measures. Studies from resource-constrained settings have demonstrated a reduction of as much as 16% unintended pregnancies among HIV-infected women to potentially reduce HIV-positive birth rates equivalent to that of the on-going PPTCT effort [28]. This coupled with a range of health benefits to women and their families can improve PLHIV health outcomes [29]. Integrated services are more efficient than vertical service provisioning [30]. Though NACP has successfully contributed to keeping the overall HIV prevalence rate in India below 1%, it faces newer challenges such as scaling up of interventions and an increase in number of infections in low prevalence states [31]. NACP has outlined a thrust on convergence and mainstreaming of HIV into general services [32]. Prospectively, undertaking India specific economic evaluation studies for linkage interventions can strengthen evidence basis for upholding reproductive and sexual rights of the vulnerable PLHIV population.

### Limitations

The effectiveness of this linkage strategy was seen in a well monitored situation. Sustenance of such an intervention at a large scale with implementation of monitoring mechanisms like MIS indicators for unmet need of contraception, referrals and acceptance by all stakeholders in the healthcare delivery system may present with its own unique challenges.

## Recommendations

Directives or SOPs for implementation of linked services between HIV and Family planning services need to be designed to strengthen programmatic response. Supportive supervision and sustained program response must be maintained to ensure documentation of crucial information on family planning services, especially for the marginalized PLHIV population. Convergence between HIV and FP planning programs must be streamlined by ensuring ease of registration through common access to both services, developing standard referral mechanism using referral slips, developing IEC materials for advocacy of dual methods, dual protection and motivation of PLHIV to access services. Service providers need to be trained and sensitized to cater to the needs of PLHIV population and male counterparts need to be involved in FP method acceptance.

## Conclusion

This study illustrates unmet need of contraception among the vulnerable PLHIV population. The study demonstrates feasibility of providing linked HIV and FP services at district hospital settings accessed by socio-economically vulnerable sections. The SOPs developed from this study can be used to upscale implementation in program settings. Dual contraception use among PLHIV in fact improves consistent condom uptake and reduces unintended pregnancies as compared to exclusive condom use. These interventions must be supported with repeated counseling and monitoring of program with well-defined MIS indicators. Training and motivation of staff is an essential component to provide holistic care to PLHIV. These interventions can help strengthen Prong 2 of the PPTCT program to help achieve the target of HIV elimination.

### Abbreviations

HIV: Human Immunodeficiency Virus; PLHIV: People Living with HIV; ART: Anti-Retroviral Therapy; OBGY: Obstetrics and Gynecology; NIRRH: National Institute for Research in Reproductive Health; AIDS: Acquired Immunodeficiency Syndrome; NACO: National AIDS Control Organization; ICMR: Indian Council of Medical Research; MDACS: Mumbai District AIDS Control Society; MSACS: Maharashtra State AIDS Control Society; FP: Family Planning; STI: Sexually Transmitted Infection; OC Pill: Oral Contraceptive Pill; IUCD: Intra-Uterine Contraceptive Device; CD4: Cluster of Differentiation 4; WHO: World Health Organization; PPTCT: Prevention of Parent to Child Transmission; TB: Tuberculosis; UN: United Nations; SRH: Sexual and Reproductive Health; MIS: Management Information System; ICTC: Integrated Counseling and Testing Center; IEC: Information, Education and Counseling; INR: Indian Rupee; USD: United States Dollar; IQR: Interquartile Range; NGO: Non-Governmental Organization; MTP: Medical Termination of Pregnancy; TL: Tubal Ligation; OPD: Out-Patient Department; OR: Odds Ratio; CI: Confidence Interval; NSV: Non-scalpel Vasectomy; SOP: Standard Operating Procedure; NOC: No Objection Certificate; NACP: National AIDS Control Programme

### Acknowledgments

We wish to acknowledge the financial and technical support rendered by NACO, India. Participants who shared personal information and committed time for study deserve a special mention. We acknowledge the enthusiastic cooperation of civil surgeons, Medical Officers and staff from HIV ART Centers and OBGYN services from study sites and project team implementing the study. We acknowledge Dr. Archana Patil (Director Health Services, Pune,Maharashtra, Dr. K.S. Sachdeva (former DDG, NACO), Dr. Shobini Rajan (Asst. DG NACO) and Dr. Smita Mahale (Former Director, ICMR – NIRRH) for their support and encouragement.

### Authors' contributions

BJ the principal investigator conceptualized, implemented, analyzed, and contributed to manuscript writing. BG participated in the study implementation and editing of the manuscript. SS developed and edited the manuscript. VV facilitated the conduct of the study and provided technical inputs. SA and PD provided technical assistance and facilitated study implementation, and contributed to manuscript editing. RK and SB provided technical assistance and edited the manuscript. All authors read and approved the final manuscript.

### Author details

[1]Indian Council of Medical Research- National Institute for Research in Reproductive Health (NIRRH), Mumbai, Maharashtra, India. [2]Family Health Department, PATH India, New Delhi, India. [3]National AIDS Control Organization, New Delhi, India. [4]Mumbai District AIDS Control Society, Mumbai, Maharashtra, India. [5]Maharashtra State AIDS Control Society, Mumbai, Maharashtra, India.

### References

1. Global HIV & AIDS statistics — 2020 fact sheet | UNAIDS. 2019 [cited 2020 Dec 1]. Available from: https://www.unaids.org/en/resources/fact-sheet
2. WHO. HIV/AIDS. [cited 2020 Mar 25]. Available from: https://www.who.int/en/news-room/fact-sheets/detail/hiv-aids
3. WHO. PMTCT strategic vision 2010-2015. Organization. 2010.
4. National AIDS Control Organisation. HIV Estimations 2017: Technical Report; 2018. p. 47. Available from: http://naco.gov.in/sites/default/files/HIVEstimations2017Report_3.pdf
5. National AIDS Control Organization. Ministry of Health and Family Welfare Government of India National AIDS Control Organisation Ministry of Health and Family Welfare Government of India National Strategic Plan for HIV/AIDS and STI "Paving Way for an AIDS Free India" 2017;168. Available from: http://naco.gov.in/national-strategic-plan-hivaids-and-sti-2017-24
6. Halperin DT, Stover J, Reynolds HW. Benefits and costs of expanding access to family planning programs to women living with HIV. AIDS. 2009; 23(SUPPL.1):1.
7. Wilcher R, Willard C, WHO. Reproductive choices for women with HIV: WHO; 2011. [cited 2019 Dec 9]; Available from: https://www.who.int/bulletin/volumes/87/11/08-059360/en/
8. WHO. Contraceptive eligibility for women at high risk of HIV. 2019. Available from: http://www.who.int/reproductivehealth/publications/family_planning/HC-and-HIV-2017/en/
9. WHO. Call to action to attain universal coverage through linked sexual and Reproductive health and rights and HIV interventions. 2018; Available from: https://www.who.int/reproductivehealth/publications/call-to-action-linked-srhr-hiv-interventions/en/
10. WHO. Providing contraceptive services in the context of hiv treatment programmes implementation tool hiv treatment and reproductive health: World Heal Organ; 2019. Available from: http://apps.who.int/bookorders

11. Dugg P, Chhabra P, Sharma A. Contraceptive use and unmet need for family planning among hiv-positive women: a hospital-based study. Indian J Public Health. 2020;64:32 Medknow Publications and Media Pvt. Ltd.; [cited 2020 Mar 20]. Available from: http://www.ijph.in/text.asp?2020/64/1/32/280762.
12. Paswan B, Singh SK, Lhungdim H, Shekhar C, Arnold F, Kishor S, et al. National family health survey (Nfhs-4) 2015–16. 2015; Available from: https://dhsprogram.com/pubs/pdf/FR339/FR339.pdf
13. Lall P. ADBI working paper series social factors affecting women's susceptibility to hiv in india asian development bank institute. 2014 [cited 2020 May 28]. Available from: http://www.adbi.org/working-paper/2014/06/12/6307.women.susceptibility.hiv.india/
14. Mahendra VS, Gilborn L, Bharat S, Mudoi RJ, Gupta I, George B, et al. Understanding and measuring AIDS-related stigma in health care settings: A developing country perspective. Sahara J. 2007;4(2):616–25 [cited 2020 Dec 1]. Available from: https://pubmed.ncbi.nlm.nih.gov/18071613/.
15. Ekstrand ML, Ramakrishna J, Bharat S, Heylen E. Prevalence and drivers of HIV stigma among health providers in urban India: implications for interventions. J Int AIDS Soc. 2013;16(3 Suppl):2 [cited 2020 Dec 1]. Available from: /pmc/articles/PMC3833193/?report=abstract.
16. Nair M, Kumar P, Pandey S, Harshana A, Kazmi S, Moreto-Planas L, et al. Refused and referred-persistent stigma and discrimination against people living with HIV/AIDS in Bihar: a qualitative study from India. BMJ Open. 2019;9(11):e033790 [cited 2020 Dec 1]. Available from: http://bmjopen.bmj.com/.
17. Joshi B, Velhal G, Chauhan S, Kulkarni R, Begum S, Nandanwar YS, et al. Linking HIV & family planning services to improve dual methods of contraception among women infected with HIV in Mumbai, Maharashtra. India Indian J Med Res. 2016;143(April):464–73.
18. Joshi B, Velhal G, Chauhan S, Kulkarni R, Begum S, Nandanwar YS, et al. Contraceptive use and unintended pregnancies among HIV-infected women in Mumbai. Indian J Community Med. 2015;40(3):168–72 [cited 2020 Dec 2]. Available from: http://www.ijcm.org.in/text.asp?2015/40/3/168/158855.
19. Ippf, Unfpa, Who U. Rapid Assessment ToOl for Sexual & Reproductive Health and HIV Linkages A Generic Guide; 2009. p. 1–88.
20. Joshi BN, Girase BA, Kulkarni RN, Begum S. Status of family planning service delivery for people living with HIV at public hospital settings in Maharashtra: opportunities and challenges. Int J Community Med Public Heal. 2017;4(7):2463.
21. Mohd SS. Modified Kuppuswamy socioeconomic scale updated for the year 2019. Indian J Forensic Community Med. 2019;6(1):1–3.
22. Official exchange rate (LCU per US$, period average) - India | Data. [cited 2020 May 28]. Available from: https://data.worldbank.org/indicator/PA.NUS.FCRF?locations=IN
23. Hogg RS, Puskas C, Parashar S, Montaner JSG. The effect of socioeconomic disadvantage on strategies to end the AIDS epidemic. Lancet Public Health. 2016;1:e6–7 [cited 2020 May 28]. Available from: www.thelancet.com/public-health.
24. Burch LS, Smith CJ, Anderson J, Sherr L, Rodger AJ, O'Connell R, et al. Socioeconomic status and treatment outcomes for individuals with HIV on antiretroviral treatment in the UK: cross-sectional and longitudinal analyses. Lancet Public Health. 2016;1(1):e26–36.
25. Baumgartner JN, Green M, Weaver MA, Mpangile G, Kohi TW, Mujaya SN, et al. Integrating family planning services into HIV care and treatment clinics in Tanzania: evaluation of a facilitated referral model. Health Policy Plan. 2014;29(5):570–9.
26. Munsakul W, Lolekha R, Kowadisaiburana B, Roongpisuthipong A, Jirajariyavej S, Asavapiriyanont S, et al. Dual contraceptive method use and pregnancy intention among people living with HIV receiving HIV care at six hospitals in Thailand. Reprod Health. 2016;13(1):1–11. https://doi.org/10.1186/s12978-016-0123-2.
27. Cates W, Steiner MJ. What is the best contraceptive approach? Sex Transm Dis. 2002:168–74.
28. Haberlen SA, Narasimhan M, Beres LK, Kennedy CE. Integration of family planning services into HIV care and treatment Services : a systematic review; 2017.
29. Reynolds HW, Janowitz B, Homan R, Johnson L. The Value of Contraception to Prevent Perinatal HIV Transmission. Sex Transm Dis. 2006;33(6):350–6.
30. Hewett PC, Nalubamba M, Bozzani F, Digitale J, Vu L, Yam E, Nambao M. Randomized evaluation and costeffectiveness of HIV and sexual and reproductive health service referral and linkage models in Zambia. BMC Public Health. 2016;16(1).
31. Sharma DC. India's BJP Government and health: 1 year on. The Lancet. 2015; 385(9982):2031–2.
32. Convergence Plan between NACP and DOHFW: National Health Mission [Internet]. Available from: https://nhm.gov.in/index1.php?lang=1&level=2&sublinkid=1079&lid=150. [cited 2020 Mar 20].

8

# Assessment of intention to use postpartum intrauterine contraceptive device and associated factors among pregnant women attending antenatal clinics in ambo town public health institutions, Ethiopia, 2018

Gurmessa Daba[1], Jembere Tesfaye Deressa[2*] and Workinesh Sinishaw[2]


## Abstract

**Background:** Maternal mortality tragedy is the issue of both developed and developing countries, especially sub-Saharan Africa including Ethiopia, which is due to poor quality of maternal health care services. Therefore family planning especially the use of Postpartum intrauterine contraceptive devices can tackle unintended pregnancy and maternal death. However,the intention to use PPIUCD and the use of IUCD in general is not well practiced in Ethiopia according to evidences of the literatures. For this reason, many mothers are exposed to unintended pregnancy and pregnancy related complications. The main purpose of the study was to assess the intention to use Post-partum intra uterine contraceptive devices and its associated factors among pregnant women attending Antenatal Clinics in Ambo Town Public Health Institutions, Ethiopia, 2018.

**Methods:** A facility-based cross-sectional study design was conducted from March – April 2018 to assess the intention of pregnant women about Postpartum intrauterine contraceptive devices and associated factors in 422 pregnant women. Study subjects were selected using systematic random sampling. Data were collected by structured questionnaire, entered into a computer using Epi-info 3.5.4 statistical program, and exported to SPSS version 20 for analysis. A Logistic regression model was used to predict the intention of pregnant women about Postpartum intrauterine contraceptive devices and associated factors. Lastly, a significant statistical association was tested using 95% confidence interval (CI) and $p$ value ($p < 0.05$).

**Results:** The response rate was 417 (98.3%) and this study showed that 145(34.9%) of pregnant women intended to use Postpartum intrauterine contraceptive device. Age of pregnant women [AOR = 8.348(CI: 3.602–19.347], educational level [AOR = 3.249(1.057–9.985)], occupational status [AOR = 4.101(CI: 1.788–9.405)], monthly income [AOR = 3.175(CI: 1.423–7.082)] and knowledge [A0R = 5.408(2.994–9.767)] have shown significant associations with intention to use Postpartum intrauterine contraceptive devices.


(Continued on next page)

* Correspondence: jembere_tesfaye@yahoo.com
[2]Addis Ababa University College of Health Science, School of Nursing & Midwifery, Addis Ababa, Ethiopia

(Continued from previous page)

**Conclusions:** The study found that 34.9% women intended to use PPIUCD. Maternal age, maternal educational level, occupational status, monthly income and knowledge were significantly associated with pregnant women intention to use PPIUCD.

**Keywords:** Antenatal care, Intention, Postpartum intrauterine contraceptive device, Pregnancy

## Introduction

An IUCD is a small, "T-shaped" intrauterine contraceptive devices, which is placed in a woman's uterus. It is also known as the IUD, loop or coil. Postpartum IUCD is an intrauterine contraceptive device which is inserted during the postpartum period (up to 48 hrs after birth, optimally within10 min of delivery of the placenta). IUCDs are prepared of flexible plastic with thin copper wire coating. It has one or two soft threads on the last part. These thin threads hang through the opening at the entrance of the uterus into the top of the vagina [1].Copper-bearing IUDs come in a variety of designs the IUD recommended by WHO for bulk obtaining is the TCu380A it works primarily by causing chemical changes that prevent fertilization. Studies show that the copper IUD effectively interrupts the reproductive process before implantation and pregnancy and it does not act by initiating an abortion, as has sometimes been suggested [2]. Renewed interest in the intrauterine device (IUD), a highly effective, long-acting reversible contraceptive (LARC) that is safe for breastfeeding women, can be inserted in a matter of minutes by a trained provider, and do not require an additional facility visit when inserted during the childbirth stay has encouraged some programs to add postpartum IUD services to their PPFP options [3–5]. Ethiopia in collaboration with Maternal and Child Health Integrated Program (MCHIP) started the PPIUCD program in 2012, PPIUCD services were initiated as one FP option for postpartum clients [6, 7].

The most successful PPFP programs will focus on providing PPFP counseling to women at every opportunity. In low-income countries, increasing emphasis on antenatal care and childbirth in a health care facility has created an opportunity to counsel women about family planning. The health benefits of contraception and birth spacing for women and their infants are remarkable and the woman is not pregnant at the time of insertion and is protected against pregnancy prior to resuming sexual activity [3].

Appropriate times for IUCD insertion in the postpartum periods include the post placental IUCD insertion, the immediate postpartum IUCD insertion and the trance cesarean IUCD insertion. The post placental IUCD insertion is done within 10 minutes after expulsion of the placenta, following a vaginal delivery. The immediate postpartum IUCD insertion is done after the post.

placental period, but within 48 hrs of delivery and the trance cesarean IUCD insertion is when the insertion takes place following a cesarean delivery, before the uterus incision is sutured [7, 8]. These periods the cervix is open and limp and an IUCD can easily be placed high in the fundus, either manually or using forceps. Furthermore it continues to be possible to insert an IUCD with an instrument for up to 48 h postpartum [8]. After birth, uterine contractions expel retained placental tissues and blood clots and may have a similar effect on any foreign body introduced into the uterus. IUCDs inserted post-placentally have a much lower expulsion risk than those inserted later in the postpartum period, although the expulsion is still higher than for interval insertions. However, the benefits of providing highly effective contraception immediately after delivery often outweigh the disadvantage of the higher postpartum expulsion rates [8]. Two reasons informed the decision to focus on contraceptive intention. First, intention has been posited in many theories of behavior change as the most proximate determinant of actual behavior. Also, many studies have found intention to be a very strong determinant of behavior. Second, in the absence of longitudinal data, the focus on the association of ideation with intention to use as opposed to actual contraceptive use allows us to better address possible reverse causality inherent in cross-sectional data. Behavioral intentions (an indication of an individual's readiness to perform a given behavior it is assumed to be an immediate antecedent of behavior) relate to how people see themselves in the future [9]. The information derived from this study would provide directions for both governmental and non-governmental bodies to implementing successful strategies that are effective in promoting use of PPIUCD in maternal health service utilization areas like ANC and FP which eventually leads to the improvement of CPR and health of the women. So, intention to use PPIUCD which is effective, safe, reversible and long acting method of contraception is going to be crucial in meeting the above needs because there is a limited study conducted to assess intention to use PPIUCD use and factors affecting intention to use PPIUCD in Ethiopia.

## Methods

### Study design and study period

Institution based cross sectional study design was used to collect data from pregnant women attending antenatal clinic from March 1, 2018- April 30, 2018.

**Source population**

All women who are in the reproductive age group (15–49 years old) and living in the Ambo town.

**Study subjects**

From the source population women those who are pregnant and attending ANC Clinics in Ambo town during data collection period.

**Inclusion and exclusion criteria**

All reproductive and pregnant women aged 15–49 years were included to the study but seriously sick and those who unable to respond like laboring mothers were excluded.

**Sample size determination**

The sample size was calculated by using single population proportion formula based on the following assumptions: Since there is no appropriate population value to calculate n from the reviewed literature and it was not only done on pregnant women the proportion was taken at 50%. Significant level at $\alpha = 0.05$, at 95% confidence interval, Margin of error is 5 and 10% nonresponsive rate, the sample size is calculated by the following formula:

$n = (Z\alpha/2)2$ P (1-p) d 2 $n = (1.96)2$ (0.5) (0.5) = 384 (0.05)2 Where: $n$ = the required Sample size $p$ = prevalence of intention to use PPIUCD (50% or $P = 0.5$) Z = the value of the standard normal curve score corresponding to the given Confidence interval 1.96 d = the permissible Margin of error (the required precision) = 5%.

By adding 10% of non-response rate, total of 422 pregnant women will be recruited as study units among pregnant women who attended ANC follow up at health facilities in Ambo town during study period.

**Sampling procedure**

In this study, all public health institutions which provide ANC service were selected. Based on these, three public health institutions, (one hospital and two health centers) was included. The total population for these health institutions (their average monthly ANC flows of previous, at least for 2 months is estimated that 928, (321 for Ambo Hospital, 396 for Ambo health center and 211 for Awaro health center) so final sample size (422) is obtained by proportionally allocating to these selected health facilities by considering their monthly ANC flows. Lastly, subjects (pregnant mother) were taken by systematic Random sampling. Based on assessment of each health facility monthly load, by systematic random sampling technique (i.e. Kth = N / sample size= > 928 /422 ≈ 2 which means K th = 2), thus every 2nd pregnant women who attended this facility was recruited as study units in each health facilities until the total sample size for this study is obtained.

**Data quality control/ assurance**

The data collection instrument was pre-tested for its relevance and clarity to address the research problems appropriately and corrected prior to the actual data collection period. Pretest was done at another health center, before conducting the major study on 5% of the sample to check consistency of questionnaire. The authors checked for completeness and consistencies of questionnaires filled by the data collector and ensured the quality of the data.

**Operational definition**

***PPIUCD***

An intrauterine contraceptive device that can be inserted post placentally, intra cesarean and within 48 hrs of delivery.

***Intention to use PPIUCD***

pregnant women who responded "yes" or "no"to use PPIUCD method after delivery within 48 hrs.

**Awareness of PPIUCD:simply information responded by the participants whether the participants ever heard of PPIUCD and the source of the information**

***Knowledge on PPIUCD***

Pregnant women's awareness of the existence of PPIUCD, its importance and effectiveness.

PPIUCD knowledge was measured by the total number of correct answers to 10 items on knowledge with a minimum score of 0 and maximum of 10. It was categorized based on the percent of knowledge of the distinct characteristics of PPIUCD as: "high" - those who scored 80% and above, "moderate" those who scored 60 - 79% and "low" those who scored less than 60%.

***Attitude on PPIUCD***

The likert scale with scores ranging from 1=strongly disagree to 5=strongly agree was used. To measure the attitude of the pregnant women's towards intention to use PPIUCD two categories were assigned. Data was checked for normal distribution normally distributed so, the mean was used to measure attitude.

Positive Attitude - those who scored above the mean on attitude items and Negative Attitude - those who scored the mean or below mean to attitude items.

### Data entry and analysis procedure

After data collection, the questionnaire was checked for completeness. The collected data was entered in to Epi-info version 3.5.4 and exported to Statistical Package for Social Science (SPSS) version 20 for analysis. To identify the existence of association between the selected dependent and independent variables, bivariate logistic regression with 95% CI at $p$-value < 0.2 and multivariate logistic regression modelling with 95% CI at $p$-value < 0.05 was used. For all of statistical test used in this study, descriptive statistics such as frequency distribution and measure of central tendency and variability (mean and standard deviation) was computed to describe variables of the study. A confidence interval of 95% was used and thus a $p$-value < 0.05 was considered significant.

## Results

### Socio-demographic characteristics of pregnant women intention to use post-partum IUCD

The complete response rate of this study was 415(98.3%). Majority of the study participants were 115 (27.7%) in the age range of greater than 27 years. The mean age of the respondent was 24.23 ± 3.91 SD years. One hundred fifty three (36.9%) of the participants have completed grade 9–12, followed by one hundred thirty four (32.3%) those who completed grade 1–8. One hundred forty two (34.2%) were getting monthly income of less than 1000 ETB (Ethiopian Birr).

### Reproductive characteristics of the participants

The mean age at marriage was 19.23 (±2.45 SD) years. Majority, 286 (68.9%), of the women had ever given birth and more than three-fourth, 298 (71.8), had less than 2 ever born children. The mean number of alive and more wanted children in life was 1.56 (±1.48 SD) and 2.3 (± 1.15 SD) respectively. Most, 336 (81%), women discussed about FP with their husbands and the number of children was decided both by the mother and father in more than three-quarters 344 (82.9%) of the families (Table 1).

**Table 1** Reproductive characteristics of intention to use post-partum IUCD in Ambo town public health institution, Ethiopia, May 2018. ($n = 417$)

| Variables | Number | Percent |
|---|---|---|
| Age at first marriage | | |
| ≤ 18 years | 154 | 37.1 |
| 19-20 years | 184 | 44.3 |
| ≥ 21 years | 77 | 18.6 |
| Ever give birth | | |
| Yes | 286 | 68.9 |
| No | 129 | 31.1 |
| Number of birth | | |
| ≤ 2 | 298 | 71.8 |
| 3+ | 117 | 28.2 |
| Number of alive children | | |
| ≤ 2 | 228 | 75.6 |
| 3+ | 101 | 24.4 |
| Number of children want to have in life | | |
| ≤ 3 | 398 | 79.7 |
| > 4 | 84 | 20.2 |
| Want to have child within two years | | |
| Yes | 49 | 11.8 |
| No | 366 | 88.2 |
| Discuss on family planning methods with partner | | |
| Yes | 336 | 81.0 |
| No | 79 | 19.0 |
| Decision on the number of children want to have | | |
| Husband | 17 | 4.1 |
| Wife | 54 | 13.0 |
| Both | 344 | 82.9 |
| Ever used family planning methods previously | | |
| Yes | 348 | 83.9 |
| No | 67 | 16.1 |
| Method you used previously | | |
| Natural family planning | 3 | 0.7 |
| Pills | 114 | 27.5 |
| Injectable | 253 | 61.0 |
| Implanon | 119 | 28.7 |
| IUCD | 11 | 2.7 |
| Condom | 12 | 2.9 |

### Participant's awareness about PPIUD

One hundred seventy six (42.6%) of the participants have good awareness about PPIUCD. Majority of the study participants, 121(29.2%), had awareness about PPIUD from a Mass media where as only 18(4.3) of the women heard about PPIUD from husband. There were 60(14.5%) women who heard about PPIUD from a family member/friend, 104(25.1%) heard from Health professionals.

### Knowledge of pregnant women to use post-partum intrauterine contraceptive

This study showed 205 (49%) of the respondents were found to have good knowledge, while210 (51%) of the respondents was not on intention to use postpartum IUCD. One hundred sixty (38.6%) of the participants know that PPIUD can prevent pregnancies for more than 10 years. One hundred forty-five (34.9%) of the participants know PPIUD is not appropriate for females at high risk of getting STIs. While only 100 (24.1%) know PPIUD has no interference with sexual intercourse or

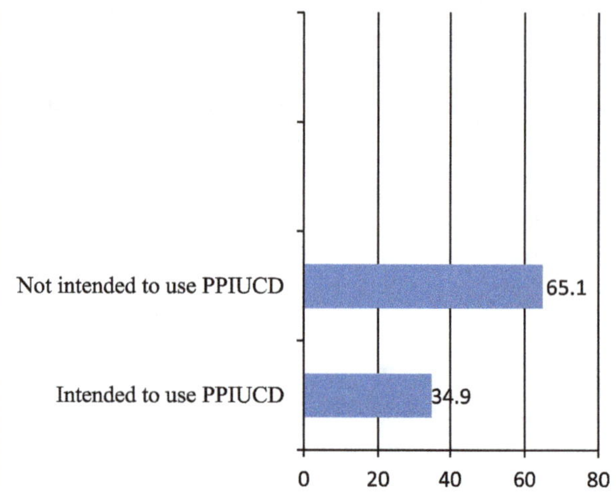


**Fig. 1** Intention to use Post-partum intra uterine contraceptive method among pregnant women attending antenatal clinics in Ambo town public health institutions, Ethiopia, 2018

desire. Majority of the respondents know PPIUD can be removed at any time they want 174 (41.9%) (Table 2).

#### Intention of pregnant women to use PPIUCD

This study showed that 145(34.9%) of pregnant women intended to use PPIUCD while more than half of the study participant 270(65.1%) was not intended to use PPIUCD (Fig. 1). The reason not intended to use post-partum intrauterine device showed (Fig. 2).

#### Participant's attitude towards PPIUD

In order to ascertain the respondent's level of attitude on pregnant women intention to use post-partum IUCD, the respondents were asked to reflect their opinion on a serious of questions concerning intention to use post-partum IUCD. Attitudes towards PPIUD were summarized through five issues related to: Insertion of PPIUCD inside the uterus does not lead to lose of privacy, Using PPIUCD does not restrict normal activities, PPIUCD doesn't move through the body after insertion, PPIUCD does not interfere with sexual intercourse and PPIUCD can harm a woman's womb. There was high disagreement about PPIUD insertion inside the uterus does not lead to lose privacy 223 (53.7%). Majority 260(62.7%) of the participants agree that using PPIUCD does not restrict normal activities. Also 254(61.2%) believe that PPIUCD does not move through the body after insertion and 147 (35.4%) felt PPIUCD can interfere with sexual intercourse. Majority 234(56.3%) of the participants disagree with PPIUCD can harm a woman's womb. Below Fig. 3 presented overall positive and negative attitude of pregnant women about intention to use postpartum intrauterine contraceptive.

#### Bivariate and multivariate logistic regression analysis of pregnant women intention to use PPIUCD and its explanatory variables

Binary Logistic regression was performed to assess the association of each independent variable with intention to use PPIUCD. After controlling the confounding factors, the multivariate revealed that the following factors have association with intention to use PPIUCD: Respondents age, educational status, respondent's occupational status, respondent's income and respondent's knowledge (Table 3).

The result revealed that age of the respondent was among the variables that were found to be associated with pregnant women intention to use PPIUCD.

**Table 2** Knowledge of pregnant women about PPIUCD in Ambo public health institution, Ambo, Ethiopia, May 2018. (*n*=417)

| Knowledge About PPIUD | LEVEL OF KNOWLEDGE | | | | Correct Response | Percent Correct |
|---|---|---|---|---|---|---|
| | Yes | | No | | | |
| | no | % | No | % | | |
| PPIUD can prevent pregnancies for more than 10 years. | 160 | 38.6 | 54 | 13 | 160 | 38.6 |
| PPIUD is not appropriate for females at high risk of getting STIs. | 145 | 34.9 | 69 | 16.6 | 145 | 34.9 |
| PPIUD has no interference with sexual intercourse or desire. | 100 | 24.1 | 100 | 24.1 | 100 | 24.1 |
| PPIUD is immediately reversible (become pregnant quickly when removed). | 151 | 36.4 | 63 | 15.2 | 151 | 36.4 |
| PPIUD does not cause cancer. | 114 | 27.5 | 99 | 23.9 | 114 | 27.5 |
| Breast feeding mothers can use PPIUD. | 153 | 36.9 | 61 | 14.7 | 153 | 36.9 |
| PPIUD may cause changes in bleeding pattern | 121 | 29.2 | 92 | 22.2 | 121 | 29.2 |
| PPIUD can be used by HIV positive patients doing well on treatment. | 100 | 24.1 | 114 | 27.5 | 100 | 24.1 |
| PPIUD is inserted free of charge in Ethiopia. | 165 | 39.8 | 48 | 11.6 | 165 | 39.8 |
| PPIUD can be removed at any time | 174 | 41.9 | 36 | 8.7 | 174 | 41.9 |

Pregnant women's who were in the age group of greater than 27 were eight times more likely to intended to use PPIUCD than those who were in the age group of less than 22 (AOR = 8.348, 95% CI: (3.602–19.347) ($P < 0.05$).

The other variables that were found to have association were the participant's educational level. Pregnant women who were college and above of education were three times more often intend to use PPIUCD when compared with those who are no formal education. (AOR = 3.249, 95%(CI: (1.057–9.985) ($P < 0.05$).

Type of job was also found to be among the factors affecting pregnant women intention to use PPIUCD. Pregnant women who were government employee are four times more likely to intention to use PPIUCD than housewife (AOR = 4.101, 95% (CI: (1.788–9.405) ($P < 0.05$).

Pregnant women monthly income was also significantly influenced intention to use PPIUCD. Pregnant women whose monthly income of greater than two thousand five hundred (> 2500) were three times more likely intend to use PPIUCD than whose monthly income of less than one thousand (< 1000) (AOR = 3.17, 95% (CI:(1.423–7.082) ($P < 0.05$).

Furthermore, knowledge of pregnant women was also found to affect the outcome variable. Respondents who had high knowledge about PPIUCD were about ten times more likely to intend to use PPIUCD than those with m knowledge (AOR = 10.338, 95% (CI: 2.59–41.49) ($P < 0.001$).

## Discussion

It was observed that the level of intention to use PPIUD among clients was low. The most appealing reason not intended to use PPIUCD was not their preferred method and fear of side effect.

This study showed the level of women intention to use PPIUCD was 34.9%, this finding was in line with findings done in Wolaita zone, (38%), Southern Ethiopia [10]. However,the present finding is inconsistent with the

**Table 3** Bivariate and multivariate logistic regression analysis of pregnant women's intention to use post-partum intrauterine contraceptive device. ($n = 417$)

| Variables | Intended To Use PPIUCD | | COR(95%CI) | AOR(95%CI) | *p*-value |
|---|---|---|---|---|---|
| | Yes | No | | | |
| Age | | | | | |
| ≥27 | 71(17.1%) | 44(10.6%) | 7.973(4.193–15.163)* | 8.348(3.602–19.347)** | 0.001 |
| 25–26 | 44(10.6%) | 61(14.7%) | 3.564(1.861–6.825)* | 2.325(1.013–5.333)** | 0.010 |
| 23–24 | 13(3.1%) | 81(19.5%) | 0.793(.362–1.737) | 0.561(0.211–1.493) | |
| ≤ 22 | 17(4.1% | 84(20.2%) | 1 | 1 | |
| Educational status | | | | | |
| College and above | 47(11.3%) | 30(7.2%) | 5.092(2.305–11.249)* | 3.249(1.057–9.985)** | 0.040 |
| Secondary (9–12) | 69(16.6%) | 84(20.2%) | 2.670(1.298–5.491)* | 1.650(0.612–4.450) | |
| Primary (1–8) | 17(4.1%) | 117(28.2%) | 0.472(.207–1.075) | 0.375(0.129–1.092) | |
| No formal education | 12(2.9%) | 39(9.4%) | 1 | 1 | |
| Occupation | | | | | |
| Goven t employee | 48(11.6%) | 25(6%) | 8.704(4.661–16.253)* | 4.101(1.788–9.405)** | 0.001 |
| Private employee | 53(12.6%) | 74(17.8%) | 3.431(2.027–5.806)* | 2.772(1.395–5.506)** | 0.004 |
| Student | 5(1.2%) | 14(3.4%) | 1.295(.481–3.485) | 2.748(0.536–14.083) | |
| Daily laborer | 6(1.4%) | 21(5.1%) | 1.619(.542–4.840) | 0.639(0.179–2.285) | |
| House wife | 30(7.2%) | 136(32.8%) | 1 | 1 | |
| Personal income | | | | | |
| > 2501 | 51(12.3%) | 45(10.8%) | 5.304(2.942–9.561)* | 3.175(1.423–7.082)** | 0.005 |
| 1501–2500 | 53(12.8%) | 77(18.6%) | 3.221(1.848–5.616)* | 1.970(0.935–4.150) | |
| 1001–1500 | 16(3.9%) | 31(7.5%) | 2.415(1.150–5.073) | 1.694(0.649–4.426) | |
| < 1000 | 25(6%) | 117(28.2%) | 1 | 1 | |
| High knowledge | 115(27.7%) | 90(21.7%) | 16.76(4.961–56.63)* | 10.338(2.59–41.49)** | .001 |
| Moderate knowledge | 30(7.2%) | 180(43.4%) | 1 | 1 | |
| Low knowledge | 38(9.2%) | 195(47.0%) | .223(.137–.362) | .288(.158–.528) | .001 |

*statistically significant at $p<0.2$ in bivariate
**statistically significant at $p<0.05$ in multivariable logistic regression

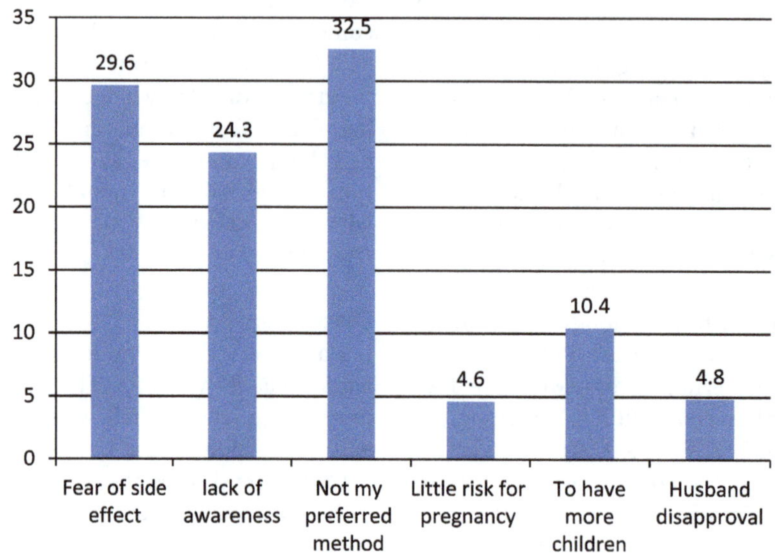


**Fig. 2** The reasons not preferring PPIUD contraceptive method among pregnant women attending antenatal clinics in Ambo town public health institutions, Ambo, Ethiopia, 2018

study done in North West Ethiopia in Adgrat town, western Ethiopia Nekemt town and Debiremarkos town were (44.6%),(47.9%) and (45.9%) of women intention to use PPIUCD respectively [11–13]. Those levels of variation may be attributed due to socio-demographic characteristic variation among study areas.

In this study, intention to use PPIUCD was significantly higher among older participants (AOR = 8.348(3.602–19.347) ($P = 0.001$) than younger participants. This finding was similar to other studies conducted in Kenya [14]. The present study is different from study done in Kenya, and Nigeria [9, 15]. This inconsistency is may be due to the variation of respondents socio demographic characteristics and may be due to time gap of the study and sample size. Educational status was found to be associated with women intention to use PPIUCD in which those who were

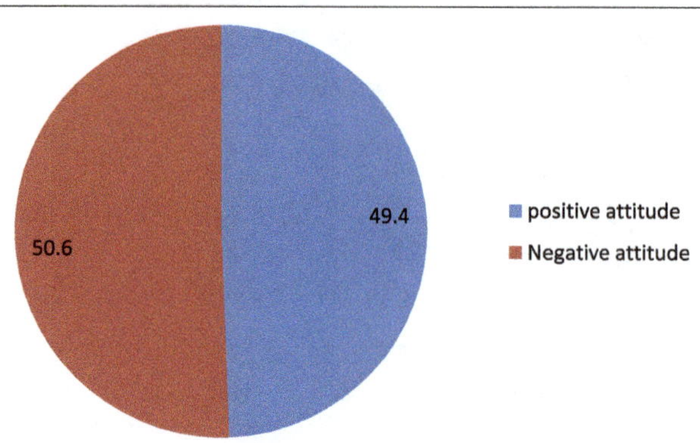


**Fig. 3** Pie chart showing Clients' Attitudes towards PPIUCD contraceptive method among pregnant women attending antenatal clinics in Ambo town public health institutions, Ambo, Ethiopia, 2018

diploma and above are three times more likely to involve than with no formal education (AOR = 3.249,95%(CI: (1.057–9.985)($P < 0.05$). This was comparable with other studies conducted in EDHS 2016 contraceptive uses increased dramatically with increase in level of education with at least 51% of women with secondary education and higher are using family planning, compared to 31% of women who had no education, Jimma, Wolaita in which women who attained secondary and higher level of education were found to be 2 and 3 times more likely to have the intention to use LAPMs compared to women who had no education, respectively and Nekemt women who had secondary school education and above were 1.82 times more likely to have intention to use LAPMs compared to those who had primary school education [10, 16–18]. This might be due to the fact that educated women might discuss more sensitive issues openly and freely they become closer and familiarized to each other. In addition women with some basic level of education can better understand the advantages and complications associated with intention to use PPIUCD.

Finding in this study indicated that pregnant mothers who were employed or government employee and private employee (AOR = 4.195% CI (1.78–9.4) $p < 0.05$and AOR = 2.7 95% CI (1.39–5.56) $p < 0.05$times more intended to use PPIUCD than daily laborer respectively. This study was consistent with the study conducted in western Ethiopia Nekemt town showed that government employed women were 2.6 times more likely express future intention to use LAPMs of contraceptive than women in other occupation [9] but inconsistent with the study done in Adgrat town [19]. This inconsistency is may be due to the variation of respondents socio demographic characteristics and may be due to sample size.

Furthermore, women intention to use PPIUCD was found to be significantly associated with personal income in which pregnant women whose monthly income was high were three times more likely involve than whose monthly income was low (AOR = 3.17,95% CI: 1.423–7.082)($p < 0.05$). This finding was similar to EDHS 2016 Use of modern contraception increases sharply with wealth, ranging from 20% for women in the lowest wealth quintile to 47% for women in the highest wealth quintile [11] and also similar to study conducted in Nigeria [9]. This could be due to exposure of women for reproductive related information and indeed employed women have better decision making power on fertility issues.

Furthermore women intention to use PPIUCD was significantly higher among participants who had good knowledge on intention to use PPIUCD (A0R = 5.4, 95% (CI: 2.99–9.76) ($P < 0.05$) than those with poor knowledge. This finding was similar to other studies conducted in, Kenya s city s slums, Adgrat town and Mekelle town mothers who had high knowledge were 8 times more likely to use LAPM as compared with those who had low knowledge (AOR = 7.8, 95% CI: 3.1, 18.3) [14, 19–23] in which participant's knowledge was a major role in determining women intention to use PPIUCD. As observed from this and other similar studies, it is evident that knowledge serves as a major determinant of women intention to use PPIUCD.

## Conclusions

It was found only 34.9% women intended to use PPIUCD. Maternal age, maternal educational level, occupational status, and monthly income, knowledge and attitude were significantly associated with pregnant women intention to use PPIUCD. Since the proportion of pregnant mothers who intend to use PPIUCD is low every effort should be made to organize and implement community based information education and communication on postpartum intrauterine contraceptive device and involving pregnant women in family planning programs is essential. This could be achieved through the development and implementation of strategies that specifically target use of PPIUCD scale up program in the area.

### Abbreviations

ANC: Antenatal care; AOR: Adjusted odd ratio; CI: Confidence interval; COR: Crude odd ratio; CWC: Child welfare clinic; EDHS: Ethiopian demographic health survey; ETB: Ethiopian birr; HC: Health center; IUCD: Intra-uterine contraceptive device; LAPMs: Long acting and permanent method; MCHIP: Maternal and child health integrated program; MDG: Millennium development goal; MMR: Maternal mortality ratio; MoH: Ministry of health; NGO: Non-governmental Organization; PPIUCD: Post partum inta-uterine contraceptive device; SD: Standard deviation; SPSS: Statistical package for social sciences; WHO: World health Organization

### Acknowledgements

The authors would like to acknowledge the contributions of research assistants, Addis Ababa University and Ambo public health institutions management bodies during this study.

### Authors' contributions

JT and GD conceptualized and designed the study. GD, WS and JT participated in the collection of data and statistical analysis. JT, GD and WS interpreted the data. JT and GD drafted the first manuscript. GD and JT revised it critically for intellectual content. All authors read and approved the final manuscript.

### Author details

[1]Ambo University College of Medicine and Health Science, Ambo, Ethiopia. [2]Addis Ababa University College of Health Science, School of Nursing & Midwifery, Addis Ababa, Ethiopia.

### References

1. Fact sheet iwstpbfucf. copper intrauterine devices (IUCD). SEPTEMBER 2008.
2. Guidance WUTSaP. TCu380A intrauterine contraceptive device (IUD) 2016.
3. Pfitzer AMD, Blanchard H, Hyjazi Y, Kumar S, LisaneworkKassa S. A facility birth can be the time to start family planning: postpartum intrauterine device experiences from six countries. Int J Gynaecol Obstet. 2015; 130(Suppl2):S54–61.
4. Singh S, Darroch JE. Adding it up: costs and benefits of contraceptive services--estimates for 2012. New York: Guttmacher Institute; 2012.
5. Lopez LM BA, Hubacher D, Stuart G, Van Vliet HA. Immediate postpartum insertion of intrauterine device for contraception. 2015.
6. CHIPMM. Program learning for postpartum intrauterine contraceptive device (PPIUCD) integration with maternal health services: programmatic experience from multiple countries. Washington: Maternal and Child Heath Integrated Program; 2012.
7. FEDERAL DEMOCRATIC REPLIC of Ethiopia MoH. Post Partum Intrauterine Contraceptive Device (PPIUCD) Participant s Handout. 2013.
8. ACQUIRE Project EH. The postpartum intrauterine device handbook. 2008.
9. Stella B NJ, Bolanle A, Ilene S. . Ideation and intention to use contraceptives in Kenya and Nigeria. 2015.
10. Meskele M. Factors affecting women's intention to use long acting and permanent contraceptive methods in Wolaita zone, southern Ethiopia: a cross-sectional study. BMC Womens Health. 2014;14:109.
11. Ethiopia. COSTED IMPLEMENTATION PLAN FOR FAMILY PLANNING 2015/ 16–2020 2016.
12. Tekelab T, Sufa A, Wirtu D. Factors affecting intention to use long acting and permanent contraceptive methods among married women of reproductive age groups in Western Ethiopia: a community based cross sectional study. MedSci. 2015;4:158.
13. Abajobir AA. Intention to use long-acting and permanent family planning methods among married 15–49 years women in Debremarkos Town, Northwest Ethiopia. Fam Med MedSci. 2014;3:145.
14. Okech TC, Wawire NW, Mburu TK. Contraceptive Use among women of reproductive Age in Kenya's city slums. Int J Bus SocSci1. 2011b;2.
15. Idowu A, Deji SA, Ogunlaja O, Olajide SO. Determinants of intention to use post partum family planning among women attending immunization clinic of a tertiary hospital in Nigeria. Am J Public Health Res. 2015;3(4):122–7.
16. The Millennium Development Goals Report, New York 2015. www.un.org/ millenniumgoals.
17. EDHS. .Central Statistical Agency, Addis Ababa, Ethiopia, ICF Rockvile, Maryland, USA, July 2016.
18. Beekle AT, McCabe C. Awareness and determinants of family planning practice in Jimma, Ethiopia. Int Nurs Rev. 2006;53:269–76.
19. Gebremariam A. Intention to use long acting and permanent contraceptive methods and factors affecting it among married women in Adigrat town, Tigray, Northern Ethiopia. Reprod Health. 2014.

20. Alemayehu M, Belachew T, Tilahun T. Factors associated with utilization of long acting and permanent contraceptive methods among married women of reproductive age in Mekelle town, Tigray region, north Ethiopia. BMC Pregnancy Childbirth. 2012;12:6.
21. Jalang'o R. Determinants of contraceptive use among postpartum women in Kisii Level Hospital, Kisii County.nairobi kenya 2015.
22. Pathfinder international technical briefApril 2016 expanding contraceptive options for postpartum women in ethiopia: introducing the postpartum iud. Expanding Contraceptive Options for Postpartum Women in Ethiopia: Introducing the Postpartum IUD pathfinder international, 2016. https://www.k4health.org.
23. Fantabun M. Comparative study of the characteristics of family planning service users and non-users in North West Ethiopia. Afr J Reproductive Health. 2006;10:54–7.

9

# Determinants of female sterilization method uptake among women of reproductive age group in Uganda

Paula Anita[1,2*], Abel Nzabona[1] and Richard Tuyiragize[1]

**Abstract**

**Background:** Despite its great effectiveness, safety and convenience for women who do not wish to have more children; female sterilization method uptake in Uganda is very low. This study aimed at establishing factors associated with female sterilization uptake in Uganda.

**Methods:** Secondary data were sourced from the 2016 Uganda Demographic and Health Survey (UDHS). We analyzed all (18,506) women aged 15–49 years who were interviewed in the 2016 UDHS. This sample was categorized into women who were sterilized and those using other modern methods. We used a Chi-square test to measure the association between the current uptake of female sterilization by the women and selected independent variables. Multivariate analysis applied the complimentary log-log model to determine the net effect of selected characteristics on female sterilization uptake in Uganda.

**Results:** The overall prevalence of female sterilization among modern contraceptive users was 2%. Female sterilization uptake was highly associated with age of 30 years and older (OR = 34.49;, 95%CI:13.33–99.88), middle wealth status (OR = 0.65, 95% CI:0.47–0.92), women who had ever given birth to at least four children (OR = 3.19, 95% CI:1.63–6.22) and decision making by either the husband/partner (OR = 2.42, 95% CI:1.55–3.78) or jointly between a woman and her husband/partner (OR = 1.38, 95% CI:1.02–1.86).

**Conclusions:** The uptake of female sterilization was very low, and this was associated with; age, household wealth, parity and contraceptive decision-maker. The uptake of Family planning programs needs to focus on male engagement to increase joint decision making on family planning issues especially those relating to fertility limitation. Government and its other implementing partners need to scale-up efforts that increase accessibility to information on female sterilization services for women who have completed their fertility.

**Keywords:** Female sterilization, Tubal ligation prevalence, Contraceptive decision-making, Uganda

## Introduction

Female sterilization is a permanent contraceptive method used by women who do not wish to have more children. Together with, long-acting methods such as Intra-Uterine Devices (IUDs) and implants, female sterilization (tubal ligation) and vasectomy are the most effective methods of contraception and would thus provide a very safe and convenient alternative [1]. Globally, female sterilization is used by 19% of married women but there are marked regional differences in its uptake among women of childbearing age. Studies show that female sterilization uptake is incomparably high in developed countries.

The prevalence of permanent contraception such as female sterilization in developing countries is only 20.6%

* Correspondence: anitapaula69@gmail.com
[1]School of Statistics and Planning, Makerere University, Kampala, Uganda
[2]Marie Stopes Uganda, Kampala, Uganda

[2]. Female sterilization is more common in Asia (23%) and Northern America Oceania and some parts of Asia, but less common in Africa (1.7%) as well as in Central Asia, South-Eastern Asia and Western Asia [3]. In developing countries, about 20 to 30% of women who use oral contraceptives or injectable stop within 2 years of starting due to side effects or other health concerns [4]. The low uptake of female sterilization in sub-Saharan Africa (SSA) is linked to poverty, limited awareness, lack of skilled personnel, limited resources to purchase and maintain sophisticated laparoscopic equipment [5]. In many countries of SSA, fertility rates and unmet need for family planning remain high [6]. Contraceptive prevalence in countries such as Uganda, Ghana, Nigeria and Rwanda among others has been reported to be influenced by partner support, approval or opposition [4].

Despite many women in SSA wanting to stop having children, the proportion using long acting and permanent methods such as female sterilization which is the most effective birth control method is very low [7]. Women and couples could achieve their desired fertility goals by using more effective, reliable and safe methods of family planning. Female sterilization is safe and effectively provides longer protection against pregnancy for women who do not wish to have more children. The 2016 Uganda Demographic and Health Survey (UDHS) report indicated that the proportion of currently married women in Uganda who have undergone sterilization increased from 2% in 2000/01 to only 3% in 2016 [8]. Due to this, women continued to have unwanted fertility as seen in the discrepancy between women's actual fertility and wanted fertility rate. The 2016 UDHS reports that whereas, total wanted fertility rate for the women in Uganda in the year 2016 was 4.3 children per woman, the actual fertility rate was 5.4 [8]. This implies that women in Uganda have about 1.1 more children than they want. This unwanted fertility can be reduced by using safe, effective methods that have higher continuation rates. Results of the 2016 UDHS indicated that use of modern contraception among currently married women increased from 14% in 2000–01 to 35% in 2016 and injectables remained the most used method [8]. The results also revealed that in the 5 years preceding the survey, 45% of episodes of contraceptive use were discontinued within 12 months and the main reason for discontinuation was method-related health concerns or side effects (35%) [8]. According to the 2016 UDHS report, 28% of currently married women and 32% of sexually active unmarried women have an unmet need for family planning. Due to their effectiveness, reliability, safety and lower (if any) side effects, permanent methods such as female sterilization can improve continuation rates and also reduce unmet need for family planning that may be associated with fears of side effects and method failures.

Most studies in Uganda examined factors that influence uptake of modern contraception methods [6, 9–17]. Some studies also explored the utilization of long acting reversible methods such as implants and intrauterine device (IUD) [7]. However, there is limited documentation on the non-reversible methods of family planning such as female and male sterilization. Female sterilization contraception method is highly effective (more than 99%), has very low failure rates and minimal serious complications [18] and due to its limited side effects may attract partner approval. Moreover, high female sterilization uptake reduces population growth rate by limiting unplanned births and like other contraceptive methods improves maternal and child health by preventing unwanted, high-risk pregnancies and reducing the need for unsafe abortions [19, 20]. This study explored the factors influencing uptake of female sterilization among women in Uganda.

## Data and methods

Secondary data from the 2016 Uganda Demographic and Health Survey (UDHS) were used. The UDHS is a nationally representative cross-sectional survey on household, socio-demographic, health status and health care data. The survey was conducted by the Uganda Bureau of Statistics (UBOS) with technical support from ICF (originally, Inner City Fund). The UDHS collected data from women, children, men and couples. This study used the women's dataset which has data on marriage, sexual activity, and the contraceptive behavior of women aged 15–49 years. A total of 18,506 women aged 15–49 years were interviewed during the 2016 UDHS. The samples were obtained using a two-stage cluster sampling process beginning with the selection of clusters followed by the selection of households from each cluster and the selection of respondents from households.

During the survey, the women were asked to report about their current use of any method of contraception to avoid or delay pregnancy. The women were specifically asked; *"Are you or your partner currently doing something or using any method to delay or avoid getting pregnant?* And this led to a follow-up question *"Which method are you using?"* These questions provided responses on various methods used by women to prevent pregnancy which helped to categorize the dependent variable for this study. This study was conducted on all the 18,506 women of reproductive age who were interviewed in the UDHS. Data were weighted to ensure representativeness and control for non-responsiveness across regions. The sample was weighed using the sampling variable and the svy command as recommended by

DHS. The weighted sample included 18,165 women who were not sterilized and 341 who were sterilized.

The dependent variable (sterilization status) was generated from the question on current use of family planning methods. We categorized the women into two categories depending on whether they were sterilized or not. The women who were using methods other than female sterilization as well as those who were not using any method of family planning were categorized as "not sterilized". The independent variables included age, education (highest education level attained by the woman), place of residence, wealth status, marital status, number of children ever born, ideal number of children, ideal number of boys and ideal number of girls, women's paid employment status, whether woman earns more than partner (based on the question; would you say that the money that you earn is more than what your (husband/ partner) earns, less than what he earns, or about the same?), decision maker on respondent's earnings (who makes the decision on how to spend the woman's earnings), and contraceptive decision maker (who makes the decision to use contraceptives). Selection of the independent variables was based on previous studies and the hypothetical relationship they have with sterilization uptake. Wealth status was a variable that we generated from the DHS wealth quintiles. In the DHS, wealth quintiles were obtained by using an asset index which grouped households into five categories (poorest, poorer, middle, richer and richest). We combined poorest and poorer to generate the category "poor" and also merged richer and richest categories to generate the "rich" category.

Data were analyzed at three levels using STATA software version 13. We first generated frequency distributions to describe the characteristics of the study sample. Using cross-tabulations and a Pearson's Chi-square test, we measured the association between female sterilization use and each of the explanatory variables. The complementary log-log model (Clog log) for multivariate analysis. Complementary log-log model is recommended for use in analysis of rare phenomena such as female sterilization use whose prevalence is very low in Uganda. Model adequacy was checked using the link test. All statistical tests were interpreted at a 5% level of significance.

**Table 1** Percentage distribution of women by socio-demographic characteristics ($n = 18{,}506$)

| Characteristic | Frequency (*n*) | Percent (%) |
|---|---|---|
| **Age** | | |
| Younger than 30 years | 11,137 | 60.2 |
| 30 years and older | 7369 | 39.8 |
| **Marital status** | | |
| Never in Union | 4783 | 25.8 |
| Currently married | 11,223 | 60.7 |
| Formerly married | 2500 | 13.5 |
| **Education level** | | |
| No education | 1781 | 9.6 |
| Primary | 10,630 | 57.4 |
| Secondary+ | 6095 | 32.9 |
| **Household wealth status** | | |
| Poor | 6643 | 35.9 |
| Middle | 3460 | 18.7 |
| Rich | 8403 | 45.4 |
| **Place of residence** | | |
| Urban | 4943 | 26.7 |
| Rural | 13,563 | 73.3 |
| **Employment status** | | |
| Not employed | 4986 | 26.9 |
| Employed | 13,520 | 73.1 |
| **Total number of children ever born** | | |
| 0–3 children | 11,511 | 62.2 |
| 4+ children | 6995 | 37.8 |
| **Ideal number of children** | | |
| None | 148 | 0.8 |
| 1–3 children | 2937 | 15.9 |
| 4+ children | 14,985 | 81.0 |
| Non-numeric | 437 | 2.4 |
| **Ideal number of boys** | | |
| None | 2278 | 12.3 |
| 1–3 boys | 14,040 | 75.9 |
| 4+ boys | 1658 | 9.0 |
| Non-numeric | 529 | 2.9 |
| **Ideal number of girls** | | |
| None | 2250 | 12.2 |
| 1–3 girls | 13,714 | 74.1 |
| 4+ girls | 2012 | 10.9 |
| Non-numeric | 529 | 2.9 |
| **Sterilization status** | | |
| Not sterilized | 18,165 | 98.2 |
| Sterilized | 341 | 1.8 |
| **Total** | **18,506** | **100** |

## Results

The analysis was undertaken on a weighted sample of 18,506 women aged 15–49 years. The findings in Table 1 indicate that 60% of the women were younger than 30 years, 61% were currently married, 57% had attained primary level of education and 45% were from rich households. Furthermore, majority of the women (73%) resided in rural areas, 73% were employed and 62% had ever given birth to 0–3 children. Also, majority (81%) of the women preferred at least 4 children, 76% preferred 1–3 boys, and 74% preferred 1–3 girls. It is important to note here that the non-response categories on ideal number of children, ideal number of boys and ideal number of girls refer to women who d made statements such as; "It depends on God", "As many as I can support", "I don't know" rather than specifying numbers when asked about their fertility preferences. Regarding the uptake of female sterilization, Table 1 indicates that only 2% of the women had been sterilized.

Table 2 indicates that although slightly less than three quarters (74%) of the women earned less than their husband/partner, 53% decided on how to spend their own earnings. The results also show majority of the women (62%) reported that contraceptive decision making was jointly made with their partners. The results also show that 99% had knowledge of any family planning method, 73% did not know the source of any family planning method while 59% obtained family planning methods from a public health facility.

**Table 2** Distribution of respondents by enabling factors

| Factor | Frequency (*n*) | Percent (%) |
|---|---|---|
| **Whether respondent earns more than husband/partner (*n* = 7096)** | | |
| Earn more than him | 671 | 9.5 |
| Earn less than him | 5244 | 73.9 |
| Earn about the same | 925 | 13.0 |
| Don't know | 256 | 3.6 |
| **Decision maker on respondent's earnings (*n* = 7096)** | | |
| Respondent | 3733 | 52.6 |
| Husband and wife | 2719 | 38.3 |
| Husband/Partner | 644 | 9.1 |
| **Decision-maker on contraception (*n* = 4373)** | | |
| Respondent | 1340 | 30.6 |
| Husband/Partner | 312 | 7.1 |
| Joint decision | 2721 | 62.2 |
| **Knowledge of any family planning method (*n* = 18,506)** | | |
| No knowledge | 187 | 1.0 |
| Has knowledge | 18,319 | 99.0 |
| **Knowledge of source of any family planning method (*n* = 18,391)** | | |
| Don't know | 13,456 | 73.2 |
| Public source | 2888 | 15.7 |
| Private source | 1914 | 10.4 |
| Other | 133 | 0.7 |
| **Source of family planning method (*n* = 4935)** | | |
| Public facility | 2888 | 58.5 |
| Private facility | 1914 | 38.8 |
| Other | 133 | 2.7 |

Table 3 presents the distribution of female sterilization by selected characteristics. The results in the table indicate that age, marital status, education level attained, employment status, total number of children ever born, ideal number of children, ideal number of boys, ideal number of girls and whether the husband earned more than the partner/husband were significantly associated with female sterilization uptake ($p < 0.05$). On the other hand, wealth status, place of residence, decision maker on respondent's earnings, decision maker on contraception and preexisting knowledge of family planning were not significant. The non-numeric responses as presented in the Table on fertility preferences whether it was with ideal number of children, ideal number of sons and daughters are for the proportion of women who did not specify the ideal numbers of children they preferred but rather made statements such as; "It depends on God", "As many as I can support", "I don't know".

### Predictors of female sterilization uptake

Table 4 presents predictors of female sterilization. Older women (> 30 years) are more likely to undergo sterilization compared to those less than 30 years. The odds of being sterilized were highest among women above 30 years (OR = 34.49, 95% CI = 13.33–99.88). On the other hand, women's highest education level attained, place of residence, employment status, the ideal number of children and ideal number of sons preferred did not have a significant influence on female sterilization uptake. The findings also revealed that being from middle households reduced the odds of being sterilized as compared to being from the poor households. The odds of being sterilized of women from middle households were approximately 0.65 times compared to their counterparts. Furthermore, the results show that the odds of being sterilized for women who reported that the contraception decision-maker was the husband/partner were 2.42 times those of their counterparts who took independent decisions (OR = 2.42, 95% CI = 1.55–3.78). Women who took joint decisions with their husbands/partners had 1.38 odds higher of undergoing sterilization compared to those that took independent decisions (OR = 1.38, 95% CI = 1.02–1.86). Education level, place of residence, employment status, ideal number of children, and ideal number of boys were not significant.

## Discussion

This study assessed factors influencing female sterilization uptake in Uganda. The study findings indicated a low uptake of female sterilization in Uganda. Female sterilization uptake was significantly associated with older age, middle wealth status, number of children ever born and joint decision making. The odds of taking

**Table 3** Association between female sterilization use and women's socio-demographic characteristics

| Characteristic | Frequency | Sterilized | | *P*- value |
|---|---|---|---|---|
| | | Not sterilized (%) | Sterilized (%) | |
| **Age** | | | | |
| Younger than 30 years | 11,000 | 100.0 | 0.0 | < 0.001 |
| 30 years and older | 7369 | 95.4 | 4.6 | |
| **Marital status** | | | | |
| Never in Union | 4783 | 99.9 | 0.1 | < 0.001 |
| Married | 11,000 | 97.3 | 2.7 | |
| Formerly married | 2500 | 98.8 | 1.2 | |
| **Education level attained** | | | | |
| No education | 1781 | 96.8 | 3.2 | < 0.001 |
| Primary | 11,000 | 97.9 | 2.1 | |
| Secondary+ | 6095 | 99.1 | 1.0 | |
| **Wealth quintile** | | | | |
| Poor | 6643 | 98.1 | 1.9 | 0.529 |
| Middle | 3460 | 98.0 | 2.0 | |
| Rich | 8403 | 98.3 | 1.7 | |
| **Place of residence** | | | | |
| Urban | 4943 | 98.5 | 1.5 | 0.120 |
| Rural | 14,000 | 98.0 | 2.0 | |
| **Employment status** | | | | |
| Not employed | 4986 | 99.1 | 0.9 | < 0.001 |
| Employed | 14,000 | 97.8 | 2.2 | |
| **Total number of children ever born** | | | | |
| 0–3 children | 12,000 | 99.8 | 0.2 | < 0.001 |
| 4+ children | 6995 | 95.4 | 4.6 | |
| **Ideal number of children** | | | | |
| None | 148 | 98.6 | 1.4 | < 0.001 |
| 1–3 children | 2937 | 99.5 | 0.5 | |
| 4+ children | 15,000 | 98.0 | 2.0 | |
| Non-numeric | 437 | 95.6 | 4.4 | |
| **Ideal number of boys** | | | | |
| None | 2278 | 98.8 | 1.2 | < 0.001 |
| 1–3 boys | 14,000 | 98.3 | 1.7 | |
| 4+ boys | 1658 | 96.3 | 3.7 | |
| Non-numeric | 529 | 96.2 | 3.8 | |
| **Ideal number of girls** | | | | |
| None | 2250 | 98.9 | 1.2 | < 0.001 |
| 1–3 girls | 14,000 | 98.4 | 1.7 | |
| 4+ girls | 2012 | 96.6 | 3.4 | |
| Non-numeric | 529 | 96.2 | 3.8 | |
| **Whether respondent earns more than husband/partner** | | | | |
| Earn more than him | 671 | 95.0 | 5.0 | 0.005 |
| Earn less than him | 5244 | 97.5 | 2.5 | |
| Earn about the same | 925 | 98.0 | 2.0 | |

**Table 3** Association between female sterilization use and women's socio-demographic characteristics *(Continued)*

| Characteristic | Frequency | Sterilized | | *P*- value |
|---|---|---|---|---|
| | | Not sterilized (%) | Sterilized (%) | |
| Don't know | 256 | 97.0 | 3.0 | |
| **Decision maker on respondent's earnings** | | | | |
| Respondent | 3733 | 97.5 | 2.5 | 0.550 |
| Husband and wife | 2719 | 97.3 | 2.7 | |
| Husband/Partner | 644 | 96.6 | 3.4 | |
| **Decision-maker on contraception** | | | | |
| Respondent | 1340 | 93.7 | 6.4 | 0.078 |
| Husband/Partner | 312 | 89.6 | 10.4 | |
| Joint decision | 2721 | 93.1 | 6.9 | |
| **Knowledge of any family planning methods** | | | | |
| No knowledge | 187 | 100.0 | 0.0 | 0.140 |
| Has knowledge | 18,000 | 98.1 | 1.9 | |

up sterilization were highest among older women (> 30 years). This is not surprising as younger women may prefer reversible methods that are suitable for spacing over those that limit childbirths. Older women are more likely to be multiparous and prefer to use long acting and permanent methods as compared to younger women. The uptake of female sterilization may be affected by issues of informed choice and availability of quality services as was reported in a study conducted in India that women did not generally opt for sterilization in equal proportion due to very poor informed choice among women [21]. None the less, these findings are consistent with evidence from a similar study in Ethiopia [22] which revealed that older women (35–49 years) had three times higher odds of using sterilization contraception than their younger counterparts. The findings also partly agree with those of a study in Nigeria on female surgical sterilization which found that more than half of the women who opted for sterilization were aged between 35 to 39 years [23]. However, the study disagrees with findings of a study done in India where sterilization method uptake and acceptance was at a much younger age (mean age 28.9 years) among women [24].

The number of children ever born was associated with female sterilization uptake. This is probably because contraception choices are based on the already achieved fertility. Since sterilization is effective and irreversible, women who have not yet attained their desired fertility are less likely to use it. Women can confidently make contraceptive choices and implement decisions such as undergoing sterilization after achieving a certain number of children. This finding may also explain the high fertility preferences among women in Uganda. In addition, for some high parity women, these may be influenced by birth related experiences to stop childbearing and thus opt for sterilization. It is perhaps not very surprising since most users of female sterilization are those who do not wish to have any more children. Furthermore, women prefer many children as a source of workforce since Uganda is largely an agrarian economy with a poorly mechanized sector compared to other developed countries. This is in agreement with study findings from Uganda, rural Rakai which revealed that women with higher number of children had a significant desire to undergo sterilization [25] and partly agree with those from Brazil and India where women with three or more living children were more likely to undergo sterilization than their counterparts who had fewer children [26]. The finding is also consistent with a study done in Malawi [27] and another one in Nigeria where higher rates of sterilization uptake were found among women of parity four and above compared to those women with lower parities [28] but partly disagrees with findings in Nepal where intention to undergo sterilization was higher among women with a lower number of children [29].

The findings indicated that the contraceptive decision maker was significantly associated with the uptake of female sterilization. This is in agreement with previous studies done in other countries and contexts. For instance, in Zambia, joint contraceptive decision making between spouses was found to be a key determinant of uptake of injectable, long acting and permanent methods [30]. Similarly, in Ethiopia, women who discussed with their husbands about modern contraceptives in a bid to make contraceptive decisions were seven times more likely to use modern contraceptive methods than women who did not discuss at all [31] while in India, women who made joint decisions with their husbands were more likely to use sterilization compared to their

**Table 4** Complementary log-log model of predictors of female sterilization uptake

| Characteristic | OR | *P*-value | 95%CI |
|---|---|---|---|
| **Age** | | | |
| Below 30 | 1.00 | | |
| 30+ | 36.49 | ***< 0.001*** | 13.33–99.88 |
| **Education level** | | | |
| None | 1.00 | | |
| Primary | 0.91 | 0.554 | 0.66–1.25 |
| Secondary+ | 0.69 | 0.102 | 0.44–1.08 |
| **Wealth status** | | | |
| Poor | 1.00 | | |
| Middle | 0.65 | ***0.014*** | 0.47–0.92 |
| Rich | 0.74 | 0.073 | 0.53–1.03 |
| **Place of residence** | | | |
| Urban | 1.00 | | |
| Rural | 0.83 | 0.329 | 0.57–1.20 |
| **Employment status** | | | |
| Not employed | 1.00 | | |
| Employed | 0.98 | 0.914 | 0.66–1.45 |
| **Total number of children ever born** | | | |
| 0–3 children | 1.00 | | |
| 4+ children | 3.19 | ***0.001*** | 1.63–6.22 |
| **Contraception decision-maker** | | | |
| Respondent | 1.00 | | |
| Husband/partner | 2.42 | ***< 0.001*** | 1.55–3.78 |
| Joint | 1.38 | ***0.034*** | 1.02–1.86 |
| **Ideal number of children** | | | |
| None | 1.00 | | |
| 1–3 children | 0.29 | 0.151 | 0.06–1.56 |
| 4+ children | 0.57 | 0.471 | 0.13–2.60 |
| Non-numeric | 0.35 | 0.420 | 0.03–4.54 |
| **Ideal number of boys** | | | |
| None | 1.00 | | |
| 1–3 boys | 1.14 | 0.578 | 0.72–1.79 |
| 4+ boys | 1.34 | 0.266 | 0.80–2.26 |
| Non-numeric | 4.34 | 0.153 | 0.58–32.68 |

*CI* Confidence interval, *OR* Odds ratio

counterparts who made independent decisions [32]. Eliason et al.(2014) asserted that women whose partners approved as decision makers of modern family planning were more likely to use modern contraceptives than their counterparts whose partners did not approve [33]. Likewise, in Bangladesh, there were higher odds of female sterilization acceptance among women whose partners approved compared to those whose partners did not approve [34]. Kabagenyi et al., (2014) found that the major barrier to use modern contraceptive methods among women in Uganda was partner disapproval [6].

This study also revealed that women who were from middle wealth households had reduced odds of being sterilized compared to their poor counterparts. Women from poor wealth class have higher birth rates and are more likely to undergo sterilization compared to women from middle wealth class. Also, women in middle wealth class enter marriages late and childbearing is relatively delayed compared to women from poor households who enter marriages early. This agrees with findings of a study conducted in India on dominance of sterilization and alternative choices of contraception which revealed that women from poor households relied on sterilization compared to their counterparts from rich households [32]. This study disagrees with findings of study done in Zambia where women from richer households had higher odds of using long acting and permanent methods compared to their counterparts from poorest households [30] and those on modern contraceptive use in Nigeria which reported that poorest women least used modern contraceptives compared to richest women [35].

Husband/partners' decision on contraception was also associated with female sterilization uptake. Women who reported that the contraceptive decision maker was husband/partner had higher odds of utilizing female sterilization compared to those who took an independent decision. This can be attributed to the patriarchal nature of our society. This points to the significant influence of husbands/partners in determining women's contraceptive choices. Women have limited decision-making power even on issues concerning their own health as a result of power dynamics from the male dominated societies. This is closely related to limited decision-making power among most women in many African societies. In addition, men have control over resources such as money and determine how they are used including facilitating a woman to undergo sterilization or not. Our findings are in agreement with the assertion that women whose partners are decision makers of modern family planning more likely to use modern contraceptives than their counterparts whose partners did not approve [6, 33, 34]. Similarly, study findings from Zambia [30], Ethiopia [31] and India [32] indicated that joint contraceptive decision making between spouses was a key determinant of uptake of family planning methods including female sterilization.

Although a woman's highest level of education has been found to significantly affect her contraceptive choice and decision, our findings revealed that education attained did not have a significant association with the uptake of female sterilization. This is partly in disagreement with a study in Ethiopia which revealed that women with secondary level education had higher odds of using sterilization compared to those with no education [36]. The findings also partly contrast study findings in Nepal where it was revealed that an increase in a woman's education reduced the probability that she will choose sterilization contraception [29]. The study also disagrees with study findings in India which revealed that women with secondary or higher education preferred temporary methods of contraception over sterilization [32] and in Ghana where women with no education were significantly less likely to use modern contraceptive including sterilization as compared to women with secondary or higher levels of education [33].

Our findings on place of residence partly disagree with other studies which indicated that place of residence significantly influenced contraceptive uptake including female sterilization. For instance, our study partly disagrees with findings from a comparative study between India and Brazil which indicated that female sterilization was generally higher among women in the rural areas compared to women in urban areas [26]. The results also disagree with a studies done in Uganda [37] and Nigeria [35] which reported that women in urban areas utilized modern contraceptives more than their counterparts in rural areas.

In this study, we found no evidence to suggest that women's employment status associated with uptake of female sterilization. This is in contrary with the assertion that women's employment status has a significant positive relationship with contraceptive use. Previous studies in India [32], Bangladesh [34, 38] asserted that women who are in paid employment were more likely to use sterilization than their counterparts who were unemployed because they are empowered to make independent reproductive health choices.

Our findings indicated that fertility preferences (ideal number of children and ideal number of boys) were not associated with the uptake of female sterilization by women of reproductive age. This finding partly disagrees with those of earlier studies such as in Uganda where contraceptive use among women is partly hindered by patriarchal family units that highly value children and encourage large family sizes [6], Ethiopia where the desire for no more children by women was significantly associated with women's demand for long acting and permanent methods in [39], Zambia where women whose husbands desired more children were less likely to use modern contraceptive methods including female sterilization [30] and Pakistan where permanent method use among women was significantly associated with the number of sons they had ever born [40].

### Study limitations

Like other cross-sectional studies, the study could not determine a causal inference about female sterilization uptake. The study was also not able to clearly determine the causes of choice to undergo sterilization by individual women. In addition, as this study was based on secondary data, we were not able to investigate all factors associated with the uptake of female sterilization. In addition, this study is unable to explain the factors associated with family planning choices. A qualitative inquiry would provide a detailed understanding and explanation of the circumstances around uptake or no uptake of female sterilization as well as other family planning choices. Also, the other limitation of this study is that it did not include male sterilization (vasectomy) which is one of poorly utilized contraceptive method in Uganda. The study thus recommends that a similar study to investigate factors influencing the uptake of voluntary male sterilization be done.

## Conclusion and implications

The findings indicate that uptake of female sterilization in Uganda is generally low. The uptake was associated with being older, having ever given birth to at least four children and making independent contraceptive decisions. Therefore, there is need for male engagement by all stakeholders and implementing partners in matters related to women's sexual and reproductive health, since it is evident that they play a key role in contraceptive decision making of service uptake.

The government of Uganda and its implementing partners of sexual and reproductive health programmes need to target higher parity (4+ children) and older (> 30 yrs) women through awareness creation campaigns and comprehensive counseling to promote female sterilization method acceptance. Also, promotion of permanent methods should target all sexually active young women to help them reach appropriate decisions on their contraceptive choices and limit their fertility if they desire to do so.

#### Abbreviations

UDHS: Uganda Demographic and Health Surveys; UBOS: Uganda Bureau of Statistics; IUD: Intra Uterine device; LAPM: Long acting and permanent methods; CI: Confidence Interval; OR: Odds Ratios; SSA: Sub Saharan Africa

#### Acknowledgements

The authors express sincere gratitude to MEASURE DHS program for granting permission to use the UDHS data.

#### Authors' contributions

Paula Anita conceptualized and designed the study, carried out data analysis, interpreted the results and drafted the manuscript. Abel Nzabona and Richard Tuyiragize guided on the conceptualization, data analysis and final manuscript development. All authors edited and approved the final manuscript.

**Authors' information**

Paula Anita is a demographer with research interests in population, family planning and reproductive health. She is a graduate of Master of Science of Population and Reproductive Health of Makerere University and works with Maries Stopes Uganda. Abel Nzabona (PhD) and Richard Tuyiragize (PhD) are lecturers at the School of Statistics and Planning, Makerere University.

## References


1. Melka AS, Tekelab T, Wirtu D. Determinants of long acting and permanent contraceptive methods utilization among married women of reproductive age groups in western Ethiopia: a cross-sectional study. Pan Afr Med J. 2015;21:246. https://doi.org/10.11604/pamj.2015.21.246.5835.
2. Patil E, Jensen JT. Permanent contraception for women. Semin Reprod Med. 2016;34:139–44.
3. United Nations. Trends in contraceptive use worldwide. New York: United Nations Department of Economic and Social Affairs, Population Division; 2015.
4. Mota K, Reddy S, Getachew B. Unmet need of long-acting and permanent family planning methods among women in the reproductive age group in shashemene town, Oromia region, Ethiopia: a cross sectional study. BMC Womens Health. 2015;15:1–8. https://doi.org/10.1186/s12905-015-0209-y.
5. Dennis O. Allagoa, Nyengidiki Tamunomie Kennedy, Kotingo E.L, Kotingo E, Allagoa D, Tamunomie N. evolving trends in female sterilization. A review article. Elit Res J Med Med Sci. 2014;2:11–6.
6. Kabagenyi A, Jennings L, Reid A, Nalwadda G, Ntozi J, Atuyambe L. Barriers to male involvement in contraceptive uptake and reproductive health services: a qualitative study of men and women's perceptions in two rural districts in Uganda. Reprod Health. 2014;11:21. https://doi.org/10.1186/1742-4755-11-21.
7. Anguzu R, Tweheyo R, Sekandi JN, Zalwango V, Muhumuza C, Tusiime S, et al. Knowledge and attitudes towards use of long acting reversible contraceptives among women of reproductive age in Lubaga division, Kampala district, Uganda. BMC Res Notes. 2014;7:153.
8. UBOS, ICF. Uganda demographic and health survey 2016. Kampala, Uganda and Rockville, Maryland USA: UBOS and ICF; 2018.
9. Thummalachetty N, Mathur S, Mullinax M, Decosta K, Nakyanjo N, Lutalo T, et al. Contraceptive knowledge , perceptions , and concerns among men in Uganda. BMC Public Health. 2017;17:1–9.
10. Asiimwe JB, Ndugga P, Mushomi J. Socio-demographic factors associated with contraceptive use among young women in comparison with older women in Uganda. Calverton, Maryland: Measure DHS; 2013.
11. Sileo KM, Wanyenze RK, Lule H, Kiene SM. Determinants of family planning service uptake and use of contraceptives among postpartum women in rural Uganda. Int J Public Health. 2015;60:987–97.
12. Lule H, Echoru I, Nnabagulanyi M, Mulumba R. Determinants of contraceptive utilisation amongst teenage mothers: a case-control study in Kyangwali refugee settlement (Uganda). Int J Curr Adv Res. 2015;4:243–57.
13. Kabagenyi A, Habaasa G, Rutaremwa G. Low contraceptive use among young females in Uganda: does birth history and age at birth have an influence ? Analysis of 2011 demographic and health survey abstract data source. iMedPub J. 2016;1(1):4 1–7.
14. Blackstone SR, Nwaozuru U, Iwelunmor J. Factors influencing contraceptive use in sub-Saharan Africa : a systematic review. Int Q Community Health Educ. 2017;37:79–91.
15. Rutaremwa G, Kabagenyi A, Wandera SO, Jhamba T, Akiror E, Nviiri HL. Predictors of modern contraceptive use during the postpartum period among women in Uganda: a population-based cross sectional study. BMC Public Health. 2015;15:1–9. https://doi.org/10.1186/s12889-015-1611-y.
16. Kabagenyi A, Ndugga P, Wandera SO, Kwagala B. Modern contraceptive use among sexually active men in Uganda : does discussion with a health worker matter? BMC Public Health. 2014;14:286.
17. Kabagenyi A, Reid A, Ntozi JPM, Atuyambe LM. Socio-cultural inhibitors to use of modern contraceptive techniques in rural Uganda: a qualitative study. PanAfrican Med J. 2016;25:78.
18. World Health Organization. Family planning: a global handbook for providers (2018 update). Baltimore and Geneva: World Health Organization; 2018.
19. Kavanaugh ML, Anderson RM. Contraception and beyond: The health benefits of services provided at family planning centers. Guttmacher Inst. 2013;July:1–39.
20. WHO. Family planning/contraception methods: World Health Organization; 2020. https://www.who.int/news-room/fact-sheets/detail/family-planning-contraception. Accessed 2 Aug 2020.
21. Pradhan MR, Ram U. Female sterilization and ethical issues: the Indian experience. Soc Change. 2009;39:365–87. https://doi.org/10.1177/004908570903900303.
22. Geta W, Abera Asseffa N, Mekonnen N. Utilization of long acting and permanent contraceptive methods and associated factors among married childbearing age women in Bombe District, Southern Ethiopia. 2018; March.
23. Salaudeen AG, Akanbi A, Jimoh G, Panti AA, Rakiya S. Female surgical sterilization at University of Ilorin Teaching Hospital, Ilorin: 10-year review original article. 2012; July 2015.
24. Bharadwaj MK, Patrikar S, Singh S. Determinant factors affecting the trends of permanent sterilization : a decadal analysis in a tertiary care institute. Int J Reprod Contracept Obstet Gynecol. 2017;6:5348–53.
25. Paul B, Ayo AS, Ayiga N. Rural-urban contraceptive use in Uganda: evidence from UDHS 2011; 2015.
26. Leone T, Padmadas SS. The proliferation of female sterilization in Brazil and India. A comparative analysis of the cohort and parity effects; 2007. p. 63.
27. Palamuleni ME. Socio-economic and demographic factors affecting contraceptive use in Malawi. Afr J Reprod Health. 2013;17:91–104.
28. Adesiyun AG. Female sterilization by tubal ligation: a re-appraisal of factors influencing decision making in a tropical setting. Arch Gynecol Obstet. 2007;275:241.
29. Dhungana A, Nanthamongkolchai S, Pitikultang S. Factors related to intention to undergo female sterilization among married women in rural Kathmandu, Nepal. Nepal J Epidemiol. 2016;6:539–47. https://doi.org/10.3126/nje.v6i1.14736.
30. Mutombo N, Bakibinga P. The effect of joint contraceptive decisions on the use of Injectables, long-acting and permanent methods (ILAPMs) among married female (15–49) contraceptive users in Zambia: a cross-sectional study. Reprod Health. 2014;11:51. https://doi.org/10.1186/1742-4755-11-51.
31. Mwaikambo L, Speizer IS, Schurmann A, Morgan G, Fikree F. What works in family planning interventions : a systematic review. Stud Fam Plan. 2011;42:67–82.
32. de Oliveira IT, Dias JG, Padmadas SS. Dominance of sterilization and alternative choices of contraception in India. An appraisal of the socioeconomic impact; 2014.
33. Eliason S, Awoonor-Williams JK, Eliason C, Novignon J, Nonvignon J, Aikins M. Determinants of modern family planning use among women of reproductive age in the Nkwanta district of Ghana: a case-control study. Reprod Health. 2014;11:65.
34. Kamal N. The influence of husbands on contraceptive use by Bangladeshi women. Health Policy Plan. 2000;15:43–51. https://doi.org/10.1093/heapol/15.1.43.
35. Johnson OE. Determinants of modern contraceptive uptake among Nigerian women: evidence from the national demographic and health survey. Afr J Reprod Health. 2017;21:89–95.
36. Zenebe CB, Adefris M, Yenit MK, Gelaw YA. Factors associated with utilization of long-acting and permanent contraceptive methods among women who have decided not to have more children in Gondar city. BMC Womens Health. 2017;17:1–7.
37. Kibira SPS, Ndugga P, Nansubuga E, Sewannonda A, Kwagala B. Contraceptive uptake among married women in Uganda: does empowerment matter? Etude la Popul Africaine. 2014;28:968–77.
38. Islam AZ, Mondal NI, Khatun ML. Prevalence and determinants of contraceptive use among employed and unemployed women in Bangladesh. Int J MCH AIDS. 2016;5:92–102.
39. Bulto GA, Zewdie TA, Beyen TK. Demand for long acting and permanent contraceptive methods and associated factors among married women of reproductive age group in Debre Markos Town, North West Ethiopia. BMC Womens Health. 2014;14:46. https://doi.org/10.1186/1472-6874-14-46.
40. Channon. Son preference and family limitation in Pakistan: a parity- and contraceptive method–specific analysis. Int Perspect Sex Reprod Health. 2017;43:99–110.

# 10

# Risk factors for postpartum intrauterine device expulsion among women delivering at a tertiary Hospital in Uganda

Joy Muhumuza[1,2], Richard Migisha[3*], Joseph Ngonzi[1], Musa Kayondo[1] and Godfrey Mugyenyi[1]

**Abstract**

**Background:** Postpartum intrauterine device (PPIUD) use refers to intrauterine device (IUD) insertion after delivery but within 48 h of birth. In Uganda, the general use of modern methods of contraception is low with < 1% of the women adopting the IUD as a method of contraception. An important limiting factor to increased uptake of immediate postpartum IUD insertion may be its expulsion rates which vary widely. There is minimal documentation PPIUD expulsion rates and factors associated with PPIUD expulsion during puerperium in Uganda.

**Objective:** We aimed to determine the proportion of TCu380A (copper) intrauterine devices expelled by 6 weeks postpartum, and identify risk factors for expulsion among women delivering at Mbarara Regional Referral Hospital (MRRH) in southwestern Uganda.

**Methods:** We conducted a prospective cohort study from September 1, 2014 to January 31, 2015 at MRRH. We administered a structured questionnaire to all participants, to capture data on their baseline demographic, clinical and obstetric characteristics. We followed up women who accepted the PPIUD insertions at 6 weeks post insertion for any IUD expulsion. We fit multivariable log binomial regression models to identify risk factors for IUD expulsion.

**Results:** We enrolled 167 women who had PPIUDs inserted. Of the144 women who returned at 6 weeks for follow up, 13 (9%; 95%CI:4.9–15%) of them had the IUDs expelled. In the multivariable model, the significant risk factors for PPIUD expulsion were: IUD insertion more than 10 min post-delivery (aRR 8.1, 95%CI 1.26–51.98, $p = 0.027$) and bloody lochia flow of ≥15 days (aRR 8.5, 95%CI 1.47–48.47, $p = 0.017$).

**Conclusion:** The cumulative expulsion rate of postpartum IUDs among women delivering at MRRH was low and comparable to expulsion rates in interval insertions. Longer duration from delivery to IUD insertions and longer duration of bloody lochia flow were key risk factors for postpartum IUD expulsion. More emphasis should be put on prenatal counseling for postpartum family planning to allow for postplacental IUD insertions, which are associated with lower expulsion rates.

**Keywords:** Copper intrauterine device, Intrauterine device, Intrauterine device expulsion, Postpartum contraception, Postpartum intrauterine device, Postplacental intrauterine device, TCu380A intrauterine device

* Correspondence: migisha85@gmail.com
[3]Department of Physiology, Mbarara University of Science and Technology, P.O Box 1410, Mbarara, Uganda

## Introduction

Globally, approximately 220 million women in need of modern family planning methods are unable to access them for various reasons [1, 2]. The unmet need for family planning in sub-Saharan Africa, including Uganda is still very high (25 and 34% respectively) [3–5]. Across sub-Saharan Africa and Uganda, the IUD remains underutilized with just 1 and 0.5% of married women using it, respectively [5, 6]. The intrauterine device (IUD) is a highly effective, safe, reversible and long-acting type of contraception [7]. The CuT380A device is the most effective of IUDs with failure rate of 0.6–0.8 pregnancies per 100 women in the first 12 months of use and has the lowest cumulative pregnancy rate (2.2 per 100 women after 8 years) [8]. Postpartum intra uterine device (PPIUD) insertion bridges the limitations to the unmet family planning need by promoting IUD use. Offering postpartum insertions is one of the reasons for high uptake of the IUD in countries like China, Egypt, Mexico and Turkey where the IUD is the most popular reversible method of contraception [9]. The unique advantage of postpartum intrauterine contraception is that contraception is initiated early with a very low failure rate. Insertion of an IUD immediately after delivery has been recommended by WHO, as one of the safest and most effective method of reversible contraception for postpartum women who wish to either space or limit births, whether they are breastfeeding or not [8].

In Uganda, 25% of total births are less than 2 years apart [5], yet birth spacing is an important maternal and child health intervention [10]. For women with limited access to medical care, the time of delivery offers a unique opportunity to address their need for contraception if the delivery takes place in a healthcare facility. In addition, PPIUD may help avoid the discomfort related to interval insertion since insertion complaints caused by bloody lochia and cramping are masked [11]. Furthermore, effective utilization of family planning could avert approximately 32% of maternal deaths worldwide, by avoiding unintended premature pregnancies and abortions [12]. As previously reported [13], optimal utilization of modern contraceptive methods could result in approximately 85% decline in induced abortions in Uganda. In the immediate post-partum period, women are highly motivated to take up an effective contraception, as opposed to waiting for 6 weeks to initiate effective contraception. On the contrary, if the women are left to wait, they may conceive unintentionally or may not even return for contraception [14]. Appropriate times for IUD insertion in the immediate postpartum period include the postplacental (within 10 min after expulsion of the placenta), the immediate postpartum (within 48 h of delivery) and trans-cesarean IUD insertion (during a cesarean delivery), before the uterine incision is sutured.

An important limiting factor to increased uptake of immediate PPIUD insertion may perhaps be due to its expulsion rates, that range from as low as 5% to as high as 70 [15, 16]. Indeed, there has been skepticism in the recent past about PPIUD among some healthcare professionals with regard to the variable complication and expulsion rates cited in literature [1, 17]. Previous studies have found several factors to be associated with PPIUD expulsion, including: age [18], parity [19], mode of delivery [20] and timing of insertion [21]. There is minimal documentation on expulsion rates and risk factors of PPIUD expulsion in Uganda. In this prospective cohort study, we sought to determine the expulsion rate of PPIUD at 6 weeks postpartum and risk factors for PPIUD expulsion, among women delivering at Mbarara Regional Referral Hospital (MRRH), southwestern Uganda.

## Methods

### Study site and setting

We conducted a prospective cohort study from September 1, 2014 to January 31, 2015 at the maternity ward (labor, postnatal and operating theatre sections) of Mbarara Regional Referral Hospital (MRRH) in southwestern Uganda. The hospital serves as a referral centre for other ten district hospitals within the south-western region. The maternity ward of MRRH records approximately 10,223 total deliveries annually, with an average of 20–25 vaginal deliveries daily and a caesarean section rate of 30%. The hospital also has a family planning clinic which offers contraceptive services to an estimated 993 women annually and about 3% of these women take up interval IUD [22].

### Study population

Our study participants were women who delivered at MRRH (both vaginal and cesarean deliveries) during the 5 months' study period, that fulfilled the inclusion criteria. We included women who met the WHO medical eligibility for PPIUD insertion [8], resided in Mbarara municipality (within 30 km radius), consented to participate in the study, and were willing to return at 6 weeks post IUD insertion for follow up. We excluded women with any of the following medical conditions: altered level of consciousness, post-partum hemorrhage (PPH), temperature > 38 °C during or after labor, pre-labor rupture of membranes > 18 h, obstructed labor, and uterine fibroids or malformations.

### Study procedures and sampling

We employed consecutive sampling technique to recruit eligible participants. We assessed eligibility by checking medical records of all women in early labor and those who had delivered vaginally a night before, to ascertain eligible participants without contraindications to PPIUD insertion, as well as checking the place of residence. We introduced the study to eligible participants through family planning health talks held daily on the maternity ward as part of routine practice.

Each eligible woman received individual counseling session about postpartum contraception where IUD was highlighted together with other options that included: mini-pills, bilateral tubal ligation, implants, lactation amenorrhea method and condoms. This enabled the women to make a voluntary and informed choice. The merits of each method, their common side effects and possible complications were explained comprehensively. Eligible participants were then approached individually to obtain an informed consent. Upon consent, the IUD was inserted within 48 h of delivery. Those who opted for an alternative method were referred to the family planning clinic at MRRH to receive the methods of their choice.

We used the following study instruments: a screening tool, a structured questionnaire and a PPIUD follow up card and form. We used the screening tool to counter check the eligibility of the women and to exclude those with contraindications to PPIUD insertion. We administered a structured questionnaire to capture data on socio-demographic, clinical and obstetric characteristics of the participants, including their data on family planning and gynecological history. The study participants were given health education on how best to recognize expulsions for example through the string length or even vivid expulsion, postpartum warning signs like bright red bleeding for which the woman needed to change her pad more than six times a day, unusual abdominal or pelvic pain (not after-birth pain) and unusual vaginal discharge or pain. The PPIUD follow-up card contained information on the date of insertion and follow up visit, date of removal of the IUD, the telephone number of the principal investigator and one of the research assistants. We used the PPIUD follow-up form to assess the postnatal experiences of the participants and it was filled at the follow-up visit. The follow up form was filled by asking questions and performing clinical examination. A speculum examination was then performed to check if the strings were visible or not and any discharge noted. The visible IUD strings were trimmed at approximately 3-5 cm. Participants whose strings were invisible at the cervical opening (os) and had not reported vivid IUD expulsion were sent for a uterine ultra sound scan to confirm expulsion. We assessed the study participants in whom the PPIUDs were inserted before discharge for comfort and followed them up at 6 weeks for expulsion. We emphasized the need for review at 6 weeks post-insertion. Participants were advised to call or comeback (any time before the set follow-up date) in case of any concern about the method. At 6 weeks, speculum or digital vaginal examination and/or abdominal/pelvic ultra sound scan were used to confirm IUD presence or expulsion. In addition, string shortening was done at the follow up visit.

#### IUD insertion technique

All necessary instruments (CuT380A, sterile ring forceps, Sims speculum, povidone- iodine, kidney dish, head lamp and gauze pieces) were prepared. Infection prevention protocols were observed at all times by use of sterile equipment and the insertion was performed by a trained healthcare professional (midwife or medical doctor) using ring forceps. The IUD was inserted to the uterine fundus as confirmed by palpation with a hand placed on the abdomen overlying the fundus. The cervical os was then gently inspected with the Sims speculum for strings before the participant left the procedure room. To ensure data quality control, all the healthcare professionals involved in IUD insertion had undertaken a training program on PPIUD and interval IUD insertion by Population Services International (PSI) and Marie stopes International (MSI) and were certified competent. In addition, every 10th PPIUD insertion was supervised by a consultant Obstetrician/gynecologist.

#### Study variables

Our primary outcome variable was IUD expulsion by 6 weeks post insertion. The independent variables were: socio-demographic factors (age, marital status, tribe, religion, level of education and occupation), obstetric and gynecologic factors (parity, birth weight of baby, duration of labor, mode of delivery, time lag from delivery to IUD insertion, menstrual flow and history of IUD expulsion), and postnatal factors (severe cramps in puerperium, resumption of sexual intercourse, breastfeeding, excessive vaginal bleeding in puerperium, use of herbs, douching, tummy tying, return of menses and heavy physical activity).

#### Sample size and data analysis

We computed the sample size using the Fleiss formula for unmatched cohort studies, with the following assumptions: power of 80%, percentage of exposed with outcome of 25.9% and percentage of unexposed with outcome of 14.3%, based on the Mexican prospective cohort study where 25.9% of women who were multiparous expelled the PPIUD and 14.3% of primeparas expelled the PPIUD [19]. This gave a total sample size of 170 participants, after inflation for 10% loss to follow-up.

We entered data in EpiData (EpiData, Odende, Denmark) and later exported to Stata (StataCorp, College Station, Texas, USA) for analysis. We described baseline socio-demographic, obstetric, gynecological and clinical characteristics of participants. We determined the expulsion rate as the cumulative incidence by dividing the number of women who had the IUDs expelled by total number of women who came for follow up and expressed as a percentage. To determine the risk factors for expulsion of IUD, we performed univariable and multivariable analysis, using log binomial regression analysis. Our measure of association was risk ratios (RRs). All factors with $p$-value < 0.2 in univariable models were included in the multivariable models through backward stepwise method to determine the adjusted risk factors for PPIUD expulsion. Corresponding adjusted risk ratios (aRRs) and their 95% confidence intervals were reported. Risk factors were considered significant at a $p$-value of < 0.05.

## Results

Of 324 women who received health education, we present results for 167 women who were enrolled into the study. The various reasons for non-participation into the study are depicted in Fig. 1.

### Baseline characteristics of study participants

Of the 167 study participants, most were aged 25–34 years (53.9%), married (91%), housewives (50.9%), had some formal education (94.6%) and were Christian (89.7%) (Table 1).

The majority of the participants were multiparas (84.4%), had delivered vaginally (74.9%) and had live babies (99.3%) with a mean birth weight of 3.3 kg (SD ± 0.6). Seventy-five participants (45.2%) had IUD inserted within 10 min of delivery. Only eleven participants (6.6%) had ever used IUD for family planning and the mean duration of use was 4.0(SD ± 1.9) years.

Postnatal characteristics of the 144 participants who returned for follow-up are presented in Table 2. About half (51.4%) of the study participants had resumed sexual activities by the time of review; 9% of the participants had returned their menses by 6 weeks' post- delivery. Few (12.5%) participants had resumed heavy physical activity by 6 weeks' postpartum. History of herbal medicine use was reported in 15.3% of the study participants.

### Expulsion rate of PPIUD by 6 weeks post-insertion

Among the 144 participants who had PPIUDs inserted, 13 had them expelled by 6 weeks post-insertion, for an expulsion rate of 9% (95%CI:4.9–15%), as seen in Fig. 1. Of the 13 participants who had PPIUD expelled, two (15.4%) had complete expulsion of the IUD within 2 weeks of insertion, while the remaining 11 (84.6%) had their IUDs partially expelled (with IUD stem visualized at the external cervical os on speculum exam) at 6 weeks (Fig. 1).

### Risk factors for PPIUD expulsion

The results for univariable and multivariable analysis for the risk factors for PPIUD expulsion are presented in Table 3. In the multivariable model, the significant risk factors for PPIUD expulsion were: IUD insertion between 11 and 59 min after delivery (aRR 8.11, 95%CI: 1.26–51.98, $p = 0.027$) and duration of bloody lochia flow> 15 days (aRR 8.45, 95%CI: 1.47–48.47, $p = 0.017$).

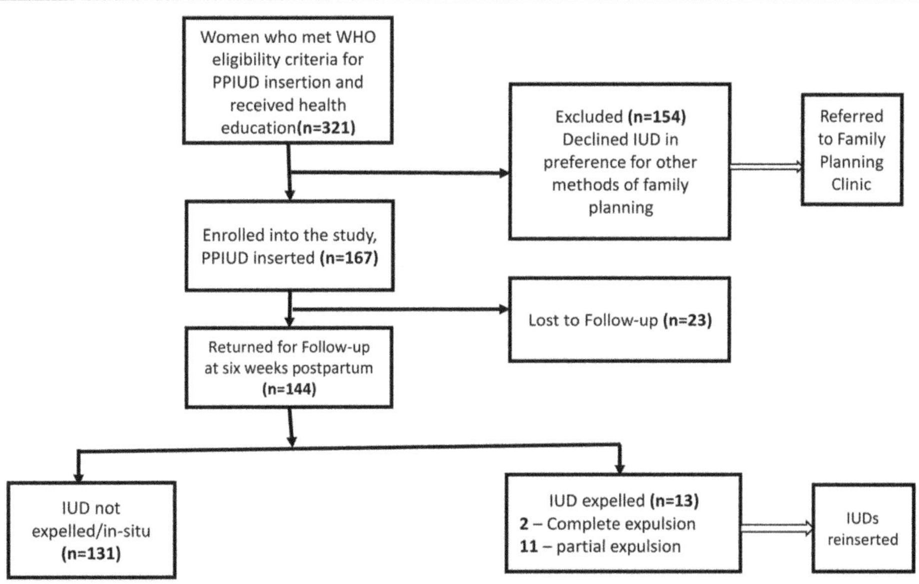


**Fig. 1** Flow diagram showing recruitment, enrollment and Intrauterine device (IUD) status at follow up of study participants

**Table 1** Baseline Socio-demographic and obstetric Characteristics of study participants ($N = 167$)

| Characteristics | Frequency (n) | Percentage (%) |
|---|---|---|
| **Age** | | |
| 18–24 | 44 | 26.3 |
| 25–34 | 90 | 53.9 |
| > =35 | 33 | 19.8 |
| **Education** | | |
| None | 9 | 5.4 |
| Primary | 64 | 38.3 |
| Secondary | 55 | 32.9 |
| Tertiary | 39 | 23.4 |
| **Marital Status** | | |
| Single /Divorced | 15 | 9 |
| Married | 91 | 91 |
| **Parity** | | |
| One | 26 | 15.6 |
| Two | 30 | 18 |
| Three | 34 | 20.4 |
| Four | 18.5 | 18.5 |
| Five & above | 46 | 27.5 |
| **Mode of delivery** | | |
| Vaginal | 125 | 74.9 |
| Caesarean section | 42 | 25.1 |
| **Baby condition at birth** | | |
| Alive | 166 | 99.3 |
| Stillbirth | 1 | 0.7 |
| **Birth weight (Bwt*) in kilograms** | | |
| < 2.5 | 12 | 7.2 |
| 2.5–3.9 | 96 | 57.5 |
| > =4.0 | 59 | 35.3 |
| **Time from delivery to IUD insertion (in minutes)** | | |
| < =10 | 75 | 45.2 |
| 15–59 | 28 | 16.9 |
| > =60 | 63 | 37.9 |
| Median | 20 (IQR,10–285) | |
| **Menstrual flow** | | |
| Heavy | 7 | 4.2 |
| Normal | 157 | 94 |
| Scanty | 3 | 1.8 |
| **Associated cramps** | | |
| Yes | 60 | 35.9 |
| No | 107 | 64.1 |
| **Ever used Intrauterine Device** | | |
| Yes | 11 | 6.6 |
| No | 156 | 93.4 |

*IQR* Inter-quartile range, *IUD* Intra-uterine device; Bwt*: Mean, 3.3 kg (SD ± 0.6).

**Table 2** Postnatal characteristics of study participants ($N = 144$)

| Characteristic | Frequency | Percentage |
|---|---|---|
| **Resumption of sexual activities** | | |
| Yes | 74 | 51.4 |
| No | 70 | 48.6 |
| **Return of menses** | | |
| Yes | 13 | 9 |
| No | 131 | 91 |
| **Tummy tying** | | |
| Yes | 70 | 48.6 |
| No | 74 | 51.4 |
| **Vaginal douching** | | |
| Yes | 18 | 12.5 |
| No | 126 | 87.5 |
| **Use of herbs** | | |
| Yes | 22 | 15.3 |
| No | 122 | 84.7 |
| **Resumption of heavy physical activity** | | |
| Yes | 18 | 12.5 |
| No | 126 | 88.5 |

**Table 3** Risk factors for PPIUD expulsion

| | Unadjusted analysis | Adjusted analysis | |
|---|---|---|---|
| Variable | RR (95% CI) | Adjusted RR (95%CI) | *p*-value |
| **Age in years** | | | |
| 18–24 | 1 | | |
| 25–34 | 1.18 (0.22–6.16) | | |
| ≥ 35 | 2.79 (0.49–15.62) | | |
| **Education Level** | | | |
| None | 1 | | |
| Primary | 0.88 (0.091–8.646) | | |
| Secondary | 1.00 (0.102–9.75) | | |
| Tertiary | 0.44 (0.035–5.522) | | |
| **Birth weight (in kilograms)** | | | |
| < 2.5 | 1 | | |
| 2.5–3.9 | 0.36 (0.35–3.71) | | |
| ≥ 4 | 1.24 (0.13–11.52) | | |
| **Parity** | | | |
| Parity 1 | 1 | | |
| Parity 2 | 2.71 (0.26–28.37) | | |
| Parity3 | 0.65 (0.04–11.11) | | |
| Parity4 | 0.70 (0.04–11.96) | | |
| 5 & above | 4.03 (0.46–35.29) | | |
| **Time from delivery to IUD insertion (in minutes)** | | | |
| ≤ 10 min | 1 | 1 | |
| 11-59 min | 8.95 (1,61–49.81) | **8.11 (1.26–51.98)** | **0.027** |
| ≥ 60 min | 4.86 (0.94–25.19) | 4.78 (0.86–26.43) | 0.070 |
| **Duration of menses in days** | | | |
| ≤ 3 | | | |
| 4 | 1 | | |
| > =5 | 1.23 (0.34–4.49) | | |
| **Past IUD use** | 1.61 (0.35–7.30) | | |
| No | 1 | | |
| Yes | 1.1 (0.13–9.53) | | |
| **Resumption of sex** | | | |
| No | 1 | | |
| Yes | 3.60 (0.95–13.69) | | |
| **Duration of bloody lochia flow in days** | | | |
| 0–7 | 1 | 1 | |
| 8 to 14 | 1.91 (0.48–7.53) | 1.35 (0.33–5.53) | 0.924 |
| ≥ 15 | 7.37 (1.45–37.45) | **8.45 (1.47–48.47)** | **0.017** |

## Discussion

The expulsion rate of 9% observed in our prospective study is consistent with findings from several studies that have reported expulsion rates that range from 5 to 15% [23–27]. A lower expulsion rate of 3.8% than ours was reported in India, probably because the study in India relied on self-report of IUD expulsion, and therefore subjectively determined. In our study we used both clinical exam and sonographic criteria to ascertain IUD expulsion. Higher expulsion rates of 17 and 16% have been reported in USA [28] and Mexico [19] respectively. The possible reason for the higher expulsion rates in these studies than ours, could be because of the longer follow-up time of 3 to 6 months. In our study, we followed up women for only 6 weeks postpartum. Similarly, higher expulsion rates than ours have been observed in studies that used levonorgestrel IUD [17, 29]. The higher expulsion rates of levonorgestrel IUD may possibly be attributed to the use of levonorgestrel-releasing IUD inserter for postplacental insertions, as opposed to our study in which we used ring forceps for IUD insertions, and therefore had higher chances for high fundal placement [30]. To decrease IUD expulsion rates, high fundal placement is recommended [30, 31].

The expulsion rate in the current study is comparable to that observed in interval IUD insertions. This has important implications for family planning uptake and reproductive health in Uganda. Given that Uganda has a high unmet need for family planning [5, 32], there is need to emphasize prenatal counseling for postpartum family planning as this will facilitate postplacental IUD uptake. In addition, the Ministry of Health should consider conducting in-service training of all health personnel who conduct deliveries, in postplacental IUD insertions, so as to ensure 24-h availability of the service providers with skills to insert postplacental IUDs.

In this study, the time lag from delivery to IUD insertion and duration of lochia flow were significantly associated with postpartum IUD expulsion, in agreement with previous findings [15, 21, 28]. We found that women who had IUDs inserted 11–59 min after delivery had a higher risk than those who had the IUDs inserted within 10 min post-delivery. This could be explained by the fact that within 10 min of delivery, the cervix is still fully open, making placement of the IUD high in the uterine fundus much easier compared to insertion at a later time [15]. This finding further underscores the need for routine prenatal counselling of women on post-partum post placental IUD insertions to reduce on expulsion rates associated with late insertions.

Women who experienced bloody lochia flow for 15 or more days had higher risk for IUD expulsion compared to their counterparts who experienced fewer days of bloody lochia flow. This is probably due to the fact that bloody lochia flow is associated with increased uterine contractions, which may be induced by the presence of a foreign body in the uterus [33], and this may lead to IUD expulsion. Although this association is a new finding, these data call for ensuring that women who experience prolonged bloody lochia flow following postpartum IUD insertion, be encouraged to return early for follow up (within 6 weeks), in order to detect any spontaneous expulsion.

## Limitations

Our study has some limitations worth mentioning. First, the main limitation for our study is loss to follow-up. Twenty-three (14%) of the 167 participants were lost to follow-up. Nevertheless, the retention rate was good enough (86%) not to affect the power of the study. In addition, there was no statistically significant difference in the baseline characteristics of participants who were lost to follow-up and those who were retained in the study. Second, our follow-up period of 6 weeks was relatively shorter compared to what is reported in background literature [9]. We recommend further longitudinal studies, with longer follow-up periods for PPIUD expulsions in our setting in Uganda. Finally, we used only CuT380A IUDs in our study because they are the ones recommended for use for PPIUD insertions, by the Ministry of Health in Uganda. Therefore, our findings may not be generalizable beyond the population of women using CuT380A IUDs, such as those using Levonorgestrel IUDs. The major strengths of our study lie in its prospective nature and the fact that we objectively assessed expulsion of PPIUDs using both clinical examinations and ultrasound scan when clinically indicated.

## Conclusion

In conclusion, the cumulative expulsion rate of postpartum IUD among women delivering at MRRH was low and comparable to expulsion rates in interval IUD insertions. Delayed time from delivery to IUD insertion and prolonged duration of bloody lochia flow were the key risk factors for postpartum IUD expulsion during puerperium, among women delivering at MRRH in south-western Uganda. Our findings support routine prenatal counseling for postpartum family planning to allow for post-placental IUD insertions, which are associated with lower expulsion rates.

#### Abbreviations

aRR: Adjusted risk ratio; CI: Confidence interval; FRC: Faculty Research Committee; IQR: Interquartile range; IUD: Intrauterine device; MRRH: Mbarara Regional Referral Hospital; MSI: Marie stopes International; MUST: Mbarara University of Science and Technology; PPH: Postpartum hemorrhage; PPIUD: Postpartum intrauterine device; PSI: Population Services International; REC: Research Ethics Committee; RR: Risk ratio; SD: Standard deviation; WHO: Word Health Organization

#### Acknowledgements

The authors are grateful to the study participants, the staff and management of Mbarara Regional Referral Hospital who provided support during the study period. We are very thankful to our research assistants (Sr.Naiga Patience and Sr. Kibesigire Scondinah). We also acknowledge Dr. Daniel Atwiine and Dr. Ronald Mayanja (R.I.P) for their technical input into the study.

#### Authors' contributions

J.M., M.K., G.M., R.M., and J.N., contributed conception of the study, wrote, reviewed and edited the manuscript. R. M and J. M analyzed the data. G.M., M.K., and J.N. supervised the research. All authors read and approved the final manuscript.

#### Author details

[1]Department of Obstetrics and Gynecology, Mbarara University of Science and Technology, Mbarara, Uganda. [2]Department of Obstetrics and Gynecology, Kampala International University, Kampala, Uganda. [3]Department of Physiology, Mbarara University of Science and Technology, P.O Box 1410, Mbarara, Uganda.

#### References

1. Makins A, Arulkumaran S. Institutionalization of postpartum intrauterine devices. Int J Gynaecol Obstet. 2018;143(Suppl 1):1–3.
2. Darroch JE, Sully E, Biddlecom A. Adding it up: investing in contraception and maternal and newborn health, 2017—supplementary tables. New York: The Guttmacher Institute; 2017.
3. Gribble J, Haffey J. Reproductive health in sub-Saharan Africa. Population Reference Bureau; 2008. p. 8.
4. Clifton D, Kaneda T, Ashford L. Family planning worldwide 2008 data sheet. Washington: Population Reference Bureau; 2008. p. 15.
5. UBOS I. Uganda demographic and health survey 2011. Kampala and Claverton: Uganda Bureau of Statistics and ICF International Inc.; 2012.
6. Pollack A, GP J. Intrauterine devices (IUDs) in developing countries: assessing opportunities for expanding access and use. Assessment prepared for the Hewlett Foundation population Program; 2006.
7. Winner B, Peipert JF, Zhao Q, Buckel C, Madden T, Allsworth JE, et al. Effectiveness of long-acting reversible contraception. N Engl J Med. 2012; 366(21):1998–2007.
8. Organization WH, Health WHOR. Medical eligibility criteria for contraceptive use: World Health Organization; 2010.
9. Grimes DA, Lopez LM, Schulz KF, Van Vliet HA, Stanwood NL. Immediate post-partum insertion of intrauterine devices. Cochrane Database Syst Rev. 2010;5:CD003036.

10. Organization WH. Report of a WHO technical consultation on birth spacing: Geneva, Switzerland 13–15 June 2005: World Health Organization; 2007.
11. Mohamed SA, Kamel MA, Shaaban OM, Salem HT. Acceptability for the use of postpartum intrauterine contraceptive devices: Assiut experience. Med Princ Pract. 2003;12(3):170–5.
12. Arulkumaran S, Hediger V, Manzoor A, May J. Group MHW. In: Saving Women' lives: transforming strategy into action: report of the maternal health working group 2012: Global Health policy summit; 2012.
13. Vlassoff M, Sundaram A, Bankole A, Remez L, Mugisha F. Benefits of meeting the contraceptive needs of Ugandan women. Issues Brief (Alan Guttmacher Institute). 2009;4:1–8.
14. Borda MR, Winfrey W, McKaig C. Return to sexual activity and modern family planning use in the extended postpartum period: an analysis of findings from seventeen countries. Afr J Reprod Health. 2010;14(4):72.
15. Morrison C, Waszak C, Katz K, Diabaté F, Mate E. Clinical outcomes of two early postpartum IUD insertion programs in Africa. Contraception. 1996; 53(1):17–21.
16. Hayes JL, Cwiak C, Goedken P, Zieman M. A pilot clinical trial of ultrasound-guided postplacental insertion of a levonorgestrel intrauterine device. Contraception. 2007;76(4):292–6.
17. Goldthwaite LM, Sheeder J, Hyer J, Tocce K, Teal SB. Postplacental intrauterine device expulsion by 12 weeks: a prospective cohort study. Am J Obstet Gynecol. 2017;217(6):674.e1–8.
18. Shukla M, Sabuhi Qureshi C. Post-placental intrauterine device insertion-a five year experience at a tertiary care Centre in North India. Indian J Med Res. 2012;136(3):432.
19. RosalesaFB, Zamudio MEA, Montero MdLC, Ortiz MEH, Ruiz MÁL. Factors for expulsion of intrauterine device Tcu380A applied immediately postpartum and after a delayed period. Revista médica del Instituto Mexicano del Seguro Social 2005;43(1):5–10.
20. Müller ALL, Ramos JGL, Martins-Costa SH, Dias RSP, Valério EG, Hammes LS, et al. Transvaginal ultrasonographic assessment of the expulsion rate of intrauterine devices inserted in the immediate postpartum period: a pilot study. Contraception. 2005;72(3):192–5.
21. Eroğlu K, Akkuzu G, Vural G, Dilbaz B, Akın A, Taşkın L, et al. Comparison of efficacy and complications of IUD insertion in immediate postplacental/ early postpartum period with interval period: 1 year follow-up. Contraception. 2006;74(5):376–81.
22. MRRH. Mbarara Regional Referral Hospital (MRRH) Annual Report-2012/2013. In: Obstetrics and Gynecology, editor. Mbarara 2014.
23. Colwill AC, Schreiber CA, Sammel MD, Sonalkar S. Six-week retention after postplacental copper intrauterine device placement. Contraception. 2018; 97(3):215–8.
24. Gurney EP, Sonalkar S, McAllister A, Sammel MD, Schreiber CA. Six-month expulsion of postplacental copper intrauterine devices placed after vaginal delivery. Am J Obstet Gynecol. 2018;219(2):183. e1–9.
25. Bhattacharya P, Linyu K, Chakraborty S. Acceptability, Uptake and safety of post-partum intrauterine contraceptive device: a case study. Population Dynamics in Eastern India and Bangladesh: Springer; 2020. p. 105–13.
26. Spagnolo A, Giussani M, Ambruzzi AM, Bianchetti M, Maringhini S, Matteucci MC, et al. Focus on prevention, diagnosis and treatment of hypertension in children and adolescents. Ital J Pediatr. 2013;39(1):20.
27. Çelen Ş, Möröy P, Sucak A, Aktulay A, Danışman N. Clinical outcomes of early postplacental insertion of intrauterine contraceptive devices. Contraception. 2004;69(4):279–82.
28. Jatlaoui TC, Marcus M, Jamieson DJ, Goedken P, Cwiak C. Postplacental intrauterine device insertion at a teaching hospital. Contraception. 2014; 89(6):528–33.
29. Chen BA, Reeves MF, Hayes JL, Hohmann HL, Perriera LK, Creinin MD. Postplacental or delayed insertion of the levonorgestrel intrauterine device after vaginal delivery: a randomized controlled trial. Obstet Gynecol. 2010; 116(5):1079.
30. O'Hanley K, Huber DH. Postpartum IUDs: keys for success. Contraception. 1992;45(4):351–61.
31. Stumpf PG, Lenker RM. Insertion technique, not design, affects expulsion rates of postpartum intrauterine device. Contraception. 1984;30(4):327–30.
32. Statistics UBo ICF. Uganda demographic and health survey 2016: key indicators report. UBOS. In: And Rockville Maryland; 2017.
33. Sheppard BL. Endometrial morphological changes in IUD users: a review. Contraception. 1987;36(1):1–10.

11

# Prevalence of anemia and its associated factors among pregnant women attending antenatal care follow up at Wollega University referral hospital, Western Ethiopia

Gemechu Kejela[1*], Aga Wakgari[2], Tariku Tesfaye[1], Ebisa Turi[1], Moa Adugna[2], Netsanet Alemu[2] and Latera Jebessa[2]

**Abstract**

**Background:** Even if anemia is a worldwide public health problem affecting numerous people in all age groups, particularly the burden of the problem is higher among pregnant women. Anemia is estimated to contribute to more than 115,000 maternal deaths and 591,000 prenatal deaths globally per year. Maternal mortality is the prime health indicator in any society. Therefore, determining the prevalence of anemia and assessing its associated factors among pregnant women might help for the intervention of the problem.

**Objective:** The objective of this study was to determine the prevalence of anemia and its associated factors among pregnant women attending Antenatal Care (ANC) at Wollega University Referral Hospital, Western Ethiopia.

**Methods and materials:** Institution based cross-sectional study was conducted at antenatal care (ANC) departments of Gynecology and Obstetrics, and MCH at Wollega University Referral Hospital from July 15–22, 2019. A systematic random sampling technique was used to select the study unit. The data were collected using questionnaires, physical examination, and laboratory investigation. After collection, the data were entered using Epi Data version 3.1 and analyzed using SPSS version 20 statistical software. Bivariate and multivariate logistic regression analysis was performed to identify predictors of anemia. Finally, the result was presented using text, tables, and charts.

**Results:** The overall prevalence of anemia using a cut off level of hemoglobin < 11 g/dl (< 33% Haematocrit) was 51 (17.8%). Out of all anemic pregnant women, 19 (37.25%) were mildly anemic, 24 (47%) were moderately anemic and 8 (15.68%) were severely anemic. Multivariable logistic regression analysis revealed that Birth interval of less than 2 years (AOR = 2.56 CI [2.84–4.52]), history of malarial attack in the past 12 months (AOR = 2.585 CI [1.181–5.656]) and engaging into daily laborer occupation (AOR = 8.33 CI [2.724–25.497]) showed significant association with maternal anemia.

**Conclusions:** The prevalence of anemia among pregnant women in this study is high. Having a birth interval of < 2 years, having a history of malarial attack in the past 12 months, and being engaged in daily laborer occupation were factors associated with anemia among pregnant women. Thus, contraceptive methods and information to space children, information, and services to prevent malaria and economically empowering women is needed to prevent anemia among pregnant women in the study area.

**Keywords:** Anemia, Pregnant women, Hemoglobin

* Correspondence: gemechukejela86@gmail.com
[1]Department of Public Health, Institute of Health Sciences, Wollega University, Nekemte, Ethiopia

## Background

Anemia is defined as a condition in which there is less than the normal hemoglobin level in the body, which decreases the oxygen-carrying capacity of red blood cells to tissues. World Health Organization (WHO) definitions for anemia differ by age, sex, and pregnancy status as follows: in children 6 months to 5 years, anemia is defined as a Hemoglobin level < 11 g/dl; in children 5–11 years, Hemoglobin < 11.5 g/dl; in adult males, Hemoglobin < 13 g/dl; in non-pregnant women, Hemoglobin < 12 g/dl and in pregnant women Hemoglobin < 11 g/dl [1].

Anemia could be classified as mild, moderate, and severe. The Hemoglobin 10.0 g/dl for each class of anemia in pregnancy is considered mild. The hemoglobin level from 7 to 9.9 g/dl is considered as moderate and if < 7 g/dl, it is considered as severe. Anemia is considered as an indicator of both poor nutrition and health status [2, 3].

Anemia is one of the most widespread public health problems, especially in developing countries. It impairs cognitive development, reduced physical work capacity, and in severe cases increased the risk of mortality particularly during the prenatal period. During pregnancy, approximately 75% of all anemia diagnosed are due to iron deficiency. Furthermore, WHO considers that women in developing countries may be pregnant for as much as one-half of their reproductive lives and therefore are at increased risk of anemia during this time [4]. About 20% of pregnant women suffer from anemia, and most of the cases are iron deficiency, folic acid deficiency, or both. The administration of iron and folic acid to pregnant women is a divisive issue, and the guiding principle regarding this remedy varies among countries [3].

Globally, anemia is the most common complication in pregnancy. The World Health Organization estimates that more than 40% of non-pregnant and over 50% of pregnant women in developing countries are affected. The majority of the cases occur in sub-Saharan Africa and Southeast Asia [5].

Anemia in pregnancy leads to premature births, low birth weight, fetal impairment, and infant deaths. It also reduces the productivity of women. The reduction in women's productivity places an economic burden on families, communities, and societies. Recently, the mental impairment of children who were anemic at the very beginning of their life has been reported. All of those showed the necessity of a special control program for anemia in vulnerable populations [6].

Food-based approaches to increase iron intake through food fortification and dietary diversification are important, sustainable strategies for preventing iron deficiency anemia in the general population. In settings where iron deficiency is not the only cause of anemia, approaches that combine iron interventions with other measures are needed. Strategies should include addressing other causes of anemia and should be built into the primary health care system and existing programs [7, 8].

In Ethiopia, the Federal Ministry of Health has laid out a policy on iron supplementation to all women attending antenatal clinics [9]. As a result, pregnant women attending antenatal clinics are routinely put on iron supplementation in their second through to the third trimester of pregnancy.

Despite all the above efforts, the burden of disease remains high as determined by anemia related to fetal and maternal mortality and morbidity. As a result, knowing the prevalence of anemia and its associated factors in pregnant women is fundamental for the planning and execution of effective interventions by health authorities. So, the main aim of this study was to assess the prevalence of anemia and its associated factors among pregnant women attending the ANC clinic of Wollega University referral hospital and the results of this study will help to put in place policies to effectively investigate and manage anemia in pregnancy and thereafter to reduce the burden of disease.

## Methods and materials

An institution-based quantitative cross-sectional study was carried out from July 15–22/2019 in Nekemte administrative city, at Wollega University Referral Hospital among 286 respondents. Nekemte town is the capital city of the East Wollega zone and it is located at 331 Km to the west of Addis Ababa. Its altitude ranges from 1960 to 2170 above sea level and the total surface area of the town is 5480 Km$^2$. The climatic condition of the town is Woina dega with an annual environmental temperature range of 14–26 degrees Celsius. The total population of the town as 2018 data is 127,380 from which 65,002(51.03%) are males and 62,378 (48.97%) are females. Pregnant women accounts for 4420(3.47%) and non-pregnant women accounts for 23,731 (18.6%). Regarding the health facilities of the town, there are two governmental Hospitals, two governmental Health centers, 21 medium clinics, 26 lower clinics, 12 pharmacies, and 26 drug stores [10].

Wollega University Referral Hospital is a teaching hospital in western Ethiopia serving millions of people. The hospital has different departments, of which the obstetrics and gynecology department is one of the main departments. This department gives ANC, pregnancy-related problem diagnosis and management, delivery, and post-delivery service.

All pregnant women attending ANC service at Wollega University Referral Hospital were the source population and all pregnant women attending ANC Service at Wollega University Referral Hospital who fulfilled the inclusion criteria and available during the data collection period were the study population for this study. All pregnant women who attended antenatal clinics at Wollega University Referral Hospital during the study period were included in the study and seriously ill patients due to other medical conditions, unable to respond, and mentally ill pregnant women were excluded from the study.

### Sample size determination and sampling procedures

The sample size was calculated by using a single population proportion formula ($n = (Z\ \alpha\ /2)^2\ p\ (1\text{-}p)/d^2$), considering the following assumptions;

$Z\alpha/2$ (significance level) at 0.05 = 1.96, d (margin of error) = 5% and P (proportion of anemia) in reproductive age group women in western Ethiopia =21.6% [11]. After adding a 10% nonresponse rate, the final sample size becomes 286. Finally, the study respondents were selected from pregnant women who visited ANC during the study period by using simple random sampling.

### Measurements

In this study, anemia in pregnancy is defined as a hemoglobin level below 11 g/dl during the first and third trimester and 10.5 g/dl during the second trimester of pregnancy. Mild anemia is defined as a hemoglobin level from 10 to 10.9 g/dl., moderate anemia is defined as a hemoglobin level from 7 to 9.9 g/dl, and severe anemia was defined as a hemoglobin level of < 7 g/dl.

### Data collection instruments, procedure, and quality assurance

Data were collected using an interviewer-administered structured questionnaire, physical examination, and laboratory investigation. The questionnaire was prepared from similar studies conducted before and modified based on the local context. It was prepared in English and translated to the local language (Afan Oromo) and then retranslated to English to check its consistency. The questionnaire addressed; socio-demographic factors, obstetric related factors, and anemia related factors. The data was collected by 4 diploma nurses and supervised by two MPH supervisors. Data were collected during an exit interview after they got service. The quality of data was assured through training of data collectors and supervisors for two days, pretesting data collection tools on 5% of the sample, and close supervision of the data collection process.

### Data processing and analysis

Data were coded, entered into Epi data version 3.1, and exported to SPSS version 20.0 for analysis. Descriptive statistics were computed to determine the frequency and percentages. Binary logistic regression was conducted and COR with 95% CI was estimated to select the candidate variables for the final model. Then, variables with a *p*-value of < 0.25 at binary logistic regression were taken into a multivariable logistic regression to control confounding. Hosmer-Lemeshow goodness-of-fit with stepwise (backward elimination) logistic regression was used to test for model fitness, and the exact value was 0.078. AOR with 95% CI was estimated to assess the presence of association at multivariable logistic regression. Finally, variables with a p-value of < 0.05 were considered as statistically significant predictors of maternal anemia.

## Results

### 5.1 Socio-demographic characteristics of the study respondents

A total of 286 pregnant women attending antenatal care were included in the study making a response rate of 100%. About 156(54.5%) of the study participants were found in the age group of 20–30. The majority, 264(92.3%) of the respondents were married and most, 114(39.9%) of them were protestant religious followers, followed by orthodox 107(37.4%), and 102(35.7%) of the respondents attended above the secondary school. Oromo ethnicity was the most widely distributed ethnic group in this study area with a frequency of 244 (85.3%) (Table 1).

### Reproductive characteristics of respondents

All (100%) of respondents had latrine and more than two-third, 202(71%) of respondents were multigravida. The majority, 210 (73.4%) of women with multigravida gave birth within an interval of < 2 years. Around half of the respondents, 120 (42%) were in the second trimester, while 86 (30.1%) of them were in the third trimester. About 177 (61.9%) of them used contraceptive methods previously. Currently, more than-two third, 221 (77.3%), of pregnant women had taken iron supplementation and 63(22%) had a history of previous abortion. Around 32 (11.2%) of the respondents had a parasitic infection and all of them took medication for it. About 3(1%) of the respondents had a history of chronic diseases (Table 2).

### Laboratory findings

The hemoglobin level of pregnant who women attended ANC at Wollega University Referral Hospital was checked. Accordingly, the majority 235 (82.2%) of them had hemoglobin levels above 11 g/dl. The result from the stool examination revealed that about 26 (9.1%) of them were found to be positive for different parasites. About 4(1.4%) of the respondents were found to be positive for malarial parasites. Few, 45 (15.7%) of the respondents had a history of malarial attacks in the past 12 months (Table 3).

**Table 1** Socio- demographic characters of pregnant women attending ANC at WURH, West Ethiopia, 2019

| Variable | Category | Frequency | Percent (%) |
|---|---|---|---|
| **Age** | 20–30 | 156 | 54.5 |
| | 30–40 | 85 | 29.7 |
| | > 40 | 45 | 15.7 |
| **Marital status** | Married | 264 | 92.3 |
| | Single | 6 | 2.1 |
| | Divorced | 7 | 2.4 |
| | Widowed | 7 | 2.4 |
| | Separated | 2 | 0.7 |
| **Religion** | Orthodox | 107 | 37.4 |
| | Protestant | 114 | 39.9 |
| | Muslim | 59 | 20.6 |
| | Catholic | 6 | 2.1 |
| **Occupation** | Housewife | 58 | 20.3 |
| | Employed | 76 | 26.6 |
| | Farmer | 75 | 26.2 |
| | Daily labor | 23 | 8 |
| | Merchant | 54 | 18.9 |
| **Ethnicity** | Oromo | 244 | 85.3 |
| | Amara | 36 | 12.6 |
| | Gurage | 6 | 2.1 |
| **Monthly income (Ethiopian birr)** | < 1000 | 11 | 3.8 |
| | 1000–2000 | 129 | 45.1 |
| | 2000–4000 | 114 | 39.9 |
| | > 4000 | 32 | 11.2 |
| **Educational status** | Uneducated | 59 | 20.6 |
| | Read and write only | 29 | 10.1 |
| | Primary | 36 | 12.6 |
| | Secondary | 60 | 21 |
| | Above secondary | 102 | 35.7 |

**Prevalence and severity of Anemia among respondents**

In this study, the overall prevalence of anemia using a cut off level of hemoglobin < 11 g/dl was 51 (17.8%) (Fig. 1). Out of all anemic pregnant women, about 19 (37.25%) were mildly anemic, 24 (47%) were moderately anemic and 8 (15.68%) were severely anemic (Fig. 2).

**Predicting factors of anemia among pregnant women**

According to bivariate analysis result; age, occupation, birth interval, parasitic infestation during pregnancy, history of malarial attack in the past 12 months, and iron supplementation during pregnancy were significantly associated with maternal anemia.

After controlling the effect of confounding, multivariable logistic regression revealed that birth interval of less than 2 years (AOR = 2.56 CI [2.84–4.52]), history of malarial attack in the past 12 months (AOR = 2.585[1.181–5.656]) and engaging into daily laborer occupation (AOR = 8.33[2.724–25.497]) showed significant association with maternal anemia.

Pregnant women who had a birth interval of less than 2 years were 2.56 times more likely to be anemic compared to those who had birth intervals of greater than or equal to 2 years (AOR = 2.56 CI [2.84–4.52]). In this study, having a history of malarial attack in the past 12 months shows a significant association with maternal anemia. Pregnant women who had a history of malarial attacks in the past 12 months were 2.6 times more likely to be anemic compared to their counterparts (AOR = 2.585[1.181–5.656]). Similarly, engaging in daily laborer occupations shows a significant association with maternal anemia. Pregnant women who engaged in daily laborer occupations were 8.33 times more likely to be anemic compared

**Table 2** Clinical and reproductive history of pregnant women attending ANC at WURH, western Ethiopia, 2019

| Variable | Category | Frequency | Percent (%) |
|---|---|---|---|
| **Gravidity** | Primigravida | 83 | 29 |
| | Multigravida | 203 | 71 |
| **Birth interval** | < 2 years | 210 | 73.4 |
| | ≥ 2 years | 76 | 26.6 |
| **Gestational age** | First trimester | 80 | 28 |
| | Second trimester | 120 | 42 |
| | Third trimester | 86 | 30.1 |
| **Use of contraceptives** | Yes | 177 | 61.9 |
| | No | 109 | 38.1 |
| **Iron supplementation on current pregnancy** | Yes | 221 | 77.3 |
| | No | 65 | 22.7 |
| **Previous history of abortion** | Yes | 62 | 22 |
| | No | 223 | 78 |
| **Parasitic infection** | Yes | 32 | 11.2 |
| | No | 254 | 88.8 |
| **Presence of chronic diseases** | Yes | 3 | 1 |
| | No | 283 | 99 |

to those who engaged in merchant occupation (AOR = 8.33[2.724–25.497]) (Table 4).

## Discussion

This study was conducted with the intention of assessing the prevalence of anemia and identifying its determinants. To describe the prevalence of anemia, WHO criteria to diagnose anemia among pregnant women was used. According to findings from this study the prevalence of anemia among studied pregnant women attending ANC was 51 (17.8%). This finding was found to be comparable with results obtained from studies conducted in Gondar [11], Tikur Ambessa specialized hospital [12], and Benchimaji, Keffa, and Shekka zone public hospitals [13] where the prevalence of anemia was 16.6, 21.3, and 19% respectively. However, this result was lower than the study conducted in Boditti Health center with a prevalence of 60% [14] and Kenya where the prevalence of anemia was 57% [15]. This difference might be due to the study period and the attention given for focused antenatal care and supplementation of iron sulfate throughout the pregnancy. The finding of the current study was higher than the study conducted in Adigrat General Hospital, which was 7.9% [16]. The reason for this discrepancy might be due to differences in methodology including sampling technique among these studies. Also, it may be a result of improvement in health service and the time gap between these studies.

Multivariable logistic regression analysis revealed that Birth interval of less than 2 years, engaging into daily

**Table 3** Laboratory result of pregnant women attending ANC at WURH, Western Ethiopia, 2019

| Variable | Category | Frequency | Percent (%) |
|---|---|---|---|
| **Hemoglobin level** | ≤ 7 | 8 | 2.8 |
| | 8–9.9 | 24 | 8.4 |
| | 10–11 | 19 | 6.6 |
| | > 11 | 235 | 82.2 |
| **Stool examination** | Yes | 26 | 9.1 |
| | No | 260 | 90.9 |
| **Blood film** | Malaria parasite present | 4 | 1.4 |
| | Malaria parasite absent | 282 | 98.6 |
| **Malarial attack within 12 months** | Yes | 45 | 15.7 |
| | No | 241 | 84.3 |

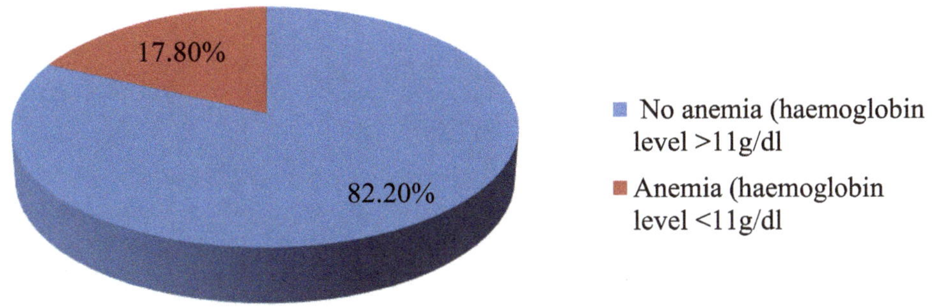


**Fig. 1** Prevalence of anemia among pregnant women attending ANC at WURH, Western Ethiopia, 2019

laborer occupations, and having a history of malarial attacks in the past 12 months showed significant association with maternal anemia.

The prevalence of anemia was seen to be increased with close birth interval. Pregnant women who had close birth intervals (less than 2 years) were 2.56 times more likely to be anemic compared to those who had greater than or equal to 2 years of birth intervals. This finding is consistent with a study conducted in Arba Minch [17], a study conducted in Bangladesh [18], a study conducted in Mogadishu [19], and a study conducted in Walayta Soddo, Otona Hospital [20]. This might be related to decreased iron stores of women due to the occurrences of pregnancy in quick succession between subsequent pregnancies. However, the study done at Trinidad and Tobago indicated a birth interval had no association with the prevalence of anemia [21]. The reason for this might be due to limited cases with a birth interval in the above study as well as due to methodological difference.

Having a history of malarial attacks in the past 12 months revealed to have a significant association with maternal anemia. Accordingly, women who had a history of malarial attacks in the past 12 months were 2.6 times more likely to be anemic as compared to their counterparts. This finding is consistent with a study conducted in Mizan Tepi University Teaching Hospital, in which women who had a history of malarial attacks were eight times more likely to be anemic as compared to those having no malarial attack [9], a study conducted in Walayta Soddo, Otona Hospital [20], a study conducted in Azezo health center of Gondar town [22] and study conducted in public Hospitals of Ilu Aba Bora [23]. This might be due to malaria causes anemia by destroying red blood cells at a rate faster than the body can replace them.

In this study, the prevalence of anemia was Eight times higher in those women who led their lives with daily labor as compared to merchants. This finding is consistent with the study conducted in India [24], a study conducted in eastern Nepal [25], and a study conducted in Arba Minch town, Gamo Gofa zone, Ethiopia [17], and a study conducted in Walayta Soddo, Otona Hospital [20]. This might be due to low income that results in a lack of adequate nutrition and poor personal hygiene which exposes them to parasitic infestations.

## Strength and limitation of the study

### *Strength of the study*

- The diagnosis of anemia was based on laboratory analysis and did not depend on only clinical assessment.

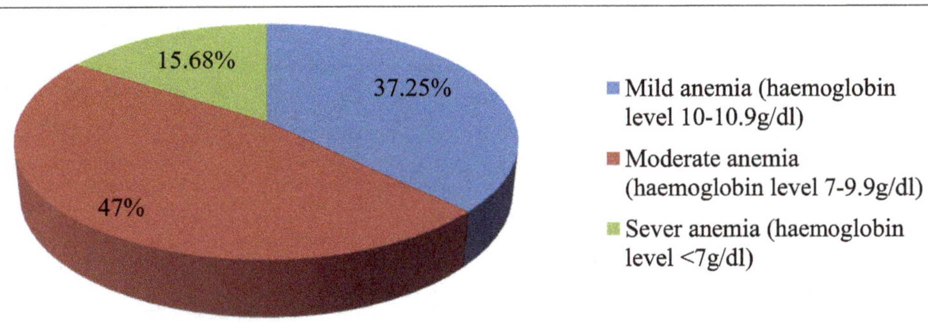


**Fig. 2** Severity of anemia among anemic pregnant women attending ANC at WURH, Western Ethiopia, 2019

**Table 4** Multivariate logistic regression analysis of factors associated with anemia among pregnant women attending ANC at WURH, Western Ethiopia, 2019

| Variable | Category | Anemia | | COR (95%) | AOR (95%) |
|---|---|---|---|---|---|
| | | Yes | No | | |
| **Age** | 20–30 | 26 | 130 | 1 | 1 |
| | 31–40 | 9 | 76 | 0.938 [0.106–8.287] | 2.145 [0.90–3.150] |
| | > 40 | 16 | 29 | 0.201 [0.023–1.736] | 1.660 [0.32–2.880] |
| **Birth interval (in year)** | < 2 | 46 | 164 | 3.98 [1.973–8.724] | 2.56 [2.84–4.52]* |
| | ≥ 2 | 5 | 71 | 1 | 1 |
| **Parasite infection** | Yes | 11 | 21 | 2.8 [0.16–0.797] | 2.211 [0.896–5.461] |
| | No | 40 | 214 | 1 | 1 |
| **Malarial attack in the past 12 months** | Yes | 19 | 26 | 4.77 [1.113–5.656] | 2.585 [1.181–5.656]* |
| | No | 32 | 209 | 1 | 1 |
| **Iron supplementation** | Yes | 28 | 193 | 1 | 1 |
| | No | 23 | 42 | 0.260 [0.17–0.997] | 0.542 [0.251–1.40] |
| **Occupation** | House wife | 8 | 50 | 0.347 [0.551–7.165] | 1.987 [0.551–7.165] |
| | Employed | 4 | 72 | 0.50 [0.569–10.923] | 2.492 [0.569–10.903] |
| | Farmer | 30 | 45 | 4.167 [0.179–3.230] | 0.760 [0.179–3.230] |
| | Daily labor | 5 | 18 | 1.736 [0.039–0.367] | 8.33 [2.724–25.497]* |
| | Merchant | 4 | 50 | 1 | 1 |

Key: * = significant association at *P*-value < 0.05

### *Limitation of the study*

- The Cross-sectional nature of the study limits the cause and effect relationship.
- There may be recall bias while subjects were requested to give information about monthly income.

## Conclusion and recommendations

The overall prevalence of anemia in this study using a cut off level of hemoglobin of < 11 g/dl was 17.8% and the majority of them were moderately anemic (Hb level from 8 to 9.9 g/dl). Less than 2 years of birth interval, having a history of malarial attacks in the past 12 months, and engaging in daily laborer occupation were factors which were significantly associated with maternal anemia.

Based on the result of this study the following recommendations were forwarded.

- Information on the importance of birth spacing and contraceptive service information and service should be provided for pregnant women.
- Concerned stakeholders (health professionals working at hospitals and health centers found in the study area) should work on the prevention of malarial attacks, through giving information about prevention methods and provision of an insecticide-treated bed net, particularly for pregnant women and children.
- Concerned bodies (Government and other stakeholders) should work in collaboration to economically empower women to prevent their engagement in risky works including a daily labor.
- Further research on risk factors of anemia which include micronutrient deficiencies, as well as laboratory studies should be conducted to identify the root cause of underlying problems in the pregnant women to guide the health care provider to alleviate the existing problem.

### Abbreviations

ANC: Antenatal care; AOR: Adjusted odd ratio; AIDS: Acquired immune deficiency syndrome; COR: Crude odd ratio; CI: Confidence interval; G/DL: Gram per deciliter; Hb: Hemoglobin; HIV: Human immunodeficiency virus; MCH: Maternal and child health; NRH: Nekemte Referral Hospital; SPSS: Statistical package for social sciences; WHO: World health organization; WURH: Wollega University Referral Hospital

### Acknowledgments

The authors would like to thank Wollega University, Institute of health sciences for initiating them to conduct this study and financial support. Deep appreciations have gone to the manager of the hospital. Also, special thanks to data collectors, supervisors, study respondents, and all peoples who are involved in the study directly or indirectly.

### Authors' contributions

GK, MA, NA, LJ wrote the proposal, participated in data collection, analyzed the data, and drafted the paper. GK, AW, TT, and ET approved the proposal with great revisions and revised subsequent drafts of the paper. GK, TT, and ET contributed to the designing of the methodology and write-up. All authors read and approved the final manuscript.

**Author details**

[1]Department of Public Health, Institute of Health Sciences, Wollega University, Nekemte, Ethiopia. [2]School of Medicine, Institute of Health Sciences, Wollega University, Nekemte, Ethiopia.

**References**

1. Haidar JA, Pobocik RS. Iron deficiency anemia is not a rare problem among women of reproductive ages in Ethiopia: a community-based cross sectional study. BMC Blood Disord. 2009;8:1–8.
2. Mclean E, Cogswell M, Egli I, Wojdyla D, De BB. Worldwide prevalence of anaemia, WHO Vitamin and Mineral Nutrition Information System, 1993–2005; 2008.
3. Banjari I. Iron deficiency anemia and pregnancy. 2016. https://doi.org/10.5772/intechopen.69114.
4. Kozuma S. Approaches to Anemia in Pregnancy. J Japan Med Assoc. 2009; 137(6):214–218.
5. Tesfaye DJ, Beshir WG, Dejene T, Tewelde T. Prevalence of intestinal Helminthiases and associated factors among pregnant women attending antenatal Clinic of Nigist Eleni Mohammed Memorial Hospital, Hossana; 2015. p. 1–11.
6. Micronutrient deficiencies, iron deficiency anemia. html who 2012. http://www.who.int/nutrition/topics/ida/en/index. Accessed 23 Oct 2019.
7. Cusick SE, Mei Z, Freedman DS, Looker AC, Ogden CL, Gunter E. Unexplained decline in the prevalence of anemia among US children and women between 1988–1994 and 1999–2002 1–3. 2008;(1);1611–7.
8. Gies S, Yassin MA, Cuevas LE. Comparison of screening methods for anaemia in pregnant women in Awassa , Comparison of screening methods for anaemia in pregnant women in Awassa, Ethiopia. 2003; (January 2019).
9. Zekarias B, Meleko A, Hayder A, Nigatu A, Yetagessu T. Prevalence of Anemia and its associated factors among pregnant women attending antenatal care (ANC) in Mizan Tepi University teaching hospital, South West Ethiopia; 2017.
10. Western Oromia, Statistical Agency. Nekemte City office eastern Wollega. Nekemte: Administrative council; 2018.
11. Mulugeta Melku, Zelalem Addis, Meseret Alem,and Bamlaku Enawgaw, Prevalence and predictors of maternal Anemia during pregnancy in Gonder, North west Ethiopia:An institution based cross-sectional study. 2014.
12. Jufar AH, Zewde T. Prevalence of Anemia among Pregnant Women Attending Antenatal Care at Tikur Anbessa Specialized Hospital, Addis Abeba,Ethiopia; 2013.
13. Gudeta TA, Regassa TM, Belay AS. Magnitude and factors associated with anemia among pregnant women attending antenatal care in bench Maji, Keffa and Sheka zones of public hospitals, southwest, Ethiopia, 2018: a cross -sectional study. PLoS One. 2019;14(11):e0225148. https://doi.org/10.1371/journal.pone.0225148.
14. Lelissa D, Yilma M, Shewalem W, Abraha A, Worku M. Prevalence of anemia among women receiving antenatal care at boditii health center, southern Ethiopia. Clin Med Res. 2015;4:79–86.
15. Okube OT, Mirie W, Odhiambo E, Sabina W, Habtu M. Prevalence and factors associated with anaemia among pregnant women attending antenatal clinic in the second and third trimesters at pumwani maternity hospital Kenya. Open J Obstet Gynecol. 2016;6:16–27.
16. Brhane B, Fitsum M, Haftom L, Aderajew G, Guesh G, Kebede T, Getachew K, Hadush N, Gebre A. Prevalence of anemia and associated factors among pregnant women in Adigrat general hospital, Tigrai, northern Ethiopia, 2018. BMC Res Notes. 2019;12:310. https://doi.org/10.1186/s13104-019-4347-4.
17. Alemayehu Bekele, Marelign Tilahun, and Aleme Mekuria: Prevalence of Anemia and its associated factors among pregnant women attending antenatal Care in Health Institutions of Arba Minch town, Gamo Gofa zone, Ethiopia: A Cross-Sectional Study. 2016.
18. Ahmed S, Mamun M, Mahmud N, Farzana N, Sathi M, Biswas B, Datta A, Ahmad T. Prevalence and associated factors of Anemia among pregnant women receiving antenatal care (ANC) at Fatima Hospital in Jashore, Bangladesh: a cross-sectional study. Food Nutr Sci. 2019;10:1056–71. https://doi.org/10.4236/fns.2019.109076.
19. Hassan D, Abdullahi H. Prevalence of Anemia and Its Associated Factors among Pregnant Women Attending Antenatal Clinic at SOS Hospital in Heliwa District, Mogadishu. Adv Soc Sci Res J. 2017;4:15.
20. Lealem G., Asrat A., Yaregal A., Andualem M. Anemia and associated factors among pregnant women attending Antenatal Care Clinic in Wolayita Sodo town, Southern Ethiopia, 2015. Ethiop J Health Sci. Vol. 25, No. 2.
21. Uche-Nwachi EO, Odekunle A, Jacinto S, Burnett M, Clapperton M, David Y, Durga S, Greene K, Jarvis J, Nixon C, Seereeram R, Poon-King C, Singh R. Anaemia in pregnancy: associations with parity, abortions and child spacing in primary healthcare clinic attendees in Trinidad and Tobago. 2010;10(1): 66–70.
22. Meseret A, Bamlaku E, Aschalew G, Tigist K, Mohammed S, Yadessa O. Prevalence of anemia and associated risk factors among pregnant women attending antenatal care in Azezo health center Gondar town, Northwest Ethiopia. J Interdiscipl Histopathol. 2013;1(3):137–44.
23. Adamu K., Efrem N., Lemi B., and Negash W. Magnitude of Anemia and Associated Factors among Pregnant Women Attending Antenatal Care in Public Hospitals of Ilu Abba Bora Zone, South West Ethiopia: A Cross-Sectional Study. Hindawi Anemia Volume 2018, Article ID 9201383, 7 doi: https://doi.org/10.1155/2018/9201383.
24. K Mujibur R., K Mohamed A., S Vijayalakshmi, S Ramkumar, Gulrukh H. Prevalence of Iron Deficiency Anaemia and its Associated Factors among Reproductive Age Women in a Rural Area of Karaikal, Puducherry, India. Journal of Clinical and Diagnostic Research. 2019 Mar, Vol-13(3): LC06-LC10.
25. Maskey M, Jha N, Poudel S, Yadav D. Anemia in pregnancy and its associated factors: a study from eastern Nepal. Nepal J Epidemiol. 2014;4(4): 386–92. https://doi.org/10.3126/nje.v4i4.11358.

# 12

# Why does uptake of family planning services remain sub-optimal among Nigerian women?

Ifeyinwa Chizoba Akamike[1,2*], Ijeoma Nkem Okedo-Alex[1,2], Irene Ifeyinwa Eze[1,2], Obumneme Benaiah Ezeanosike[3] and Chigozie Jesse Uneke[2]

## Abstract

**Background:** Over the years, family planning uptake in Nigeria has remained low and this is as a result of the various challenges and barriers faced by women. The aim of this study was to systematically review studies on family planning services undertaken in Nigeria in order to understand the challenges to uptake of the services and the policy implications.

**Methods:** A PubMed search was performed in June 2020 and studies that investigated challenges of family planning uptake in Nigeria published in English between 2006 and 2020 were sought. A combination of the search terms family planning, contraceptives, challenges, barriers, Nigeria was used. Review articles, case reports, and case studies were excluded. Studies that did not report barriers or challenges to family planning or contraceptives were excluded.

**Result:** Twenty seven studies carried out in Nigeria which provided sufficient information were identified and used for this review. The Uptake of family planning recorded in the reviewed studies ranges from 10.3 to 66.8%. Challenges that are client related include education, desire for more children, uncertainty about its need, partner disapproval, previous side effects, religious beliefs, culture disapproval, age, marital status, and wealth index, residence, ignorance, embarrassment, domestic violence and sexual factor. Health service related factors identified include cost, difficulty accessing services, and procurement difficulties. Recommendations for family planning propram and policy include targeting of health service delivery for improvement, focus on gender issues and male involvement, involvement of religious leaders, targeting of younger women for better education and counseling, and continuous awareness creation and counseling among others.

**Conclusion:** The review has shown that uptake of family planning remains low in Nigeria and challenges abound. We recommend that strategies that are multi-sectoral should be applied to address the multi-pronged challenges facing uptake of family planning services.

**Keywords:** Family planning, Contraception, Challenges, Barriers, Policy implications

* Correspondence: ifeyakamike@gmail.com
[1]Department of Community Medicine, Alex Ekwueme Federal University Teaching Hospital, Abakaliki, Nigeria
[2]African Institute for Health Policy and Health Systems, Ebonyi State University, Abakaliki, Nigeria

## Introduction

Maternal health outcomes in Nigeria have continued to be of great concern. According to the 2018 NDHS, there were 512 maternal deaths per 100,000 live births, which is still high when compared to the developed countries [1]. Family planning is one of the ways through which maternal deaths can be reduced. The interval between pregnancies can be prolonged by providing family planning services for postpartum women and this can help protect their health and that of their newborns [2]. Efforts have been ongoing to ensure that contraceptives are available to women in Nigeria [3, 4] however, uptake is still low with only 12% of women using a modern method of family planning [1]. There is also high unmet need for family planning in Nigeria with about 19% of married women having an unmet need for family planning [1]. This can subsequently lead to high fertility rates and increased population growth in the face of economic instability facing developing countries [5]. Additionally, maternal mortality and morbidity can be unfavourable to economic development.

In Nigeria, there is a high level of knowledge about family planning but most women still do not make use of family planning services [1]. There are still a number of factors that women point at as reasons for not using a method. Challenges to the uptake of family planning services as identified by previous studies include factors such as spousal disapproval, religious beliefs, cultural disapproval, fertility desires and fear of side effects, long distances of sources, poor services of family planning clinics, limited knowledge and skills of providers, workload at the clinic, inconvenience at the family planning clinic, and cost among others [6–9].

It is necessary to identify and compare these studies based on location and the most frequent factors so as to aid in designing interventions that will be most effective for particular settings.

The purpose of this study was to systematically review studies on family planning services undertaken in Nigeria in order to understand the challenges to uptake of the services and the policy implications.

## Methods

The Preferred Reporting Items for Systematic Reviews and Meta-Analysis checklist for reporting a systematic review or meta-analysis protocol was used for this review [10].(See Additional file 1).

### Search strategy

A systematic review of published quantitative and qualitative literature was carried out. A PubMed search was performed in June 2020. Additional search was also carried out in AJOL. Studies that investigated challenges to uptake of family planning services in Nigeria from 2006 to 2020 were sought. Search terms used include Uptake, family planning, family planning services, contraceptives, challenges, barriers, Nigeria.(See Additional file 2).

### Inclusion criteria

Studies were eligible for inclusion if they were carried out in Nigeria and published in English language, published between the years January 2006 and June 2020, measured barriers/challenges to any form of family planning/contraceptive method; and used any quantitative/qualitative study design.

### Exclusion criteria

Review articles, case reports, and case studies were excluded. Also studies that did not report barriers or challenges to family planning or contraceptives were excluded.

The search yielded a total of 385 publications. Citations identified through the search strategy were initially reviewed for inclusion based on information contained in titles, abstracts, citation information, and keywords. Full text articles were obtained for all eligible studies and for those requiring further review to determine eligibility. Those articles that fulfilled the inclusion criteria were critically appraised and included in the review. Figure 1 shows the article selection and inclusion process.

### Data extraction

A data extraction form was developed and used for data extraction. Mendeley reference manager was used to keep track of references. The data extraction form included the following domains: the name of first author and year of publication, study location and setting, study design, contraceptive prevalence rate/uptake, challenges/barriers, and policy implications.

### Quality appraisal

Quality appraisal of the studies included in this review was carried out by two review authors. The Quality Assessment Tool for Observational Cohort and Cross-Sectional Studies was used to assess the quality of the quantitative studies. This quality assessment tool has been used in other systematic reviews [11, 12] (See additional file 3) The tool is made up of 14 questions assessing different aspects of a study including but not limited to definition of objectives, study population, sampling strategy, sample size and statistical analyses. Each question in the tool is scored as Yes (1) or No (0), and others (CD, cannot determine; NA, not applicable and NR, not reported). All the studies included in this review were assessed for quality using the appropriate criteria.

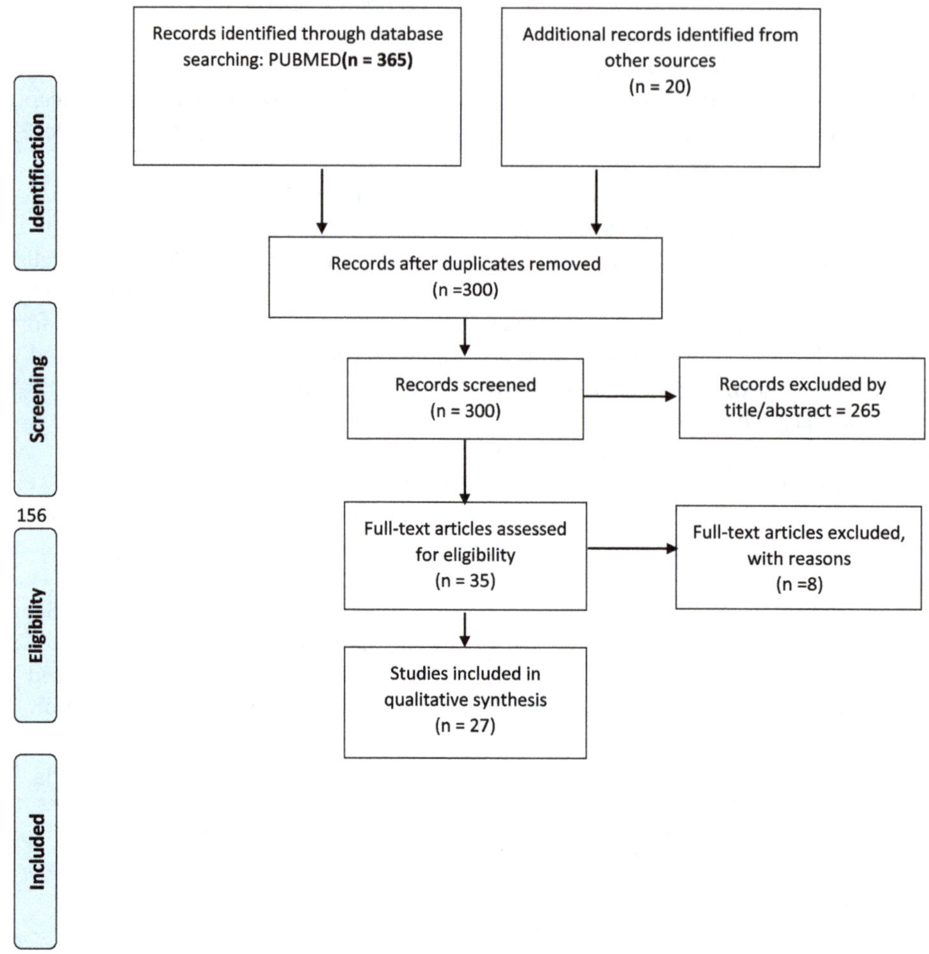


**Fig. 1** Article selection and inclusion process

All the studies fulfilled the quality criteria except that four studies did not describe how sample size was calculated [13–16] and eleven studies did not measure and adjust for the impact of key confounding variables [13–15, 17–24].

The CASP qualitative checklist was used to assess the quality of the qualitative studies [25]. The tool has been used in previous studies [26]. The tool has 10 questions assessing different aspects of a qualitative study including research design, recruitment strategy, data collection method, ethical issues, data analysis, and reporting of findings. Each question has three options which are "Yes", "No", and "Can't tell". All the qualitative studies included in this review fulfilled the CASP criteria. (See additional file 4).

## Result

### Search results

Twenty Seven studies carried out in different states in Nigeria which provided sufficient information were identified and used for this review. Three of the studies were carried out in northern part of the country [21, 27, 28], four were carried out in the Southern part [16, 19, 29, 30], four were carried out in Eastern part [13, 15, 31, 32], seven were carried out in the western part[17, 18, 23, 24, 33–35]while nine studies were carried out in more than one region of the country [14, 20, 22, 36–41]. All the studies reviewed were cross sectional studies, among which were two secondary data analyses [36, 37] and four qualitative studies [27, 28, 40, 41](Table 1).

### Study characteristics

For the purpose of this review, the studies were divided into three categories. The first category consisted of studies that identified only client related challenges to family planning. The second category are studies that identified health service related challenges while the third category identified both client and health service related challenges to uptake of family planning.(Table 1).

Nineteen studies [13, 16–21, 24, 29–31, 33–39, 41] identified only client related factors, seven studies

**Table 1** Summary of all studies

| Author/Year of publication | Type of study | Location of study | Uptake/contraceptive prevalence | Factors/challenges to uptake |
|---|---|---|---|---|
| Oye-Adeniran/2006 [22] | Cross-sectional study | Anambra, Oyo, Kaduna & Bauchi | 22.1% | Client and Health service related |
| Okanlawon/2010 [23] | Cross-sectional | Ogun | 31.6% | Client and Health service related |
| Nwachukwu/2008 [15] | Cross sectional | Imo | 29.7% | Client related and Health service related |
| Umoh/2011 [29] | Cross-sectional | Akwa-Ibom | 52.6% | Client related |
| Idris/2013 [21] | Crosss-sectional | Kaduna | 14% | Client related |
| Asekun-Olarinmoye/2013 [24] | Cross-sectional study | Osun | 13.1% | Client related |
| Eluwa/2016 [20] | Cross-sectional | Anambra, Abia, Delta, Ebonyi, Edo, Enugu | 41% | Client related |
| Ugboaja/2011 [31] | Cross-sectional | Anambra | 44% | Client related |
| Egede/2015 [13] | Cross-sectional | Ebonyi | 28.3% | Client related |
| Adebayo/2016 [35] | Cross-sectional | Ondo | 66.8% | Client related |
| Durowade/2017 [17] | Cross-sectional | Ekiti | 50.5% | Client related |
| Solanke/2017 [37] | Cross-sectional study (secondary data analysis) | Nigeria | 19.8% | Client related |
| Etokidem/2017 [30] | Cross-sectional | Cross-River | 17.2% | Client related |
| Okigbo/2014 [16] | Cross sectional | Cross River | 25.9% (among ART clients), 15.8%(among HCT clients) | Client Related |
| Adebowale 2011 [36] | Cross sectional (Secondary data analysis) | Nigeria | 26% | Client Related |
| Schwandt/2017 [14] | Cross-sectional | Abuja, Benin, Ibadan, Ilorin, Kaduna, Zaria | NA | Health service related |
| Akamike/ 2019 [32] | Quasi-experimental | Ebonyi | 9.9% in intervention arm, 12.8% in control arm | Client and Health Service related |
| Abiodun /2015 [33] | Cross sectional | Ogun | 54.1% (EC) | Client related |
| Adefalu/2019 [27] | Qualitative | Kebbi and Sokoto | NA | Client and Health service related |
| Adeyemi/2016 [34] | Cross sectional | Oyo | 25.4% | Client related |
| Bishwajit/2018 [38] | Secondary data Analysis | Nigeria | 16% | Client Related |
| Chimah/ 2016 [18] | Cross sectional | Lagos | 31.1% | Client related |
| Johnson 2/017[39] | Secondary data analysis | Nigeria | 10.3% | Client related |
| Omo-Aghoja/2009 [19] | Cross sectional | Delta | 29% | Client related |
| Sinai /2019 [28] | Qualitative | Kaduna | NA | Client and health service related |
| Ankomah /2013 [40] | Qualitative | 13 States in Nigeria | NA | Client and Health worker related |
| Aransiola /2014 [41] | Qualitative | Ibadan and Kaduna | NA | Client related |

*EC* Emergency contraception, *ART* Antiretroviral, *HCT* HIV counseling & Testing.

identified client and health service related factors [15, 22, 23, 27, 28, 32, 40] while one study identified only health service related factor [14].

#### *Uptake of family planning services*

Uptake of family planning ranged from 10.3% to 66.8%. Only three studies reported uptake of greater than 50% [17, 29, 35]. (Table 1).

#### Health service related title

**Health service related factors** identified include cost of services in four studies [15, 28, 32, 40], and difficulty accessing services in two studies [14, 23]. Procurement difficulties, long distances of sources, and poor service of family planning clinics were all reported in one study. Prior counseling was reported in one study [22]. Prior counseling was shown to significantly improve the continuation rate of contraception. Health facility dependence on donor organizations for supply of FP materials and women being responsible for purchasing required consumables were also identified as factors that affect uptake of family planning [27]. Stock out and providers adherence to cultural practices were reported in one of the studies [28].(Table 2).

### Client related factors

Challenges that are client related include education, desire for more children, uncertainty about the need for family planning, partner disapproval, previous side effects, religious beliefs, culture disapproval, age, marital status, wealth index, residence, ignorance, shyness, domestic violence and sexual factor. (Table 2).

#### *Misconceptions about side effects*

Twelve studies reported fear of side effects or misperception that family planning is dangerous as reasons for non-use of family planning services [13, 15, 17–19, 22–24, 29, 31, 32, 40].

#### *Education*

Nine studies revealed lower education as a barrier to use of family planning services [17, 20, 22, 29, 34–37, 39].

#### *Number of children*

The desire to have more children was shown to affect use of family planning services. Some studies reported having not completed their family size as a factor [13, 17, 19, 21, 24, 28, 30, 32] while some reported that people with more children were more likely to use a family planning method [20, 24, 37]. Number of male children was also reported in one study to affect uptake of family planning. Having desired number of male children encouraged uptake of family planning [27].

#### *Uncertainty about its need*

Two studies reported uncertainty about the benefits of family planning as a reason for not using a method [29, 30].

#### *Partner disapproval*

Fifteen studies reported spousal/partner disapproval as a barrier to the use of family planning services [13, 15–17, 19, 21, 24, 27–32, 40, 41].

#### *Religious beliefs*

Religious belief was reported in 14 studies as a barrier to uptake of family planning [13, 15, 17, 19, 21, 22, 24, 27, 28, 30–32, 36, 40].

#### *Cultural disapproval*

Cultural and moral disapproval were reported in six studies [15, 17, 19, 30–32].

#### *Influence of relatives/lack of social support*

Influence of relatives was documented as a barrier to uptake of family planning in two studies [27, 40], while poor support of community or lack of social support was reported as a factor that affects uptake of family planning in two studies [28, 40].

#### *Ignorance of family planning/where to access services*

Ignorance about family planning was reported in six studies [15, 17, 18, 24, 27, 32]. Three studies reported lack of awareness of where to access family services as a barrier to use of family planning methods [24, 31, 32].

#### *Sexual factor*

Reduction in sexual enjoyment [30] and promotion of unfaithfulness/infidelity [30, 40] were also documented as barriers to use of family planning methods. Another study reported unexpected timing of sexual intercourse as a barrier to use of contraceptives [18].

#### *Age*

Some of the studies reported age as a factor that affects uptake of family planning services. Three studies found that older women were more likely to use a method of family planning [22, 34, 39], while another study among university students reported that younger women were more likely to use emergency contraceptives [33]. Age at marriage was documented by one study as a factor that affects uptake of family planning. Women who married at an early age were said to be more likely to use contraceptives [27].

#### *Marital status*

Four studies reported that people who were married were likely to use a method of family planning [17, 22, 24, 34]. Two studies reported being single as a barrier to family planning uptake [20, 37]. One study also showed perceived low-risk of getting pregnant or not being sexually active as a barrier to uptake of family planning methods [24].

#### *Wealth index*

Wealth index was reported in two studies [36, 39]. Poorer women were reported to be less likely to use a method of family planning.

#### *Region/residence*

Region was reported as a factor that affects family planning uptake. In two studies, rural residence was a barrier to uptake [36, 39], while in another study, rural residence was a predictor of uptake [33].

**Table 2** Challenges of uptake of family planning services

| Author/Year of publication | Location of study | Factors/challenges to uptake |
|---|---|---|
| Oye-Adeniran/2006 | Anambra, Oyo, Kaduna & Bauchi | **Client related factors**:fear of side effects, religious belief, older age, marital status and education.<br>**Health service related factor:** Prior counseling significantly improved the continuation rate of contraception) |
| Okanlawon/2010 | Ogun | **Health service related**: difficulty in accessing family planning services. **Client related:** misperceptions that contraceptives are dangerous) |
| Umoh/2011 | Akwa-Ibom | **Client related factors**: education, side effect, uncertainty about its need, partner objection |
| Idris/2013 | Kaduna | **Client related factors**: desire for more children, religion, partner disapproval, lack of privacy |
| Asekun-Olarinmoye/2013 | Osun | **Client related factors:**<br>Desire for more children Fear of side effects/complications, ignorance, perceived low-risk of getting pregnant/not sexually active,<br>Religion, Partner disapproval, marital status, number of living children, loss of a child and awareness of place of family planning services |
| Eluwa/2016 | Anambra, Abia, Delta, Ebonyi, Edo, Enugu | **Client related:** lower education, higher number of children, being single |
| Ugboaja/2011 | Anambra | **Client related:**(fear of side effects, not aware of where to access services, husband's disapproval, cultural unacceptability, religious disapproval |
| Egede/2015 | Ebonyi | **Client related factors**: desire for more children, religious prohibition, spousal disapproval, perceived side effects |
| Adebayo/2016 | Ondo | **Client related factors:** education, health condition |
| Durowade/2017 | Ekiti | **Client related factors:** desire for more children, partner disapproval, fear of side-effects, culture, ignorance, marital status, educational level and religion. |
| Schwandt/2017 | Abuja, Benin, Ibadan, Ilorin, Kaduna, Zaria | **Health service related factors:** Restriction of access due to age, parity, marital status |
| Solanke | Nigeria | **Client factors**: lower education, higher number of living children, being single |
| Etokidem/2017 | Cross-River | **Client related factors:** religious beliefs, cultural barrier desire for more children, partner disapproval, family<br>planning does not work, it reduces sexual enjoyment, it<br>promotes unfaithfulness/infidelity |
| Okigbo, 2014 | Cross River | **Client Related:** Partner opposition |
| Adebowale 2011 | Nigeria | **Client Related:** Education, wealth index, region, religion, completed fertility, |
| Nwachukwu 2008 | Imo | **Client related:**<br>fear of the unknown<br>effects, spouse's disapproval, religious belief, cultural disapproval, shyness, moral disapproval, ignorance.<br>**Health service related**: cost, procurement<br>difficulties, long distances of sources, and<br>poor service of Family Planning Clinics |
| Akamike 2019 | Ebonyi | **Client related:**<br>Desire for more children, fear of side effects, partner opposition, religious opposition, ignorance, cultural unacceptability, unaware of where to access services<br>**Health service related:** cost |
| Abiodun 2015 | Ogun | **Client related:**<br>Age<br>Region/Residence |
| Adeyemi 2016 | Oyo | **Client Related:** younger age group, less educated, singles, |
| Bishwajit 2018 | Nigeria | **Client related:** Domestic violence |
| Chimah 2016 | Lagos | **Client Related:** Lack of fund, Too embarrassed to source for it, fear of side effects, fear of adult disapproval, Ignorance, Unexpected timing of sexual intercourse |
| Johnson 2017 | Nigeria | **Client related:** Education, wealth quintile, age, residence |
| Omo-Aghoja 2009 | Delta | **Client related:** Fear of side effects, lack of knowledge, spousal disapproval, culture, Religion, Desire for more children |
| Adefalu 2019 | Kebbi and Sokoto | **Client related:** Influence of relatives, Religion, Ignorance, Number of male children, Age at marriage, Educational attainment, spousal rejection of family planning. |

**Table 2** Challenges of uptake of family planning services *(Continued)*

| Author/Year of publication | Location of study | Factors/challenges to uptake |
|---|---|---|
| | | **Health service related**: health facility dependence on donor organizations for supply of FP materials, women seeking to accept contraceptive are responsible for purchasing required consumables |
| Sinai 2019 | Kaduna | **Client related**: Religion, Desire for more children, poor community support, partner disapproval<br>**Health service related:** Cost, Stockout, providers adhering to cultural practices |
| Ankomah 2013 | 13 States in Nigeria | **Client related**<br>Fear of side effects, causes promiscuity, religion, lack of social support, lack of family support, lack of husband's support<br>**Health service related:** Cost |
| Aransiola 2014 | Ibadan and Kaduna | **Client related**: Lack of partner support |

***Domestic violence***

One study reported an association between domestic violence and use of contraceptives [38].

***Embarrassment***

Two studies reported that respondents did not use a method of contraception because they felt embarrassed to go for it [15, 18].

**Implications for family planning program and policy**

A number of recommendations for improving uptake of family planning services were highlighted in the included studies.. (Table 3) These include:

1. Awareness creation through training [22], education [15, 23], institution of community based behavioural change communication program [24], and targeted campaign for counseling [13, 29, 31]
2. Programs targeting service delivery such as improving quality of maternal health services [21], and scaling up services [20]. One study recommended that more primary health centers, with strong family planning facilities should be made available in the rural areas [15]. It was also recommended that Policies that allow larger pool of providers to be available in all channels, such as task shifting should be positioned to address the problem of inadequate manpower plaguing the public health system in the Northern part of the country and the power of social networks in influencing reproductive health should also be explored [27].
3. Engagement of religious leaders. One Study recommended that religious leaders should be targeted for more education on the benefits of Modern Birth Control Method use [15].
4. Programmes targeting gender issues, male involvement and culture: One of the studies recommended that programs/policies that consider gender and cultural influence on family planning service utilization and method uptake should be modified. There is also a need to increase the self-efficacy of the clients towards contraceptive use and spousal communication about family planning in general [16, 30]. Some of the studies recommended that the influence of the male partner should also be considered, and more male friendly services should be incorporated into the practice of family planning [17, 32, 34, 41].It was also recommended in one study that policy makers place special emphasis on developing strategies to protect women from any form of perpetration of domestic violence and to integrate gender issues to matters that concern women's reproductive health [38]
5. Increased political and financial buy-in, especially at the state and local government levels was also recommended in one study [27]. One of the studies recommended that family planning interventions should concentrate on the benefits of family planning at the family level and not at the state or national level [40].
6. Programmes targeted at younger women/youths: Two studies recommended that efforts should be intensified to improve knowledge about contraceptives and to promote safe sexual practice including effective contraceptive use among young people in secondary schools and tertiary institutions [18, 33].

## Discussion

The review has shown the uptake of family planning services and the challenges and barriers associated with poor uptake of services. Scaling up of family planning services has been a major challenge to reproductive health service providers in Nigeria. The country's contraceptive prevalence rate (CPR) is still low at 17% [1]. Both health service and consumer factors have contributed in keeping the CPR low resulting in a huge unmet need for family planning and consequently, high unintended pregnancy rate [42]. The Uptake of family planning recorded in the reviewed studies ranges from 10.3 to 66.8%. Only three of the studies reviewed

**Table 3** Policy implications

| Author/Year | Policy implications |
|---|---|
| **Oye-Adeniran/2006** | Health-care providers should be trained to offer counseling services to all clients in general, and young, unmarried and uneducated women in particular in order to improve their acceptance of contraceptives. |
| **Okanlawon/2010** | Findings may aid in development of targeted interventions to educate refugee youths in order to dispel misconceptions about the safety of contraceptives and ensure adequate access to family planning services |
| **Umoh/2011** | There's need to tackle known obstacles to contraceptive uptake. Also targeted campaign and every available opportunity should be used to provide reproductive counselling to women especially on contraception |
| **Idris/2013** | It is recommended that while there is need to raise awareness on the utilisation of maternal health services, bring it closer to the mothers and make it more affordable, there is a more pressing need to improve its quality, especially through the alleviation of negative attitude of health care providers. |
| **Asekun-Olarinmoye/ 2013** | It is recommended that a community-based behavioral-change communication program be instituted, aimed at improving the awareness and perceptions of women with respect to desire for more children, at bridging the knowledge gaps about contraceptive methods, and at changing the deep-seated negative beliefs related to contraceptive use in Nigeria |
| **Eluwa/2016** | Scale-up of postpartum IUD services is a promising approach to increasing uptake of long-acting reversible contraceptives among women in Nigeria. |
| **Ugboaja/2011** | The use of more reliable methods should be encouraged through sensitization campaigns |
| **Egede/2015** | More education and campaigning is still needed to improve the presently low prevalence and utilization of contraception |
| **Adebayo/2016** | Concerted effort at increasing uptake is advocated to bridge the gap between client counselling and uptake. |
| **Durowade/2017** | The campaigns for family planning services should aim at the misconceptions in order to drive the demand and remove the barriers. The influence of the male partner should also be considered, and more male friendly services should be incorporated into the practice of family planning |
| **Schwandt/2017** | A constellation of creative interventions aimed at reducing, and eventually eliminating provider imposed restrictions to family planning use in Urban Nigeria are needed urgently to make family planning truly accessible |
| **Solanke** | The scope, content, and coverage of existing BCC messages should be extended to cover the contraceptive needs and challenges of women of advanced reproductive age in the country. |
| **Etokidem/2017** | The findings of this study suggest that family planning uptake would increase if couples make joint decision in this regard. There is also a need to ensure a change of behavior and attitude. |
| **Okigbo, 2014** | There is need to modify existing programs or to develop new programs/policies that consider gender and cultural influence on family planning service utilization and method uptake. There is a need to increase the self-efficacy of the clients towards contraceptive use and spousal communication about family planning in general |
| **Adebowale 2011** | Understanding the mechanisms that underline the relationships between contraceptive use and demographic characteristics are crucial in designing effective public policies aimed at improving maternal health. |
| **Nwachukwu 2008** | Governments and NGOs should provide more educational opportunities in the rural areas for the purpose of teaching birth control methods. More primary health centers, with strong family planning facilities should be made available in the rural areas. It is also necessary for religious leaders to be targeted for more education on the benefits of Modern Birth Control Method use. |
| **Akamike 2019** | Community-based interventions such as training of community resource persons particularly men is of great importance in improving uptake of health services |
| **Abiodun 2015** | There is a need for targeted health education campaign to promote consistent and proper condom use among young people. It is important that programmes and policies should be engendered to improve the knowledge of university students and address misconception about EC. There is also a need to deliberately engage health workers in the promotion of EC and in making the commodities readily accessible to university students and young people in general |
| **Adeyemi 2016** | There needs to be a conscious effort to educate women about contraception and encourage its use. Reproductive health programs and policies should adequately involve male partners/men. Researchers should seek to explore all avenues to make contraception a "couple thing" from inception |
| **Bishwajit 2018** | It is recommended that policy makers place special emphasis on developing strategies to protect women from any form of perpetration and to integrate gender issues to matters that concern women's reproductive health |
| **Chimah 2016** | Efforts should be intensified to promote safe sexual practice including effective contraceptive use among secondary school students. |
| **Johnson 2017** | Measures should be taken to improve female literacy and employment |

**Table 3** Policy implications *(Continued)*

| Author/Year | Policy implications |
|---|---|
| **Omo-Aghoja 2009** | Effective educational and counseling interventions are likely to improve knowledge and uptake |
| **Adefalu 2019** | Increased political and financial buy-in, especially at the state and local government levels, needs to be developed. Policies that allow larger pool of providers to be available in all channels, such as task shifting should be positioned to address the problem of inadequate manpower plaguing the public health system in the North.The power of social networks in influencing reproductive health, may serve as an effective route of effecting FP behavioral change. |
| **Sinai 2019** | Programmatic interventions at home, in the community and at the facility should capitalise on the changing cognitive and emotional ideation to increase demand for contraception and address barriers to contraceptive uptake |
| **Ankomah 2013** | Family planning interventions should concentrate on the benefits of family planning at the family level and not at the state or national level |
| **Aransiola 2014** | To significantly improve family planning adoption rates among urban slum dwellers in Nigeria, there is the need to specifically and specially target men alongside their female partners as well as other stakeholders who have significant influences at family and community level |

*IUD* Intrauterine device, *BCC* Behavioural change communication, *EC* Education Campaign

recorded an uptake of 50% or more. This is still poor and calls for targeted strategies to improve uptake.

Several challenges and barriers to uptake were reported by the studies included in this review. Both client and health service related factors were identified. Health service related factors identified include cost, prior counselling and difficulty accessing services. Others include procurement difficulties, long distances of sources, and poor service of Family Planning Clinics. Prior counseling was shown to significantly improve the continuation rate of contraception. A similar systematic review to determine the barriers of family planning and contraception services in sub-Saharan Africa identified similar challenges [7].

The issue of cost of family planning methods is an important challenge that must be addressed to improve the uptake of family planning services. Also, access to family planning services is another factor affecting uptake of services that was identified in this review. Ensuring access to and availability and affordability of good-quality methods of contraception is a major determinant for achieving universal access to sexual and reproductive health [43]. The findings of this review about the factors influencing uptake of family planning services offer some guidance for health planners about strategies that should be prioritized. The health service factors such as cost, and poor access to health services highlight the need for planners to implement strategies that reduce these access barriers. It is recommended that there is need to raise awareness about maternal health services, bring it closer to the mothers and make it more affordable.

The client factors identified such as misconceptions, fear of side effects, low education, uncertainty about its need, and ignorance of family planning and its sources shows the need for provision of information about family planning methods. Strategies to ensure that clients are supplied with necessary information about the different methods, and their potential side effects are important to improve uptake of family planning services [13, 29, 31]. Religious belief was identified by some of the studies as one of the challenges to uptake of family planning services. Program planners should develop strategies that target religious groups through engaging the religious leaders, this will go a long way in overcoming this barrier [15]. Partner disapproval was also pointed out by some of the studies. Strategies that target the men should be adopted by program implementers since men are the major decision makers in the African culture and specifically in Nigeria. It is also important to encourage spousal communication and joint decision making on health matters [16, 30]. This will contribute in addressing the challenges to use of family planning services. In addition, male friendly services should be included as part of family planning services [17].

A number of studies highlighted culture as a challenge to uptake of family planning services. This explains why most studies reported desire for more children as a challenge to family planning use. African women are considered responsible for increasing the family size and failure to do so attracts negative judgment from the society. In Africa, family planning is viewed as a means of restricting growth and economic productivity. Interventions in sub-Saharan Africa and in Nigeria specifically must consider the complex cultural and social norms of each group of individuals so as to identify strategies that will fit into each situation. Community attitude towards modern family planning is an important factor that may influence adoption of family planning by married women. Social and community support of family planning may help to promote adoption of family planning. Therefore, traditional rulers can be targeted to serve as advocates to address these deep seated beliefs.

Study limitation includes the use of few databases for search. However, this review draws its strength from the fact that it focused on a particular context and will therefore be of benefit for policy making in the specific regions.

## Conclusion

Challenges that were identified include lower education, desire for more children, side effect, uncertainty about its need, partner disapproval, previous side effects, religious beliefs, cost of services, and difficulty accessing services. A multi-sectoral approach including the traditional leaders, religious leaders, education sector, reproductive health professionals, and women affairs department among others is needed to address the multi pronged challenges facing uptake of family planning services.

### Abbreviations

EC: Emergency contraception; ART: Antiretroviral; HCT: HIV counseling & Testing; CPR: Contraceptive Prevalence Rate


### Acknowledgements

Not applicable.


### Authors' contributions

ICA: conceptualisation and study design, data extraction, analysis and interpretation of results, manuscript drafting and approval of the final manuscript for publication. INO: study design, data extraction, interpretation of results, manuscript drafting and approval of the final manuscript for publication. IIE: study design, data extraction, manuscript drafting and approval of the final manuscript for publication. OBE: study design, data extraction, manuscript drafting and approval of the final manuscript for publication. CJU: study design, analysis and interpretation of results, manuscript drafting and approval of the final manuscript for publication.


### Author details

[1]Department of Community Medicine, Alex Ekwueme Federal University Teaching Hospital, Abakaliki, Nigeria. [2]African Institute for Health Policy and Health Systems, Ebonyi State University, Abakaliki, Nigeria. [3]Department of Paediatrics, Alex Ekwueme Federal University Teaching Hospital, Abakaliki, Nigeria.


### References


1. National Population Commission. Nigerian Demographic And Health Survey 2018. 2018.
2. OlaOlorun F, Tsui A. Advancing family planning research in Africa. Afr J Reprod Health. 2014;14(4 0 0):9–12.
3. Every woman Every Child. Family Planning 2020 – Every Woman Every Child.2017. Available from: http://www.everywomaneverychild.org/commitment/family-planning-2020/. Accessed December 2019.
4. Muhammad Ali Pate. Family Planning 2020 Commitment. 2017. Available from: http://ec2-54-210-230-186.compute-1.amazonaws.com/wp-content/uploads/2016/10/Govt.-of-Nigeria-FP2020-Commitment-2012.pdf. Accessed December 2019.
5. Olise P. Primary Health Care for Sustainable Development. 2nd ed. Abuja: Ozege Publications; 2012. p. 207–9.
6. Decker M, Constantine NA. Factors associated with contraceptive use in Angola. Afr J Reprod Health. 2011;15(4):68–77.
7. Haider TL, Sharma M. Barriers to family planning and contraception uptake in sub-Saharan Africa: a systematic review. Int Q Community Health Educ. 2012;33(4):403–13.
8. Aryeetey R, Kotoh AM, Hindin MJ. Knowledge, perceptions and ever use of modern contraception among women in the Ga East District, Ghana. Afr J Reprod Health. 2010;14(4 Spec):26–31.
9. Teye JK. Modern contraceptive use among women in the Asuogyaman district of Ghana: is reliability more important than health concerns? Afr J Reprod Health. 2013;17(2):58–71.
10. Shamseer L, Moher D, Clarke M, Ghersi D, Liberati A, Petticrew M, et al. Preferred reporting items for systematic review and meta-analysis protocols (PRISMA-P) 2015: elaboration and explanation. BMJ. 2015;349(jan032):g7647.
11. Njagi P, Arsenijevic J, Groot W. Understanding variations in catastrophic health expenditure , its underlying determinants and impoverishment in Sub- Saharan African countries : a scoping review. Syst Rev. 2018;7:136.
12. Okedo-Alex IN, Akamike IC, Ezeanosike OB, Uneke CJ. Determinants of antenatal care utilisation in sub-Saharan Africa: a systematic review. BMJ Open. 2019;9:e031890.
13. Egede JO, Onoh RC, Umeora OUJ, Iyoke CA, Dimejesi IBO, Lawani LO. Contraceptive prevalence and preference in a cohort of south-east Nigerian women. Patient Prefer Adherence. 2015;9:707–14.
14. Schwandt HM, Speizer IS, Corroon M. Contraceptive service provider imposed restrictions to contraceptive access in urban Nigeria; 2017. p. 1–9.
15. Nwachukwu I, Obasi OO. Use of modern birth control methods among rural communities in Imo state, Nigeria. Afr J Reprod Health. 2008;12(1):101–8.
16. Okigbo CC, Mccarraher DR, Chen M, Gwarzo U, Chabikuli O. Partner Opposition and Contraceptive Use Unmet Need for Contraception among Clients of FP / HIV Integrated Services in Nigeria : The Role of Partner Opposition . 2014;18(June):134–143.
17. Durowade KA, Omokanye LO, Elegbede OE, Olomofe CO, Ajiboye AD, Makinde A, et al. Barriers to contraceptive Uptake among women of reproductive age in a semi-Urban Community of Ekiti state , Southwest Nigeria.
18. Chimah UC, Lawoyin TO, Ilika AL, Nnebue CC. Contraceptive knowledge and practice among senior secondary schools students in military barracks in Nigeria. Niger J Clin Pract. 2016;19:182–8.
19. Omo-aghoja L, Omo-aghoja V, Aghoja C, Okonofua F, Aghedo O, Umueri C, et al. Factors associated with the knowledge, practice and perceptions of contraception in rural southern Nigeria. Ghana Med J. 2009;43(3):115–21.
20. Eluwa GI, Atamewalen R, Odogwu K, Ahonsi B. Success Providing Postpartum Intrauterine Devices in Private-Sector Health Care Facilities in Nigeria: Factors Associated With Uptake. Glob Heal Sci Pract [Internet]. 2016; 4(2):276–83 Available from: http://www.ncbi.nlm.nih.gov/pubmed/27353620, [cited 2017 Dec 19].
21. Idris S, Sambo M, Ibrahim M. Barriers to utilisation of maternal health services in a semi-urban community in northern Nigeria: The clients' perspective. Niger Med J [Internet]. 2013;54(1):27 Available from: http://www.ncbi.nlm.nih.gov/pubmed/23661896, [cited 2017 Dec 19].
22. Oye-Adeniran BA, Adewole IF, Umoh A, Oladokun A, Gbadegesin A, Ekanem EE, et al. Community-based study of contraceptive behaviour in Nigeria. Afr J Reprod Health. 2006;10(2):90–104.
23. Okanlawon K, Reeves M, Agbaje OF. Contraceptive use: knowledge, perceptions and attitudes of refugee youths in Oru refugee camp, Nigeria. Afr J Reprod Health [Internet]. 2010;14(4 spec):16–25 Available from: http://www.ncbi.nlm.nih.gov/pubmed/21812194, [cited 2017 Dec 19].
24. Asekun-Olarinmoye EO, Adebimpe W, Bamidele J, Odu O, Asekun-Olarinmoye I, Ojofeitimi EO. Barriers to use of modern contraceptives among women in an inner city area of Osogbo metropolis , Osun State Nigeria. Int J Women's Health. 2013:647–55.
25. Critical Appraisal Skills Programme. CASP qualitative checklist. 2018; Available from: https://casp-uk.net/wp-content/uploads/2018/01/CASP-Qualitative-Checklist-2018.pdf. ACcessed June 2020.
26. Makanjuola T, Taddese HB, Booth A. Factors associated with adherence to treatment with isoniazid for the prevention of tuberculosis amongst people living with HIV/AIDS: a systematic review of qualitative data. PLoS One [Internet]. 2014;9(2):e87166 Available from: http://www.ncbi.nlm.nih.gov/pubmed/24498298, [cited 2016 Nov 1].
27. Adefalu AA, Ladipo OA, Akinyemi OO, Popoola OA, Latunji OO, Iyanda O. Qualitative exploration of factors affecting uptake and demand for contraception and other family planning services in north-West Nigeria. Afr J Reprod Health. 2019;23(4):63–74.
28. Sinai I, Omoluabi E, Jimoh A, Jurczynska K. Unmet need for family planning and barriers to contraceptive use in Kaduna, Nigeria: culture, myths and perceptions. Cult Heal Sex [Internet]. 2019; Available from: https://doi.org/10.1080/13691058.2019.1672894.
29. Umoh AV, Abah MG. Contraception awareness and practice among antenatal attendees in Uyo, Nigeria. Pan Afr Med J [Internet]. 2011;10:53 Available from: http://www.ncbi.nlm.nih.gov/pubmed/22384299, [cited 2017 Dec 19].
30. Etokidem AJ, Ndifon W, Etowa J, Asuquo EF. Family planning practices of rural community dwellers in Cross River state, Nigeria. Niger J Clin Pract. 2017:707–15.

31. Ugboaja JO, Nwosu BO, Ifeadike CO, Nnebue CC, Obi-Nwosu AI. Contraceptive choices and practices among urban women in southeastern Nigeria. Niger J Med. 2011;20(3):360–5 Available from: http://www.ncbi.nlm.nih.gov/pubmed/21970219.
32. Akamike IC, Mbachu C, Onwasigwe C, Okedo-Alex I, Eze I, Eze N. Role of community resource persons in improving use of modern family planning methods among women of reproductive age in a rural area in Ebonyi state, Nigeria. Int J Health Plann Manag. 2019:1–10.
33. Abiodun O. Use of emergency contraception in Nigeria: an exploration of related factors among sexually active female university students. Sex Reprod Health. 2015; Available from: https://doi.org/10.1016/j.srhc.2015.10.004. Accessed June 2020.
34. Adeyemi A, Olugbenga-Bello AI, Adeoye O, Salawu M, Aderinoye A, Agbaje M. Contraceptive prevalence and determinants among women of reproductive age group in Ogbomoso, Oyo state, Nigeria. Open Access J Contracept. 2016;7:33–41.
35. Adebayo AM, Ojo TO, Omotoso BA, Ayodeji OO. Family planning services in a tertiary hospital in a semi-urban area of South-Western Nigeria: Uptake and determinants of contraceptive use. J Obstet Gynaecol (Lahore). 2016; 36(7):904–8.
36. Adebowale SA, Fagbamigbe FA, Bamgboye EA. Contraceptive use: implication for completed fertility, parity progression and maternal nutritional status in Nigeria. Afr J Reprod Health. 2011;15(4):60–7.
37. Solanke BL. Factors influencing contraceptive use and non-use among women of advanced reproductive age in Nigeria. J Health Popul Nutr. 2017: 1–14 Available from: https://doi.org/10.1186/s41043-016-0077-6.
38. Bishwajit G, Yaya S. Domestic violence: a hidden barrier to contraceptive use among women in Nigeria. Open Access J Contracept. 2018;9:21–8.
39. Johnson OE. Determinants of modern contraceptive uptake among Nigerian women: evidence from the national demographic and health survey. Afr J Reprod Health. 2017;21(3):89–95.
40. Ankomah A, Anyanti J, Adebayo S, Giwa A. Barriers to Contraceptive Use among Married Young Adults in Nigeria : A Qualitative Study 2013;3(July 2010):267–282.
41. Aransiola JO, Akinyemi AI, Fatusi AO. Women's perceptions and reflections of male partners and couple dynamics in family planning adoption in selected urban slums in Nigeria: a qualitative exploration. BMC Public Health. 2014;14(1):869 Available from: http://www.ncbi.nlm.nih.gov/pubmed/25148699.
42. World Health Organisation. High rates of unintended pregnancies linked to gaps in family planning services: New WHO study 2019. Available from: https://www.who.int/news-room/detail/. Accessed June 2020.
43. Mbizvo MT, Phil D, Phillips SJ. Best Practice & Research Clinical Obstetrics and Gynaecology family planning : choices and challenges for developing countries. Best Pract Res Clin Obstet Gynaecol. 2014;28(6):931–43 Available from: http://dx.doi.org/10.1016/j.bpobgyn.2014.04.014.

# 13

# Effectiveness of a mobile phone application to increase access to sexual and reproductive health information, goods and services among university students in Uganda

Elly Nuwamanya[1,2*], Robinah Nalwanga[1], Afra Nuwasiima[1], Janet U. Babigumira[1], Francis T. Asiimwe[1], Joseph B. Babigumira[3] and Vitalis P. Ngambouk[2]

**Abstract**

**Background:** University students are one of the most vulnerable groups to sexual reproductive health [SRH] threats like sexually transmitted infections [STIs], unwanted pregnancies, and unsafe abortions and often have limited access to SRH information, goods, and services. This study assessed the effectiveness of using a mobile phone application (APP) to increase access to SRH information, goods, and services among university students in Uganda.

**Methods:** Using data from a double-blinded randomized controlled trial, participants were randomly assigned to both the intervention (APP) and control (standard of care) arms. We executed descriptive analyses for baseline demographic characteristics by intervention, difference in difference (DID), and quantile regression analyses for both primary and secondary outcomes.

**Results:** The median age of participants was 21 years of age, and the majority were female (over 60%), unemployed (over 85%) and Christian (90%). Over 50% were resident in off-campus hostels and in a relationship. Between baseline and end-line, there was a significant increase in SRH knowledge score (DID = 2, $P < 0.001$), contraceptive use (DID = 6.6%, $P < 0.001$), HIV Voluntary testing and counselling (DID = 17.2%, $P < 0.001$), STI diagnosis and treatment (DID = 12.9%, $P < 0.001$), and condom use at last sex (DID = 4%, $P = 0.02$) among students who used the APP. There was a significant 0.98 unit increase in knowledge score (adjusted coefficient = 0.98, $P < 0.001$), a significant 1.6-fold increase in odds of contraceptive use (adjusted coefficient = 1.6, $P = 0.04$), a significant 3.5-fold increase in HIV VCT (adjusted coefficient = 3.5, $P < 0.001$), and a significant 2-fold increase in odds of STI testing and treatment (adjusted coefficient = 1.9, $P < 0.001$) after adjusting for demographic characteristics among APP users compared to the control group.

(Continued on next page)

* Correspondence: nuwellie37@gmail.com
[1]GHE Consulting, P.O Box 27011, Kampala, Uganda
[2]Department of Community Medicine and Public Health, Sahlgrenska Academy, University of Gothenburg, P. O Box 414, 40530, Gothenburg, Sweden

(Continued from previous page)
**Conclusion:** A mobile phone application increased sexual and reproductive health information (knowledge score), access to goods (contraceptives), and services (HIV voluntary testing and counseling and sexually transmitted infection diagnosis and management) among sexually active university students in Uganda. Further technical development, including the refinement of youth-friendly attributes, extending access to the app with other platforms besides android which was pilot tested, as well as further research into potential economic impact and paths to sustainability, is needed before the app is deployed to the general youth population in Uganda and other low-income settings.

**Keywords:** Mobile phone application, Mobile health, Sexual and reproductive health, University, Students

## Background

Many of the low-income countries of sub-Saharan Africa have predominantly young populations. Uganda is one such country with 78% of the general population below 30 years of age and adolescents aged 15–19 years, accounting for a quarter of the female population [1]. Given this age distribution, youth-friendly health services in Uganda and other low-income countries are a current and ongoing public policy imperative. One critical aspect of youth-friendly health services is in the area of sexual and reproductive health (SRH): young, often unmarried people are often excluded from SRH services (and research reporting) despite being sexually active [2]. This means that access to SRH information, goods, and services is a right that remains unrealized by the youth due to myriad factors, including economic hardship, social stigma, and community norms [3]. Consequently, youth access to SRH information, goods, and services is poor, and is reflected by high rates of teen pregnancy and pregnancy-related health problems, high unmet need for contraception, and low access to modern contraception [4, 5].

Nearly all low-income sub-Saharan African countries have also undergone a rapid increase in mobile and broadband internet coverage; the region is projected to have 1 billion sim connections and 500 million broadband connections by 2020 [6]. Additionally, there is an increasing penetration of technology hubs and internet developers, and an emerging tech-driven economy driven by young entrepreneurs [6]. In Uganda, there are 18 million unique mobile subscribers, well over half of the population has access to a mobile phone, network coverage is high (67%), and there have been significant increases in 4G and mobile internet connections [7].

The confluence of SRH needs for a predominantly young population and high and increasing access to mobile internet presents a unique opportunity for the development of youth-friendly, innovative digital health intervention (DHIs), particularly interventions in mobile health (mHealth). A review of mHealth projects in Uganda identified over 20 applications, including use for health worker and patient training, healthcare delivery, treatment and patient management support, and health facility improvement [8]. These interventions tended to use predominantly voice and text messaging or apply devices, such as tablet computers, directly at the point of use or service [8].

One area of potential growth in mHealth is in the use of mobile phone apps (MPAs) to increase access to health services in general and SRH information, goods, and services, in particular. DHIs, particularly mHealth, are associated with key youth-friendly attributes, including confidentiality, convenience, and entertainment/information value. The leap from text messaging-based mHealth to internet-based MPAs maintains the confidentiality and convenience attributes and magnifies the information and entertainment value of mHealth interventions. It also allows the development of multiple platforms and connections that expand their utility from information-only use to use for connecting to goods and services. This enables complex, multifaceted interventions with multiple potential avenues of impact and a wide variety of client or consumer choice. Additionally, entertainment value and appeal portend the ability to advertise, a key determinant of market success and potential sustainability at scale of a commercial MPA.

As part of a broader project conducted over an 18-month period, we developed and pilot-tested a MPA to increase access to SRH information, goods, and services in a population of university students in Kampala's capital, Uganda [9]. A detailed description of the development of the MPA has been described elsewhere (Development of a mobile phone application for access to sexual and reproductive health information, goods, and services in a low-income setting, Forthcoming). After MPA-development and as part of the impact evaluation, we conducted a study of acceptability and utilization of the MPA in which we assessed the proportion of eligible participants that accepted the MPA by downloading it and utilization as the proportion of eligible participants that used the app to access SRH information, goods and services in a six-month follow-up period (Acceptability and utilization of a mobile phone application to increase access to sexual and reproductive health information, goods, and services by university students in Uganda, Forthcoming). Acceptability was high at 84, and 82% of participants that downloaded the app used it to access SRH information, goods, and services over a six-month period (Acceptability and utilization of a mobile phone application to increase access to sexual and reproductive health information, goods, and services by university students in Uganda, Forthcoming).

Given satisfactory acceptability and utilization estimates, we hypothesized that access to the MPA would lead to an increase in SRH knowledge and lead to an increase in access to SRH goods and services among university students.

## Methods

### Study design

The study was a randomized controlled trial in which access to SRH information, goods, and services using a MPA (MPA-SRH) was compared to the standard of care of access to SRH information, goods, and services (SOC-SRH). A protocol of the trial, which was a part of a broader app development and impact evaluation project, has been published previously [9]. The trial was approved by the Mbarara University of Science and Technology Ethical Review Committee and the Uganda National Council of Science and Technology and was registered at MUREC1/7 No. 07/05–18 on 29th June 2018.

### Participants

The trial included students of Kyambogo University (KYU), the second-largest university in Uganda, which is situated in the capital city, Kampala. Eligibility criteria for inclusion into the trial were: (1) age 18 to 30 years, (2) self-reported sexual activity in the last six months, (3) more than 12 months to graduation, (4) access to an internet-enabled Android smartphone, and (5) informed consent. Trial participants were recruited in KYU halls of residence and KYU-affiliated hostels. Data were collected by in-person interviews in students' rooms.

### Intervention

In the intervention group, trial participants were granted access to a MPA to enable their access to SRH information, goods, and services over a period of six months. Details of the development and features of the app are described elsewhere (Development of a mobile phone application for access to sexual and reproductive health information, goods, and services in a low-income setting, Forthcoming). Briefly, the MPA was developed in partnership with Gershom Technologies Ltd. using the Android operating system and archived on the Google Play store. The MPA was designed to link the different goods and services providers: healthcare facilities which provided SRH goods and services; Beyonic Uganda (https://beyonic.com/), a payments company which managed payments and co-payments; SafeBoda (https://safeboda.com/ug/), a transport company which managed the transportation of ordered goods and app users to receive services; and GHE Consulting (https://www.gheuganda.com/) for coordination, management, and oversight.

The MPA included the following features: (1) sign-up and sign-in; (2) a user module for ordering SRH goods (sanitary pads, male condoms, contraceptives, pregnancy tests, and pain killers) and services (HIV voluntary testing and counseling (VTC), STI diagnosis and treatment (D&T), family planning counseling, and general SRH consultation); (3) an SRH information module (menstrual period tracker, frequently-asked questions (FAQs), SRH tips, and a live chat); (4) a payments module to enable provider payments by GHE Consulting, copays by clients, and payments for transportation; (5) a delivery module to enable clients to track shipments, set up pickups for in-facility visits, and set up pick up points for products; and (6) a security module for authentication and password protection. Embedded in the MPA was an advertising interface to test potential sustainability at the scale of in-MPA advertising. While the study provided a major subsidy for SRH goods and services as well as transportation, there was a modest co-pay that was paid by app users through a link between mobile money and the Beyonic payment system. The co-pay was designed to test the utility of client payments in potential future iterations of the MPA after the pilot period.

### Procedures

Intervention group participants received a text message with a link to download the MPA, including directions on the set up of a MPA account and instructions on the use of the MPA. Upon download of the MPA, participants could gain access to SRH information through the four in-app portals. Participants could order SRH goods and have them delivered to their rooms or to a designated spot for pick up. Participants could also connect with health service providers to book SRH services and connect with transport providers to organize transportation to and from healthcare facilities. Participants in the SOC-SRH group received no intervention, i.e., accessed SRH information, goods, and services as they did before the onset of the trial.

### Outcomes

There were four primary outcomes in the trial all reflecting changes from baseline to end-line (end of six months follow-up period): SRH knowledge score (SRH information), use of contraceptives (SRH goods), use of HIV VTC (SRH services), and use of STI D&T (SRH services). There were two secondary outcomes in the trial, both reflecting changes from baseline to end-line: use of condoms and use of alcohol during the last sexual encounter (both behavioral and attributable to SRH information).

### Sample size

The sample size was calculated to detect a change between baseline and end-line in use of modern contraceptive goods. The prevalence of modern contraceptive use among sexually active youth aged 18 to 30 years at the time of study planning was 30.2%. Using the formula for the use of the Z-test for two sample proportions in studies with behavioral components, we calculated a sample size of 435 participants per group in order to obtain 90% power to detect a 15% change in modern contraception use in this population at a two-sided significance level of 5%. The sample size calculation assumed no design effect (d = 1) and was adjusted for a 10% non-response rate to obtain a minimum sample size of 479 per group (a total of 958 participants).

### Randomization and masking

After recruitment and informed consent, participants were informed that there was a 50–50 chance that they would be randomly assigned to gain access to the MPA (MPA-SRH) or be a part of the control group (SOC-SRH). The participants' telephone numbers and unique study identification numbers were given to the app developer, who was responsible for randomization. Participants were randomized 1:1 to MPA-SRH and SOC-SRH using computer-generated random numbers. The research team, including providers at health facilities, transport providers, and payment technicians, and participants were blind to the intervention group, but the app developer was not.

### Statistical analysis

Data were double-entered and cross-validated, and all analyses were conducted in Stata version 16 (College Station TX, USA). We compared outcomes between participants randomly assigned to MPA-SRH versus SOC-SRH, ignoring potential changes in access to SRH information, goods, and services in the SOC-SRH group that may have been triggered by the use of the app by participants in the MPA-SRH group.

SRH knowledge scores were summed from correct responses from 17 different attributes and ranged from 0 to 17 (each question was awarded 1 point). Contraceptive use, HIV VTC, STI D&T, condom use during last sexual encounter, and alcohol use during the last sexual encounter were binary variables. We estimated the difference in changes from baseline to end-line (with 95% confidence intervals (CIs) and *p*-values) using differences-in-differences. We used the Wilcoxon rank-sum test for the knowledge score and the Z-test for proportions.

Using quantile regression (knowledge score) and a logit link function (access to modern contraceptive use, HIV voluntary counseling and testing, and STI testing and treatment), we estimated a mean differences-in-differences effect, adjusting for demographic characteristics. Models were estimated using maximum likelihood.

## Results

We enrolled participants from Oct 23rd, 2018, to 13th November 2018, and the last participant completed the six-month follow-up period on 25th May 2019. We

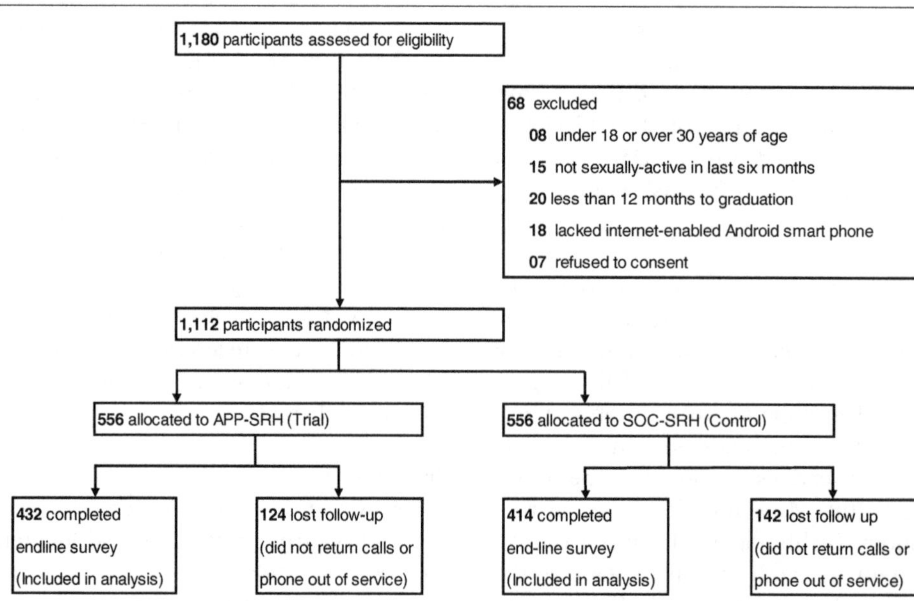


**Fig. 1** Trial profile

enrolled (and assessed for eligibility) 1180 students and randomized 1112 students, 556 to the MPA-SRH (trial arm), and 556 to the SOC-SRH (control arm). Of the participants randomized, 846 (76.1%) completed the end-line survey, 432 (76.1%) in the APP-SRH arm, and 414 (74.5%) in the APP-SOC arm, constituting the sample for the analysis (Fig. 1).

The participants were predominantly women, resident in off-campus hostels, from urban hometowns, in relationships, in their first or second years of study, unemployed, and Christian. The loss to follow-up was predominantly due to participants not answering and returning calls or out-of-service telephone numbers. The baseline characteristics of the study participants are shown in Table 1. The

**Table 1** Baseline characteristics of study participants by intervention

| Characteristic | APP-SRH | SOC-SRH | All |
|---|---|---|---|
| | (*n* = 556) | (n = 556) | (*n* = 1112) |
| **Age at entry, years** | 21 (2 [10, 11];) | 21 (2 [10, 11];) | 21 (2 [10, 11];) |
| **Sex** | | | |
| Male | 214 (38.5) | 193 (34.7) | 407 (36.0) |
| Female | 342 (61.5) | 363 (65.3) | 705 (63.4) |
| **Residence** | | | |
| Campus hall | 137 (24.6) | 133 (23.9) | 207 (24.3) |
| Off-campus hostel | 301 (54.1) | 317 (57.0) | 618 (55.6) |
| Rental home | 104 (18.7) | 86 (15.5) | 190 (17.1) |
| Own home | 02 (0.36) | 03 (0.5) | 05 (0.45) |
| Parent/ Guardian home | 12 (2.16) | 17 (3.1) | 29 (2.6) |
| **Hometown** | | | |
| Urban | 231 (41.6) | 228 (41.0) | 459 (41.3) |
| Peri-urban | 184 (33.1) | 189 (33.9) | 373 (33.5) |
| Rural | 141 (25.4) | 139 (25.0) | 280 (25.2) |
| **Marital status** | | | |
| Relationship | 298 (53.6) | 299 (53.8) | 594 (53.7) |
| Single | 239 (42.9) | 241 (43.4) | 480 (43.2) |
| Cohabiting | 13 (2.3) | 08 (1.4) | 21 (1.89) |
| Married | 04 (0.7) | 08 (1.4) | 12 (1.08) |
| Divorced | 01 (0.2) | 00 (0.0) | 01 (0.09) |
| Widowed | 01 (0.2) | 00 (0.0) | 01 (0.09) |
| **Year of study** | | | |
| First | 174 (31.3) | 195 (35.1) | 369 (33.2) |
| Second | 209 (37.6) | 201 (36.2) | 410 (36.9) |
| Third | 147 (26.4) | 134 (24.1) | 281 (25.3) |
| Fourth | 24 (4.3) | 26 (4.68) | 50 (4.5) |
| Fifth | 02 (0.36) | 00 (0.0) | 02 (0.18) |
| **Employment** | | | |
| Unemployed | 475 (85.4) | 495 (89.0) | 970 (87.2) |
| Employed | 46 (8.3) | 37 (6.7) | 83 (7.5) |
| Volunteer | 01 (0.18) | 02 (0.4) | 03 (0.27) |
| Self-employed | 34 (6.1) | 22 (3.9) | 56 (5.04) |
| **Religion** | | | |
| Christian | 500 (89.9) | 486 (87.4) | 986 (88.7) |
| Muslim | 43 (7.7) | 45 (8.1) | 88 (7.9) |
| Others | 13 (2.3) | 25 (4.5) | 38 (3.4) |

**Table 2** Differences-in-differences analysis of primary and secondary outcomes

| | MPA-SRH | | | SOC-SRH | | | DID [*P*-value: 95% CI] |
|---|---|---|---|---|---|---|---|
| | **Baseline** | **End-line** | **Difference** | **Baseline** | **End-line** | **Difference** | |
| Knowledge score | 13 (11–15) | 16 (15–16) | 03 (z = −20.64, 0.02) | 13 (11–14) | 14 (13–15) | 01 (z = − 9.01,0.01) | 02 (z = 4.69,0.00)* |
| Contraceptive use | 69.1% | 82.2% | 13.1%[0.00: 7.8–18.4] | 73.7% | 80.2% | 06.5% [0.02:1.2–11.8] | 06.6% [0.00:3.0–10.4]* |
| HIV VTC | 68.0% | 90.5% | 22.5%[0.00:17.8–27.3] | 64.2% | 69.6% | 05.4% [0.09: −0.6-11.3] | 17.2% [0.00:13.0–21.4]* |
| STI D & T | 52.3% | 82.2% | 29.8%[0.00:24.3–35.3] | 52.3% | 69.3% | 17.0%[0.00:10.9–23.1] | 12.9% [0.00:7.6–18.1]* |
| Condom use | 66.2% | 76.8% | 10.4% [0.00: 5.1–16.3] | 66.6% | 73.0% | 06.4% [0.03: 0.6–12.2] | 04.0% [0.02:0.8–7.8]* |
| Alcohol use | 7.6% | 10.9% | 03.3% [0.07: −0.3-7.0] | 04.0% | 07.5% | 03.5%[0.02: 0.5–6.5] | − 00.2% [0.86:-.0.2–2.1] |

*implies statistical significance at less than 5%

median age of participants was 21 years of age, and the majority were female (over 60%), unemployed (over 85%) and Christian (90%). Over 50% were resident in off-campus hostels and in a relationship.

Data are median (IQR; [range]), or n (%). APP = mobile phone application. SRH = sexual and reproductive health. SOC = standard of care.

Between baseline and end-line, there was a significant increase in SRH knowledge score, contraceptive use, HIV VTC, STI D &T, and condom use at last sex among APP users compared to the SOC-SRH (Table 2). There was a modest non-significant reduction in alcohol use at last sexual encounter among APP users compared to the SOC-SRH (Table 2). There was a significant 0.98 unit increase in knowledge score, a significant 1.6-fold increase in odds of contraceptive use, a significant 3.5-fold increase in HIV VCT, and a significant 2-fold increase in odds of STI testing and treatment after adjusting for demographic characteristics among APP users compared to the SOC-SRH (Table 3).

## Discussion

We assessed the effectiveness of a MPA to increase access to SRH information (measured as an increase in knowledge score and use of condoms and alcohol during the last sexual encounter), goods (measured as the proportion of participants using modern contraception), and services (a proportion that used HIV VCT and STI D&T) in a population of university students in Uganda. The MPA had a statistically significant benefit in increased SRH knowledge and increased access to SRH goods and services. MPAs are increasingly used in low- and middle-income countries for a wide range of applications, although applications in this setting are far exceeded by applications in high-income settings [12]. In sub-Saharan Africa and in the area of SRH, apps have been deployed to the public to support family planning [13] and to health-care workers for improving provider quality of maternal and neonatal care [10, 14–19]. To our knowledge, this is the first report of an app deployed to members of the public to increase access to SRH information, goods, and services in the low-income setting.

Internet-enabled mobile phones and MPAs, including social media platforms, are popular among the youth around the world. In some settings, access to MPAs is associated with negative behavioral outcomes: as an example, a study in South Africa found increased odds of multiple sexual partners in the last year and higher prevalence of hazardous alcohol use with access to social media and messaging apps [20]. The configuration of MPAs to deliver health improving information is a potential avenue to counter the potential negative impact of other more generic apps such as social media and messaging apps on youth behavior while increasing

**Table 3** Regression analyses

| | Knowledge score | | Contraceptive use | | HIV VTC | | STI testing and treatment | |
|---|---|---|---|---|---|---|---|---|
| | **Unadj.** | **Adj.** | **Unadj.** | **Adj.** | **Unadj.** | **Adj.** | **Unadj.** | **Adj.** |
| **Constant** | 13.00 [0.00(12.73,13.26)]* | 10.26 [0.00(7.63,12.69)]* | 2.81 [0.00(2.32,3.39)]* | 0.45 [0.41(0.06,3.11)] | 1.79 [0.00(1.51,2.13)]* | 0.33 [0.25(0.52,2.15)] | 1.10 [0.27(0.03,1.30)] | 0.27 [0.15(0.46,1.58)] |
| **Intervention** | 0.00 [1.00(− 0.38,0.38)] | 0.35 [0.07(− 0.03,0.734)] | 0.81 [0.09(0.61,1.03)] | 0.73 [0.02(0.56,0.96)]* | 1.18 [0.18(0.92,1.52)] | 1.55 [0.27(0.90,1.49)] | 1.00 [1.00(0.79,1.27)] | 1.02 [0.86(0.80,1.3)] |
| **End-line** | 0.10 [−0.59,1.14)] | 1.90 [0.00(1.42,2.37)]* | 1.44 [0.02(1.06,1.96)]* | 1.56 [0.01(1.1,2.22)]* | 1.27 [0.08(0.97,1.67)] | 1.44 [0.03(1.05,1.98)]* | 2.16 [0.00(1.58,2.69)]* | 2.48 [0.00(1.74,3.26)]* |
| **Intervention * End-line** | 2.00 [0.29(1.42,2.58)] | 0.98 [0.00(0.29,1.46)]* | 1.43 [0.10(0.93,2.21)] | 1.58 [0.04(1.02,2.46)] | 3.53 [0.00(2.23,5.57)]* | 3.57 [0.00(2.24–5.68)]* | 2.04 [0.00(1.37,3.04)]* | 1.99 [0.00(1.26,2.86)]* |
| **N** | 1958 | 1958 | 1958 | 1954 | 1958 | 1946 | 1958 | 1954 |
| **Log-likelihood** | – | – | – 1072.59 | – 1043.67 | – 1101.17 | – 1077.2 | – 1227.27 | – 1181.64 |
| **AIC** | – | – | 2153.17 | 2147.33 | 2210.34 | 2212.41 | 2462.55 | 2423.27 |

* implies statistical significance at less than 5%: Coefficients and P-values and 95% confidence intervals in parenthesis

access to health services such as SRH services. Our study demonstrated a significant increase in condom use during the last sexual encounter, suggesting a potential impact of a MPA on short-term behavioral change.

Research has established that the youth in low-income settings have significant SRH needs and face barriers to access to SRH goods and services, including physical access, legal and societal proscriptions, and societal barriers [11, 21]. There is substantial evidence that increasing youth-friendly information and access to SRH information and services are effective in fulfilling needs and alleviating barriers [11]. In our study, the MPA led to increased SRH knowledge and increased use of contraception, HIV VCT, and STI D&T, suggesting that the MPA was sufficiently youth-friendly to derive impact. Although there were some technical difficulties in the use of the MPA, these can be solved in future iterations of the MPA as plans are made for the transition to scale. And although our current focus was on a usable, deployable product, future prototypes will focus on refining youth-friendly attributes.

One weakness of the study was that the length of access to most components of the intervention (live chat and subsidies for goods, services, and information) were available for a short time (six months). As such, we are blind to the presence or absence of a sustained effect of increased knowledge or increase access to SRH goods and services on account of access to the MPA. Additionally, the trial was conducted among university students who are not generalizable to the general youth population in Uganda or other low-income countries. In fact, access to SRH information, goods, and services was high at baseline (13/17 knowledge score, over 70% access to contraception, 65% ever undergone HIV VCT, and 50% ever undergone STI diagnosis and treatment). This is compared to a general population contraceptive use prevalence of 29% among women of reproductive age [22] or 47% among unmarried women [1], and the prevalence of HIV testing among 15–19-year-olds of 44% in women and 53% in men [1]. University students are also different from the general population in their increased access to both smartphones and internet connections. Although the results of this study are not generalizable to the general youth population, we anticipate increasing access to smartphones and internet access [6, 23, 24] and plan to explore the feasibility and effectiveness of SRH MPAs in the general population in future studies.

The demonstration of the effectiveness of the MPA to increase access to SRH information, goods, and services, along with lessons learned in the pilot implementation and impact evaluation is a necessary precursor to the further development of the MPA with the goal of developing a sustainable product that can be rolled out to the general public. Before this goal is realized, further studies of the cost-effectiveness of the MPA and its potential economic impact at scale are needed, as are studies on the perception of potential advertisers, key partners in a possible future product, on the potential of the MPA to drive revenue.

## Conclusion

A mobile phone application increased sexual and reproductive health information (knowledge score), access to goods (contraceptives), and services (HIV voluntary testing and counseling and sexually transmitted infection diagnosis and management) among sexually active university students in Uganda. Further technical development, including the refinement of youth-friendly attributes, as well as further research into potential economic impact and paths to sustainability, is needed before the app is deployed to the general youth population in Uganda and other low-income settings. This will enable uniform access to the app by allowing users from other platforms other than the android platform, which was pilot tested.

### Abbreviations

APP: Mobile Phone Application; CIs: Confidence Intervals; D&T: Diagnosis and Treatment; DHIs: Digital Health Interventions; FAQs: Frequently Asked Questions; IQR: Inter Quartile Range; KYU: Kyambogo University; mHealth: Mobile Health; MPAs: Mobile Phone Apps; SOC: Standard of Care; SRH: Sexual and reproductive health; STI: Sexually Transmitted Infections; VTC: Voluntary Testing and Counseling

### Acknowledgements

We want to thank all partner clinics, notably NIM medical Centre, Alpha medical Centre and Kyambogo Medical Centre. We would also like to thank the KYU administration and students for their cooperation during the study period. We immensely appreciate all other partners that contributed to the success of this study.

### Authors' contributions

All authors conceived the study. EN wrote the first draft of the manuscript. All authors revised and approved the final version of this manuscript.

### Author details

[1]GHE Consulting, P.O Box 27011, Kampala, Uganda. [2]Department of Community Medicine and Public Health, Sahlgrenska Academy, University of Gothenburg, P. O Box 414, 40530, Gothenburg, Sweden. [3]Global Medicines Program, Department of Global Health, University of Washington, P.O. Box 357630, Seattle, WA 98195, USA.

### References

1. Uganda Bureau of Statistics (UBOS) and ICF. Uganda demographic and health survey 2016. Kampala, Uganda and Rockville, Maryland, USA: UBOS and ICF; 2018.
2. Darroch JE, et al. Research gaps in adolescent sexual and reproductive health. New York: Guttmacher Institute; 2016. https://www.guttmacher.org/report/research-gaps-in-sexual-and-reproductive-health.
3. Rijsdijk LE, Lie R, Bos AER, Leerlooijer JN, Kok G. Sexual and reproductive health and rights: implications for comprehensive sex education among young people in Uganda. Sex Educ. 2013;13:409–22.
4. Kassa GM, Arowojolu AO, Odukogbe AA, Yalew AW. Prevalence and determinants of adolescent pregnancy in Africa: a systematic review and meta-analysis. Reprod Health. 2018;15:195.

5. Adding It Up: Investing in Contraception and Maternal and Newborn Health for Adolescents in Uganda, 2018. Accessed on 22 Oct 2019 at https://www.guttmacher.org/fact-sheet/adding-it-up-contraception-mnh-adolescents-uganda.
6. The Mobile Economy. Sub-Saharan Africa 2017. Accessed on 16 Oct 2018 at https://www.gsmaintelligence.com/research/?file=7bf3592e6d750144e58d9dcfac6adfab&download.
7. Calum Handforth and Matthew Wilson. Digital Identity Country Profile: Uganda. Accessed on 22 Oct 2019 at https://www.gsma.com/mobilefordevelopment/wp-content/uploads/2019/02/Digital-Identity-Country-Report-Uganda.pdf.
8. Kiberu VM, Mars M, Scott RE. Barriers and opportunities to implementation of sustainable e-health programmes in Uganda: a literature review. African J Primary Health Care Family Med. 2017;9:e1–e10.
9. Nuwamanya E, Nuwasiima A, Babigumira JU, Asiimwe FT, Lubinga SJ, Babigumira JB. Study protocol: using a mobile phone-based application to increase awareness and uptake of sexual and reproductive health services among the youth in Uganda. Reproductive Health. 2018;15:216.
10. Tsai AC, Tomlinson M, Dewing S, le Roux IM, Harwood JM, Chopra M, Rotheram-Borus MJ. Antenatal depression case finding by community health workers in South Africa: feasibility of a mobile phone application. Arch Womens Ment Health. 2014;17:423–31.
11. Chandra-Mouli V, McCarraher DR, Phillips SJ, Williamson NE, Hainsworth G. Contraception for adolescents in low and middle income countries: needs, barriers, and access. Reprod Health. 2014;11:1.
12. Abaza H, Marschollek M. mHealth Application Areas and Technology Combinations*. A comparison of literature from high and low/middle income countries. Methods Inf Med. 2017;56:e105–22.
13. Shelus V, Ashcroft N, Burgess S, Giuffrida M, Jennings V. Preventing pregnancy in Kenya through distribution and use of the CycleBeads Mobile application. Int Perspect Sex Reprod Health. 2017;43:131–41.
14. Thomsen CF, Barrie AMF, Boas IM, Lund S, Sorensen BL, Oljira FG, Tersbol BP. Health workers' experiences with the safe delivery app in west Wollega zone, Ethiopia: a qualitative study. Reprod Health. 2019;16:50.
15. Willcox M, Moorthy A, Mohan D, Romano K, Hutchful D, Mehl G, Labrique A, LeFevre A. Mobile Technology for Community Health in Ghana: is maternal messaging and provider use of technology cost-effective in improving maternal and child health outcomes at scale? J Med Internet Res. 2019;21:e11268.
16. Shiferaw S, Workneh A, Yirgu R, Dinant GJ, Spigt M. Designing mHealth for maternity services in primary health facilities in a low-income setting - lessons from a partially successful implementation. BMC Med Inform Decis Mak. 2018;18:96.
17. Hackett K, Lafleur C, Nyella P, Ginsburg O, Lou W, Sellen D. Impact of smartphone-assisted prenatal home visits on women's use of facility delivery: results from a cluster-randomized trial in rural Tanzania. PLoS One. 2018;13:e0199400.
18. Shiferaw S, Spigt M, Tekie M, Abdullah M, Fantahun M, Dinant GJ. The effects of a locally developed mHealth intervention on delivery and postnatal care utilization: a Prospective Controlled Evaluation among Health Centres in Ethiopia. PLoS One. 2016;11:e0158600.
19. McNabb M, Chukwu E, Ojo O, Shekhar N, Gill CJ, Salami H, Jega F. Assessment of the quality of antenatal care services provided by health workers using a mobile phone decision support application in northern Nigeria: a pre/post-intervention study. PLoS One. 2015;10:e0123940.
20. Kaufman ZA, Braunschweig EN, Feeney J, Dringus S, Weiss H, Delany-Moretlwe S, Ross DA. Sexual risk behavior, alcohol use, and social media use among secondary school students in informal settlements in Cape Town and Port Elizabeth, South Africa. AIDS Behav. 2014;18:1661–74.
21. Renzaho AM, Kamara JK, Georgeou N, Kamanga G. Sexual, reproductive health needs, and rights of young people in slum areas of Kampala, Uganda: A Cross Sectional Study. PLoS One. 2017;12:e0169721.
22. Ba DM, Ssentongo P, Agbese E, Kjerulff KH. Prevalence and predictors of contraceptive use among women of reproductive age in 17 sub-Saharan African countries: a large population-based study. Sexual & Reproductive Healthcare. 2019;21:26–32.
23. Deloitte. Global mobile consumer trends, 2nd edition Mobile continues its global reach into all aspects of consumers' lives. Accessed at https://www2.deloitte.com/content/dam/Deloitte/us/Documents/technology-media-telecommunications/us-global-mobile-consumer-survey-second-edition.pdf on 21 Sept 2019.
24. National Information Technology Survey 2017/18 Report Study conducted by: The Collaboration on International ICT Policy for East and Southern Africa (CIPESA). Accessd at https://www.nita.go.ug/sites/default/files/publications/National%20IT%20Survey%20April%2010th.pdf on 21 Sept 2019.

14

# Assessment of women's satisfaction with family planning service at public health facilities in Northwest Region of Ethiopia

Woineshet Asrat[1], Teferi Mekonnen[2*] and Melkamu Bedimo[3]

**Abstract**

**Background:** Ethiopia is a Sub Saharan African country with an estimated contraceptive prevalence rate of 36% and 22% unmet need for family planning service among married women. Client satisfaction influences the use of Family Planning and other reproductive health services. There is limited information on satisfaction with family planning service among Family planning users particularly in the northern part of Ethiopia. Hence, this study aimed to provide information on client satisfaction and its determinant among women in Public Health facilities of Northwestern Ethiopia.

**Methods:** A Facility based cross-sectional study was conducted from March 1, 2017, to March 30, 2017. An exit interview using structured pretested questionnaire was conducted on randomly selected 490 women attending family planning service in Bahir Dar city, Public Health facilities of Northwest, Ethiopia. The data was cleaned, coded and entered into Epi info™ 7 statistical software and then exported and analyzed using SPSS Version 20 statistical software. A multivariable binary logistic regression model was fitted to identify factors associated with Client satisfaction. Adjusted Odds Ratio (AOR) with the corresponding 95% Confidence Interval (CI) was calculated to show the strength of association.

**Results:** A total of 490 family planning service users were approached for an interview and making a response rate of 99.8%. The overall client satisfaction with the family planning services was found to be 66.1%. Clients who were merchants were more likely to be satisfied with the family planning service than government employees [AOR = 2.5, *P*-value = 0.007). In addition, house wife's more likely to be satisfied with the family planning service than government employees AOR = 2.4, *P*-value = 0.007). Daily laborers were also found to be more likely to be satisfied with the FP service as compared with governmental employees AOR = 3.9, *P*-value = 0.007). New Family Planning user clients were more likely to be satisfied with the family planning service than repeat users [AOR = 2.3, *P*-value = 0.004).
Family planning service waiting time also affects client satisfaction, in which those having awaiting time of less than half an hour's (AOR = 9.7, (*P*-value =001), One to half an hour (AOR = 6.4, (P-value =001), One hour to two hours (AOR = 4.6, (*P*-value =001) were more likely to be satisfied with the family planning service delivered at the facility than those who had waited for more than two hours. In addition, those whose privacy was maintained during counseling were more likely to be satisfied with the family planning service delivered than whose privacy was not maintained (AOR = 3. 2, *P*-Value = < 0.001). Those having convenient service hour were more likely to be satisfied with the family planning

(Continued on next page)

* Correspondence: tmekonnen16@yahoo.com; teferim@bdu.edu.et; tmkeonnnen16@yahoo.com
[2]Public Health Nutrition department, School of Public Health, Bahir Dar University, P.O.Box 79, Bahir Dar, Ethiopia

(Continued from previous page)
service delivered than those who don't have convenient service hour (AOR = 2.4, *p*-value = 0.002).

**Conclusion:** The finding of this study concludes that nearly two -third of the clients were satisfied with the family planning service delivered at Public Health facilities of Northwest of Ethiopia. New family planning service users, waiting time for the service, Maintaining privacy during counseling, having convenient service hour and occupational status of the clients were the predictors for client satisfaction with family planning service delivered at Public Health facilities in Bahir Dar city.

**Keywords:** Family planning, Client satisfaction, Public health facility, Bahir Dar Ethiopia

## Background

In developing countries, maternal mortality is a major concern [1]. According to the 2015 United Nations report, around 303,000 maternal deaths were reported globally with a maternal mortality ratio of 216 per 100,000 live births [2]. Although it is noted that there is 43% decrease in maternal mortality from 1990, the death rate is still high. In Ethiopia, according to 2016 Ethiopian Demographic Health Survey report 412 pregnancy -related deaths per 100,000 live births were occurred [3]. Previous evidences revealed that family planning service utilization positively contributes to the reduction of maternal deaths. The World Health Organization (WHO) defines family planning as something that "allows individuals and couples to anticipate and attain their desired number of children and the spacing and timing of their births which can be improved by family planning counseling which deals about continuous process that the counselor as the counselor provide to help clients and people to make and arrive at informed choices about the size of their family" [4, 5]. According to lancet report, use of contraception prevents nearly 32% of maternal deaths and 10% of infant deaths [6]. After recognition of satisfaction of sexual and reproductive rights as a human rights in 1994, global efforts were made on recognition of the importance of family planning for maternal and child survival [7].

Despite these efforts, the use of modern methods as measured by the contraceptive prevalence rate (CPR) remains low in many developing countries, with a growth of 1% per year, over the last 30 years [8]. In sub-Saharan African countries the lowest contraception and highest unmet need were observed due to a mainly due to low level of knowledge and existence of variety of barriers [9, 10].

In Ethiopia, the contraceptive prevalence rate is 36% and 22% of married women have unmet need for family planning which is affected by education level, Partner education, religion, household wealth status, number of living children and media exposure [3, 11, 12]. Family planning service utilization is also affected by client satisfaction [13]. According to different studies, client satisfaction might be affected by the service waiting time [14–17], age, maternal education, cleanliness of the facility, frequency of visit, proper and adequate explanation on how to use contraceptive were factors affecting client satisfaction [18–21].

In order to improve family planning service utilization, it is better to assess levels of client satisfaction with the service delivered and its determinants. There is limited information on levels of client satisfaction with the family planning service delivered at Public Health facilities in Bahir Dar City, Northwest Ethiopia. Hence, this study will provide information on the levels of client satisfaction and its determinants delivered at public health facilities which will be used as an input for improving family planning service delivery in Northwestern part of Ethiopia.

## Methods

### Study area

This study was conducted in Bahir Dar City which is located 565 km northwest of Addis Ababa, the capital city of Ethiopia. According to Planning and Economy Bureau of Amhara Regional State report in 2016, the total population of Bahir Dar city administration was 308,877 of which 245,770 were resided in Bahir Dar town, while 63,107 are living in rural part. Out of the total population 158,824 females are eligible for family planning service use. According to 2016 zonal health department report, of the total family planning service user 55% were used family planning service from Public Health facilities.

### Study design, period, source population and study population

A Facility based cross-sectional study was conducted from March 1, 2017, to 30, 2017.. All women who were using family planning service in Bahir Dar city administration were the source population. Women's who were using family planning service at Public Health Facility at Bahir Dar City were the study population. All women who were on family Planning service during the data collection period were included in the study.

The dependent variable was client satisfaction with family planning service delivered ("satisfied" and "Not satisfied") and the independent variables were service waiting time, age, maternal educational status, cleanliness of the facility, frequency of visit, proper and adequate explanation on how to use contraceptive, occupational status, frequency of family planning visit, having convenient service hour, privacy during counseling were the independent variables assessed in this study.

According to this research, a client will be satisfied, if client had a mean satisfaction score of ≥3.22 which is used as a cut of to declare as a client is satisfied with the family planning service delivered. This categorization was made by dichotomizing clients satisfaction based on a mean satisfaction score after data collection during the analysis stage.

#### Sample size determination and sampling procedure

The sample size was determined using Epi info™ 7 after considering the following assumptions; taking 75.3% proportion of satisfaction obtained from previous studies [18], 95% confidence limit and 4% margin of error (d) and an expected non-response rate of 10%. Finally, 491 women's who were using family planning service were included in the study.

#### Sampling procedure

A systematic random sampling technique was used for selection of the clients. The proportional allocation was made for 12 Health facilities providing family planning service at Bahir Dar city. Finally, every third family planning users were included in the study.

#### Data collection technique, tools, and procedures

The Data collection was done using validated and structured pretested questionnaire through face-face interview of women at the exit of the family planning service department by trained Female data collectors. In this study, the satisfaction of clients with the Family Planning service was assessed using fourteen Likert scaled question items. Each item of the question had 5 points ranging from 1(very unsatisfied) to 5 (very satisfied) and finally, the mean score was computed.

#### Data quality control

Two- day training was given for data collectors and supervisors. The pre-test was made on 5% of the total sample and the questionnaire was developed in English and then translated into the local language, Amharic and back to English by language experts. Trained 12th Grade complete female data collector were recruited and regular supervision was made by supervisors.

#### Data processing and analysis

The data was cleaned,coded and entered into Epi info™ 7 Statistical Software and then exported and analyzed by using SPSS version 20 statistical software. Descriptive statistics such as frequencies and percentages were used to describe the study population in relation to relevant variables. Normality assumptions were checked and the satisfaction score was normally distributed. Stepwise multivariable logistic regression model was used to identify predictors' of client satisfaction. The goodness of fitness of the model was checked by Hosmer and Lemeshow assumption test (i.e *P*-Value 0.56). The association between dependent and independent variables were assessed using odds ratio with 95% confidence interval and *p*-value ≤0.05 was considered statistically significant.

#### Ethical approval

Ethical approval was obtained from the Ethical review board of Bahir Dar University, College of Medicine and Health Sciences. Permission letters were obtained from Amhara regional Health office and Bahir Dar City Health Administration. Verbal consent was obtained from the study participants after explaining the study objectives and procedures. Finally, the date collection was made after they agreed and signed for an agreement to participate in the study. Their right to refuse from being participated was considered. Names of the participants were kept anonymous.

## Results

#### Socio-demographic characteristics of study participants in Bahir Dar city

A total of 490 family planning service users were approached for an interview and making a response rate of 99.8%.

The mean (±SD) age of respondents was 27 (±5.2) years. One hundred seventy -seven (36%) of the respondents were within the age group of 25–29 years of age and four hundred seven (83.1%) of the respondents were married and more than three fourths (77.8%) of the respondents were urban residents. One hundred seventeen (23.9%) of the respondents were unable to read and write. With regarding occupational status of the respondents, one hundred sixty four (33.5%) were a housewife About 366 (88.8%) family planning users were orthodox Christian by religion (Table 1).

#### Family planning service- related characteristics among family planning service users in Bahir Dar city administration public health facility, 2017

Out of 490 respondents, 389(79.4%) respondents' had received the service from the health center and chi squire test of association was done there no more significant association between hospitals and health centers in our setup ($P = 0.19$). Three hundred sixty eight (76%) of the respondents were repeat users and about three hundred three (61.8%) of participants had used Injectables. Three

**Table 1** Socio-Demographic characteristics of Family planning user's at the public health facility in Bahir Dar city administration, from March 1,2017, to 30, 2017($n = 490$)

| Variable | Category | Number | Percent (%) |
|---|---|---|---|
| Age in years | 15–19 | 37 | 7.6 |
| | 20–24 | 110 | 22.4 |
| | 25–29 | 177 | 36.1 |
| | 30–34 | 110 | 22.4 |
| | 35 & above | 56 | 11.4 |
| Residence | Rural | 109 | 22.2 |
| | Urban | 381 | 77.8 |
| Educational status | Unable to read and write | 117 | 23.9 |
| | Read and write only | 90 | 18.4 |
| | Grade 1 to 8 | 58 | 11.8 |
| | Grade 9 to 12 | 117 | 23.2 |
| | Certificate and above | 108 | 22.7 |
| Occupational Status | Government employee | 96 | 19.6 |
| | Private employee | 58 | 11.8 |
| | Merchant | 67 | 13.7 |
| | Housewife | 164 | 33.5 |
| | Unemployed | 17 | 3.5 |
| | Student | 23 | 4.7 |
| | Daily laborer | 65 | 13.3 |
| Religion | Orthodox Christian | 394 | 80.4 |
| | Muslim | 68 | 13.9 |
| | Other | 28 | 5.7 |
| Marital status | Married | 407 | 83.1 |
| | Single | 62 | 12.7 |
| | Divorced | 17 | 3.5 |
| | Widowed | 4 | 0.8 |

hundred forty three (70.0%) of the family service users had at least one child and 68.2% of respondents had received their method of choice.

Majority 448(91.4%) of respondents have to walk less than 1 h walking distance to get the service, 302(61%) of respondents reported that, the waiting time to receive the service was short and 407(83.1%) of respondents reported the service hour was convenient for them to use family planning service (Table 2).

**Client-provider interaction and information given by family planning service provider characteristics among family planning service users at public health facility in Bahir Dar city,2017**

Majority of respondents, 439(89.6%) reported that, they can get information when they need about family planning from their service provider. About 420 (85.7%) of respondents could understand the family planning service provider easily during their contact time. About 233(47.6%) of the family planning user reported that, the family planning service provider were given a chance to ask questions and 256(32%) of respondents had received family planning service information through teaching aids (Fig. 1).

**Family planning service satisfaction among family planning user's at the public health facilities in Bahir Dar city, 2017**

The overall client satisfaction with the family planning services was found to be 66.1% (95% CI: 61.2%, 70.1%). Majority of the respondents (89%) reported as they were satisfied and very satisfied with the choice of method availability, 88% respondents were satisfied and very satisfied with the cleanness of procedures, and 87% were

**Table 2** Family planning service utilization, health facility related characteristics' among family planning user's at public health facility in Bahir Dar city administration, from March 1,2017 to March 30, 2017($n = 490$)

| Variable | Category | Number | Percent |
|---|---|---|---|
| Types of Health facility visited | Health Center | 389 | 79.4 |
| | Hospital | 101 | 20.6 |
| Frequency of visit | New | 122 | 24.9 |
| | Repeat | 368 | 75.1 |
| Number of children | Have no child | 122 | 24.9 |
| | 1–4 children | 343 | 70.0 |
| | > 4 children | 25 | 5.1 |
| Clients receiving their method of choice | Yes | 334 | 68.2 |
| | No | 156 | 31.8 |
| Method that the client was using | Pills | 32 | 6.5 |
| | Inject able | 303 | 61.8 |
| | Implant | 126 | 25.7 |
| | IUCD | 29 | 5.9 |
| Time it takes to reach the health facility for FP service | Less than half hour | 314 | 64.1 |
| | Half hour to 1 h | 134 | 27.3 |
| | 1 to 2 h | 24 | 4.9 |
| | More than 2 h | 18 | 3.7 |
| Waiting time to received the service | Less than half hour | 226 | 46.1 |
| | Half hour to 1 h | 210 | 42.9 |
| | 1 to 2 h | 33 | 6.7 |
| | More than 2 h | 21 | 4.3 |
| Perceived waiting time for the FP service | Short waiting time | 302 | 61.6 |
| | Long waiting time | 61 | 38.4 |
| FP service hour convenient for you | Convenient | 407 | 83.1% |
| | Inconvenient | 83 | 16.9% |

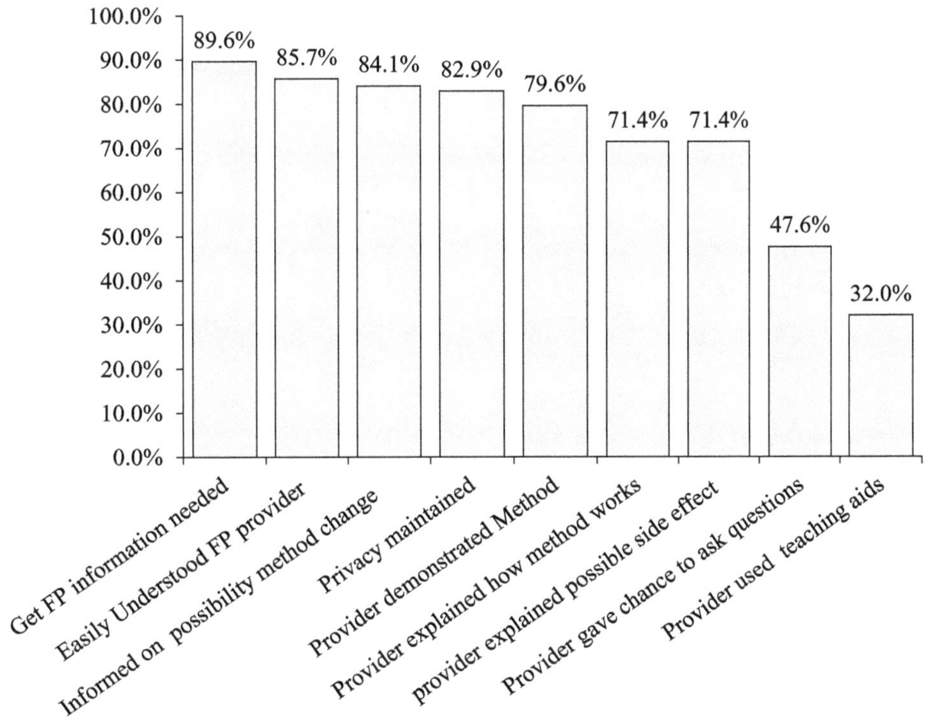


**Fig. 1** Client-provider interaction and information given by family planning service provider characteristics of family planning user's at public health facility in Bahir Dar city administration, from March 1 to 30, 2017(n=490)

**Table 3** Proportion of client Satisfaction among family planning users at public health facility at public health facility in Bahir Dar city, from March, 2017($n = 490$)

| Characteristics | Very dissatisfied [No (%)] | Dissatisfied [No(%)] | Neutral [No(%)] | Satisfied [No. (%)] | Very satisfied [No. (%)] |
|---|---|---|---|---|---|
| Registration staff warmly welcomed you | 31(6.3) | 126(25.7) | 152(31.0) | 128(26.1) | 53(10.8) |
| Professionals* informed you where FP service department | 10(2.0) | 102(20.8) | 171(34.9) | 152(31.0) | 55(11.2) |
| Professionals* were available when required | 10(2.0) | 39(8.0) | 126(25.7) | 241(49.2) | 74(15.1) |
| Professionals* introduce their name to you | 181(36.9) | 182(37.1) | 57(11.6) | 52(10.6) | 18(3.7) |
| Professionals* spent enough time in consultation | 19(3.9) | 44(9.0) | 177(36.1) | 203(41.4) | 47(9.6) |
| Professionals* were respectful | 9(1.8) | 67(13.7) | 192(39.2) | 166(33.9) | 56(11.4) |
| Professionals* performs the procedure with cleanliness and sanitation | 5(1.0) | 4(0.8) | 50(10.2) | 287(58.6) | 144(29.4) |
| Professionals* explanation was clear and straightforward | 3(0.6) | 11(2.2) | 51(10.4) | 266(54.3) | 159(32.4) |
| Choice of methods available | 14(2.9) | 6(1.2) | 32(6.5) | 219(44.7) | 219(44.7) |
| Professionals* gave adequate information | 16(3.3) | 43(8.8) | 123(25.1) | 206(42.0) | 102(20.8) |
| Health facility easily accessible | 13(2.7) | 23(4.7) | 119(24.3) | 237(48.4) | 98(20.0) |
| Location of family planning service department | 7(1.4) | 37(7.6) | 160(32.7) | 198(40.4) | 88(18.0) |
| Waiting room has enough sitting chairs | 33(6.7) | 27(5.5) | 115(23.5) | 180(36.7) | 135(27.6) |
| Cleanliness of the health facility | 5(1.0) | 18(3.7) | 128(26.1) | 228(46.5) | 111(22.7) |

* Professionals* in this table indicated that those who provide family planning service in Public Health facilities of Bahir Dar city administration

**Table 4** Factors associated with client satisfaction with family planning service among respondents at public health facilities in Bahir Dar city administration, North West Ethiopia, March, 2017 ($n = 490$)

| Variables | | Family planning Service User | | COR(95% CI) | AOR (95% CI) | p-value |
|---|---|---|---|---|---|---|
| | | Satisfied (%) | Not satisfied (%) | | | |
| Marital status | Married | 275(67.6%) | 132(32.4%) | 1.4(0.9, 2.3)* | 1.76(0.9,3.3) | 0.080 |
| | Others | 49(59%) | 34(41%) | 1 | 1 | |
| Occupational status | Government employee | 46(47.9%) | 50(52.1%) | 1 | 1 | 0.007 |
| | Private employee | 29(50.0%) | 29(50.0%) | 1.1(0.7,2.1) | 1.2(0.6,2.5) | |
| | Merchant | 48(71.6%) | 19(28.4%) | 2.7(1.4,5.3)** | 2.5(1.2, 5.2)** | |
| | Housewife | 21(73.8%) | 43(26.2%) | 3.1(1.8,5.2)** | 2.4(1.3, 4.4)*** | |
| | Unemployed | 13(76.5%) | 4(23.5%) | 3.5(1.1,11.6)** | 3.3(0.8,12.8) | |
| | Student | 15(65.2%) | 8(34.8%) | 2.0(0.8,5.3 | 1.9(0.7, 5.8) | |
| | Daily laborer | 52(80.0%) | 13(20.0%) | 4.3(2.1, 9.0) | 3.9(1.8,8.6)*** | |
| FP visit | New | 88(72.1%) | 34(27.9%) | 1.2(0.9, 2.3)* | 2.3(1.3,4.0)*** | 0.004 |
| | Repeat | 236(64.1%) | 132(35.9%) | 1 | 1 | |
| Service hour convenience | No | 35(42.2%) | 48(57.8%) | 1 | 1 | 0.002 |
| | Yes | 289(71.0%) | 18(29.0%) | 3.4(2.1,5.5) | 2.4(1.4, 4.3)*** | |
| Waiting time | < 1/2 h | 166(73.5%) | 60(26.5%) | 6.9(2.6,18.7)** | 9.7(3.2, 29.3)*** | .001 |
| | ≥1/2to 1 h | 132(62.9%) | 78(37.1%) | 4.23(1.6,11.2) | 6.4(2.1, 19.2)*** | |
| | > 1 to 2 h | 20(60.6%) | 13(39.4%) | 3.85(1.2,12.5) | 4.6(1.3, 16.7)** | |
| | > 2 h | 6(28.6%) | 5(71.4%) | 1 | 1 | |
| Privacy | No | 33(39.3%) | 51(60.7%) | 1 | 1 | < 0.001 |
| | Yes | 291(71.7%) | 115(28.3%) | 3.9(2.4,6.37)*** | 3.2(1.8, 5.5)*** | |

NB: *P-Value < 0.2, **P-Value < 0.05, ***p-value < 0.01

satisfied and very satisfied with the service provider knowledge and skill (Table 3).

### Factors associated with client satisfaction among family planning service users at the public health facilities in Bahir Dar city administration, 2017

The variable such as, occupational, type of Family Planning visit, service hour convenient, privacy during counseling and waiting time for receiving the service were significantly associated with client satisfaction by using stepwise multivariable logistic regression.

Clients who were merchants were 2.5 times more likely to be satisfied with Family planning service delivered at Public Health facilities than government employees [AOR = 2.5(95% CI =1.2, 5.2)].

Clients those who are housewife were 2.4 times more likely to be satisfied with FP service delivered than government employees AOR = 2.4 (95% CI = 1.3, 4.4). Daily laborers were also found to be 3.9 times more likely to be satisfied with the FP service as compared with governmental employees AOR = 3.9(95% CI =1.8,8.6).

New family planning user clients were 2.3 times more likely to be satisfied with FP service than repeat users [AOR = 2.3 (95% CI =1.3–4.0)] (Table 4).

## Discussion

The result of this study revealed that 66.1% (95% CI: 61.2%, 70.1%) which is nearly two -third of respondents were satisfied with family planning services rendered by public health facilities in Bahir Dar city administration.

The overall satisfaction is low when it is compared with studies done in Jimma, south -west Ethiopia which was 77% [14] and the study done in Mozambique 86% [22]. The discrepancy might be due to the fact that the study which was conducted in Jimma, south-west Ethiopia was conducted in a specialized teaching hospital which has a relatively adequate number of health professionals and better diagnostic facilities. But for the study done in Mozambique, there is a difference in socio-demographic characteristics' of the study participants.

In this study, occupational status was found to be the factor which affects family planning service satisfaction in which being merchant, housewife, and, daily laborer were more likely to be satisfied with the family planning service as compared to the government employee. Similar results have been reported by other authors [22–24]. The possible reason might be in our study area, the governmental working hour and family planning service hour was the same and an overlapping of this might lead to governmental employees to be dissatisfied with the family planning service.

Service hour for family planning service was also found to be one of the factors which affects client satisfaction with family planning service, in which those having convince service hour were more likely to be satisfied with family planning service as compared to those who don't have convenient service hours. The possible reason might be due to the fact that having convenient service hour will help the women to utilize the service appropriately without overlapping of family planning service delivery and office work hour. This evidence is supported by studies done before [25].

A woman who comes for family planning service for the first time were more likely to be satisfied with the family planning service rendered by public facilities in Bahir Dar city than who had two and more family planning visits. This might be due to the fact that the doses of service given for first family planning service users is more comprehensive than those clients who are frequently using on it.

In this study, Service waiting time was also found to be the factors which affects the family planning service satisfaction in which clients having short waiting time were more likely to be satisfied as compared to those having long waiting time and this evidence was supported by other studies [26–28]. The possible reason might be, due to the fact that in the study area, the working hour is specific due to limited number of family planning serves providers [29], which might cause the service users to wait for long time.

Clients whose privacy was maintained during family planning counseling and procedures were more likely to be satisfied with the family planning service than those whose privacy was not maintained. The possible reason might be family planning is a very personal subject and people do not like to openly discuss their problems. Therefore, privacy is very much important in providing family planning services clients feel more comfortable if providers respect their privacy during counseling sessions, examinations, This evidence was supported by previous studies [18, 30].

### Limitations of the study

Since the study was cross- sectional study it is not far from pitfalls of cross -sectional study. We didn't found comparable findings to compare our findings for discussion and we are forced to compare with studies which done in the specialized hospitals. We have used a mean satisfaction score which is not far from the limitations of using mean. There might be courtesy bias too.

## Conclusions and recommendation

The finding of this study concludes that only nearly two -third of the clients are satisfied with the family planning service delivered at Public Health facilities of Northwest Ethiopia. Frequency of visit, waiting time, privacy during counseling, having convenience of service hour and occupation of the clients were the predictors of client satisfaction with family planning service.

Hence, in order to improve client satisfaction with family planning service in northwestern Ethiopia, it is better to give attention to repeat family planning service visitor, for those government employees, maintaining privacy during counseling to family planning service, shortened service waiting time and facilitating convenience service hour for family planning service delivery. Finally, Researchers are recommended to assess determinants of family planning service satisfaction using a strong study design.

**Acknowledgments**

The Authors would like to acknowledge Data collectors, study participants, supervisors and Bahir Dar University for financial support and Amhara National Regional State Health Bureau.

**Author details**

[1]Amhara Regional Health Office, Bahir Dar, Ethiopia. [2]Public Health Nutrition department, School of Public Health, Bahir Dar University, P.O.Box 79, Bahir Dar, Ethiopia. [3]Department of Epidemiology and Biostatistics', School of Public Health, Bahir Dar University, Bahir Dar, Ethiopia.

**References**

1. World Health Organization. Maternal mortality Geneva 2018 [updated April 2018]. 2018. Available from: http://www.who.int/news-room/fact-sheets/detail/maternal-mortality.
2. Alkema L, Chou D, Hogan D, Zhang S, Moller A-B, Gemmill A, et al. Global, regional, and national levels and trends in maternal mortality between 1990 and 2015, with scenario-based projections to 2030: a systematic analysis by the UN maternal mortality estimation inter-agency group. Lancet. 2016; 387(10017):462–74.
3. Central Statstical Agency(CSA). Central Statistical Agency (CSA) [Ethiopia] and ICF. In: Ethiopia Demographic and Health Survey 2016: Key Indicators Report. Addis Ababa, Ethiopia, and Rockville, Maryland, USA: CSA and ICF; 2016.
4. Federal Democratic Republic of Ethiopia Ministry of Health. Family Planning Module: Ethiopian Federal Ministry of Health. Planning F, 2017.
5. World Health Organization. Family planning/Contraception key fact sheet. Geneva; 2018. updated 8 February 2018. Available from: http://www.who.int/news-room/fact-sheets/detail/family-planning-contraception.
6. Cleland J, Bernstein S, Ezeh A, Faundes A, Glasier A, Innis J. Family planning: the unfinished agenda. Lancet. 2006;368(9549):1810–27.
7. Glasier AGA, Schmid G, et al. Sexual and reproductive health: a matter of life and death. Lancet. 2006;368(9547):1595–607.
8. World Health Organization. The World Health Report 2005 - make every mother and child count. Geneva: World Health Organizatio; 2005.
9. Moreland S, Smith E, Sharma S. World population prospects and unmet need for family planning, vol. 62. Washington, DC: Futures Group; 2010.
10. Ashford L. Unmet need for family planning: recent trends and their implications for programs: population reference bureau Washington, DC; 2003.
11. Wondimu Ayele HT, Gebreyes R, Tesfayi Gebreselassie Trends and Determinants of Unmet Need for Family Planning and Programme Options, Ethiopia. Further analysis of the 2000, 2005 and 2011 Demographic and health surveys. In: 81 DFARN. Calverton, Maryland, USA: ICF International; 2013.
12. Mekonnen W, Worku A. Determinants of low family planning use and high unmet need in Butajira District, South Central Ethiopia. Reproductive Health. 2011;8(1):37.
13. Baraitser P, Pearce V, Blake G, Collander-Brown K, Ridley A. Involving service users in sexual health service development. J Fam Plann Reprod Health Care. 2005;31(4):281–4.

14. Fikru TTF, Woldie M, Megerssa B. Quality of family planning service in primary health center of Jimma zone, south West Ethiopia. EthioJHealSci. 2013; 23(3):245–54.
15. CFAFWD. Satisfaction with focused antenatal care and association factors among pregnant women attending focused antenatal care at health center in jimmatowon ,Jimma zone South West Ethiopia ;a facility based cross sectional study triangulated with qualitative study. BMC Res. 2014;7(1):1–8.
16. AFMAM Y. Assessment client satisfaction with health service deliveries at Jimma University specialized hospital. Ethiopia JHealithSci. 2011;21(2):101–9.
17. A. H. Petient satisfaction with maternal and chaild health service among mothers attending maternal and chaild health training institution in Dhaka, banglandesh: Mahidol; 2007.
18. Tsegaye Gebre Argago KWH, Sena Belina Kitila. Clientssatisfaction with family planning services. 2015.
19. Tesfaye H T. Arbaminch statistical analysis of patient's satisfaction with hospital services: Acase study of shashemene and Hawassa university Ethiopia Arbaminch. 2009:1–6.
20. Agha S, Do M. The quality of family planning services and cliensatisfaction in the public and private sector in Kenya. IntJQualHealthcare. 2009;21(2):87–96.
21. N-AE. Determinants of customer satisfaction of health care in Ghana 2009; 1(2):50–61.
22. Chavane LDM, Bailey P, et al. Assessing women's satisfaction with family planning service in Mozambique. J Fam Plann Reprod Health Care. 2016;0:1–7.
23. Hekkert KD, Cihangir S, Kleefstra SM, van den Berg B, Kool RB. Patient satisfaction revisited: a multilevel approach. Soc Sci Med. 2009;69(1):68–75.
24. Birhanu Z, Assefa T, Woldie M, Morankar S. Determinants of satisfaction with health care provider interactions at health centres in central Ethiopia: a cross sectional study. BMC Health Serv Res. 2010;10(1):78.
25. Williams T, Schutt-Aine J, Cuca Y. Measuring family planning service quality through client satisfaction exit interviews. Int Fam Plan Perspect. 2000;26(2):63-71.
26. Simbar MAM, Ahmadi G. Quality assessment; birth control; customer satisfaction; individual perception; Iran. Int J Health Care Qual Assur. 2000;19(5):430–42.
27. Evaluation M. Quick investigation of quality (QIQ): . 2001.
28. Singh S, Darroch Michael EJ, Nadeau VJ. Investing in Contraception and Maternal and Newborn Health, 2017 [Internet]. New York: Guttmacher Institute; 2017 [cited 2017 July 26]. USA: GUTTMACHER INSTITUTE; 2014.
29. Tsegawe W. Assessment of quality of family planning service, Bahar Dar Special Zone, Amhara Regional State Addis Ababa; 2005.
30. Creel LC SJ, Yinger JV. . Client-centered quality: clients' perspectives and barriers to receiving care 2002.

# 15

# Factors associated with long acting and permanent contraceptive methods use in Ethiopia

Gedefaw Abeje Fekadu[1,2*], Akinyinka O. Omigbodun[3], Olumuyiwa A. Roberts[3] and Alemayehu Worku Yalew[4]


## Abstract

**Background:** Long acting and permanent contraceptives methods are more effective, save cost and enable women to control their reproductive lives better. Although the Ethiopian government is promoting its use through various mechanisms, the level of use is low. Therefore, this study was designed to identify factors associated with long acting and permanent contraceptive methods use in Ethiopia.

**Methods:** Four Ethiopian demographic and health survey data were used to examine trends of long acting and permanent contraceptive methods use. To identify factors associated with long acting and permanent contraceptive methods use, the 2016 Ethiopian demographic and health survey data was used. The data was accessed from the demographic and health survey program data base. Data analysis was done using Stata 15.1. Descriptive analysis was used to describe socio-economic and other variables of the study participants. Data were weighted and design effect was considered during analysis. Multicollinearity was assessed using variance inflation factor. Finally, multinomial logistic regression model was used to identify factors associated with long acting and permanent contraceptive methods use.

**Results:** Long acting and permanent contraceptive methods use increased significantly from 0.6% in 2000 to 11.6% in 2016. The odds of long acting and permanent contraceptive methods use was higher among richer women (AOR 2.6; 95%CI 1.2–5.4), women who were sales workers (AOR 2.1; 95%CI 1.1–3.9) and women whose ideal number of children was high (AOR; 4.2, 95%CI 1.4–13.0). But the odds of long acting and permanent contraceptive methods use was lower among female headed households (AOR 0.2: 95%CI 0.1–0.5) and women who had history of abortion (AOR 0.2: 95%CI 0.1–0.5).

**Conclusion:** Long acting and permanent contraceptive methods use increased significantly in Ethiopia. Wealth index, women's occupation, ideal number of children, sex of head of the household and history of abortion were factors associated with long acting and permanent contraceptive methods use in Ethiopia. Improving economic status of women may help improve long acting and permanent contraceptive methods use in Ethiopia.


**Keywords:** Ethiopia, Long acting and permanent contraceptives, Demographic and health survey

* Correspondence: abejegedefaw@gmail.com
[1]Pan African University, Institute of Life and Earth Sciences (including health and Agriculture), University of Ibadan, Ibadan, Nigeria
[2]College of Medicine and Health Sciences, School of Public Health, Bahir Dar University, Bahir Dar, Ethiopia

## Background

About 50% of women in developing regions of the world want to avoid pregnancy but only three quarters could do so. This causes unintended pregnancies [1]. Births from unintended pregnancies are more likely to suffer from many conditions [2]. In addition, unintended pregnancy increases unnecessary burden on public spending [3].

Long acting and permanent methods (LAPMs) are better options to reduce unintended pregnancies because these methods are more effective, save cost and enable women to control their reproductive lives better [4–6]. Use of long acting and permanent contraceptive methods can significantly increase contraceptive prevalence rate in countries with low contraceptive coverage [7]. Women using short acting contraceptives are 21 times more likely to have unintended pregnancy than women using long acting reversible and permanent methods [8]. A projection in SSA countries indicated that more than1.8 million unintended pregnancies would had been averted within 5 yrs period if 20% of women using oral contraceptives and injectable shift to implant [9].

On 2015, long acting and permanent contraceptive methods (Intra uterine device (IUD), implants and sterilization) accounted for 56% of contraceptive use globally. Nineteen percent of married or in-union women relied on female sterilization and 14% used IUD. Yet most contraceptive users in Africa depend on short term methods [7].

Lack of knowledge, myths, misconceptions and negative attitude about long acting and permanent contraceptive methods are the main barriers for long acting and permanent contraceptive method use in Ethiopia [10]. A study done at Adigrat town, Northwest Ethiopia reported that participants' knowledge of long acting and permanent contraceptive methods was limited to recognizing the names of the methods. The study added that women had fears and rumors about these methods and prefer methods which do not require procedure [11]. Another study conducted in Dangila town, Ethiopia showed that men had low knowledge about vasectomy [12].

Ethiopia's health service is structured into three-tier system: primary, secondary and tertiary. The primary level of care includes primary hospitals, health centers (HCs) and health posts (HPs). The primary health care unit (PHCU) comprises five satellite HPs (the lowest-level health facility at village level) and a referral HC. The secondary and tertiary level of care refers to the general hospitals and specialized hospitals respectively [13]. Both long acting and short acting contraceptive methods can be given at all levels of health care [14]. In addition, the government launched an implanon scale up program by task shifting; enabling health extension workers to insert implanon [15]. Family planning is also one of the packages of the health extension program, one of the flagship program in the Ethiopian health system [16].

The Ethiopia government planned to increase contraceptive prevalence rate to 55% in 2020. The government planned to increase implant and IUD to 33 and 15% respectively in the method mix [17]. All contraceptives including long acing and permanent contraceptive methods are provided free in Ethiopia [18]. Many governmental and nongovernmental organizations are providing long acting methods by outreach programs [14, 19]. Regardless of all these efforts, long acting and permanent contraceptive methods use is low. There is huge gap between total demand and demand satisfied. The current contraceptive method mix is dominated with short acting methods [7, 20]. Therefore, this study was designed to examine trends of long acting and permanent contraceptive methods use and identify factors associated with its use in Ethiopia.

## Methods

### Data

To identify factors associated with long acting and permanent contraceptive method use, the 2016 Ethiopian demographic and health survey (EDHS) data was used. The EDHS data was collected by the Central statistical Agency (CSA) at the request of the Federal Ministry of Health (FMoH). It was cross-sectional survey collected from January 18, 2016 to June 27, 2016.

The EDHS followed two stage stratified random sampling technique. Enumeration areas were selected in the first stage while households were selected in the second stage. The EDHS collected information about contraceptive use from all non-pregnant, fecund reproductive age women using structured and pretested questionnaire. From 15,683 reproductive age women interviewed for the 2016 EDHS, 9824 (62.6%) were married or in union at the time of survey. One thousand ninety women were excluded from the analysis because they reported being pregnant at the time of survey. Finally, 8734 married reproductive age women were included to identify factors associated with long acting and permanent contraceptive methods use. The data collectors were trained and had experience in data collection either in previous EDHS or other similar surveys. In addition, team supervisors, field editors, interviewers and secondary editors were recruited and trained by CSA. Data was collected and transferred to the CSA electronically via a secure Internet file streaming system (IFSS) and were stored on a password-protected computer. Then secondary editor resolves computer identified inconsistencies, code open ended questions and perform other activities. All four EDHS (EDHS 2000, 2005, 2011 and 2016) data were used to examine trends of long acting and permanent contraceptive method use.

*Measurement*

**Outcome variable** The outcome variable for this study was contraceptive use. For this analysis, contraceptive use was grouped in to three categories; not using any method, using long acting and permanent contraceptive methods (IUD, female sterilization and implant) and using other methods (short acting and traditional).

**Independent variables** The independent variables of the study were categorized in to three groups; socio-demographic, fertility and decision making related, and exposure to family planning programs. Some variables were recoded to have meaningful and small categories.

The main socio-demographic variables include;

- Age, region, place of residence, educational status, religion, occupation, working status and ethnicity of the woman, household wealth index, sex of head of the household, age, educational status and occupation of partner

Fertility and decision making related variables were;

- Fertility preference, desire for more children, ideal number of children, husband's desire for more children, number of children ever born, age at first cohabitation, history of abortion
- Decision on how to spend earning, on health care, on large household purchase, to visit family and on first marriage

Family planning program exposure variables were

- Knowledge of the ovulatory period, knowledge of time of fertility, frequency of reading newspaper, frequency of listening radio, heard family planning messages on radio, heard family planning messages on TV, read family planning messages on newspaper, heard family planning messages by mobile phone, visited by health worker, health worker talked about family planning, visited health facility, told about family planning in the health facility.

**Analytical methods** After getting permission, the data was downloaded from the DHS program official data base. Analysis was done using Stata 15.1. Open EPI software was used to examine whether there was significant linear trend in long acting and permanent contraceptive methods use in Ethiopia over time. Descriptive analysis was used to describe socio-economic and other variables of the study participants. Tables and graphs were used to present results. The data were weighted to consider the disproportionate sampling and non-response. In addition, the effect of sample design was handled when computing confidence intervals and standard errors. Before running the final model, multicollinearity was assessed using variance inflation factor. Variables highly correlated with other independent variables were excluded from the final multinomial logistic regression model. Permission to use data was obtained from the DHS programs.

## Result

### Socio-demographic characteristics of women

Majority of women were aged 20–34 years. Similarly, most of the participants (83.8%) were rural residents. About two third of mothers did not attend formal education. About 69 % of mothers were not working at the time of survey (Table 1).

### Fertility and decision making

The mean ages at first cohabitation and first sex were 17.2 (±4.0) and 16.8 (±3.3) years respectively. The mean number of children ever born was 3.8 (±2.8). The survey indicated that women in Ethiopia had limited knowledge about fertile period. Among all married reproductive age women, only 22.9% correctly know the ovulatory period and only 56.8% knew a woman can get pregnant after birth and before period. A little more than half of the mothers desired to have other children. Majority of women cohabited at age less than 20 years. About two third (60.7%) women reported that their marriage was arranged by parents. About 66 % of women reported that their health care was decided jointly (by partner and themselves) (Table 2).

### Exposure to family planning programs

Majority of women did not read newspaper at all (91.7%) did not listen radio at all (69.7%) and did not watch TV at all (76.7%). About 79% women did not own mobile phone. Almost all (97.6%) women never used internet. Only 22.2, 14.1 and 3.3% women reported that they had heard family planning messages on radio, watched on TV and read on newspaper/magazine respectively on the last few months. Only 2.1% women reported that they had received family planning related text message on mobile on the last few months. Many women (70.3%) reported that they were not visited by health worker in the last 12 months (Table 3).

### Contraceptive use

About 59 % (95%CI: 55.9–63.0%) women reported that they had ever used or tried something to delay or avoid pregnancy. About one-fourth of mothers (95%CI 26.4–30.9%) reported that they were using short acting or traditional contraceptives methods while 11.6% (95%CI 10.2–13.1%) were using long acting or permanent contraceptive methods. Specifically, 8.8% (95%CI: 7.7–

**Table 1** Socio-demographic characteristics of reproductive age married or in union women in Ethiopia, 2016

| Variable | Frequency | Percent |
|---|---|---|
| Age | | |
| 15–19 | 501 | 5.5 |
| 20–24 | 1425 | 15.6 |
| 25–29 | 2075 | 22.7 |
| 30–34 | 1828 | 20.0 |
| 35–39 | 1487 | 16.3 |
| 40–44 | 1021 | 11.2 |
| 45–49 | 790 | 8.7 |
| Place of residence | | |
| Urban | 1505 | 16.5 |
| Rural | 7622 | 83.5 |
| Highest education attended | | |
| No education | 5666 | 62.1 |
| Primary | 2517 | 27.6 |
| Secondary | 563 | 6.2 |
| Higher | 381 | 4.2 |
| Religion | | |
| Orthodox | 3793 | 41.6 |
| Protestant | 3066 | 33.6 |
| Muslim | 2050 | 22.5 |
| Other | 218 | 2.4 |
| Wealth index | | |
| Poorest | 1708 | 18.7 |
| Poorer | 1814 | 19.9 |
| Middle | 1854 | 20.3 |
| Richer | 1806 | 19.8 |
| Richest | 1946 | 21.3 |
| Husband/partner's educational level | | |
| No education | 4203 | 46.1 |
| Primary | 3361 | 36.8 |
| Secondary | 846 | 9.3 |
| Higher | 643 | 7 |
| Do not know | 74 | 0.8 |
| Husband's/partner occupation | | |
| Not working | 729 | 8.0 |
| Sales worker | 623 | 6.8 |
| Skilled agriculture | 835 | 9.1 |
| Subsistence farming | 4604 | 50.4 |
| Other | 2336 | 25.6 |
| Currently working | | |
| Yes | 6250 | 68.5 |
| No | 2877 | 31.5 |
| Women's occupation | | |
| Not working | 4664 | 51.1 |
| Agriculture | 2131 | 23.4 |
| Sales | 1225 | 13.4 |
| Other | 1106 | 12.1 |
| Sex of head of the household | | |
| Male | 7941 | 87.0 |
| Female | 1186 | 13.0 |

*Table 1 (Continued)*

10.1%) and 2.3% (95%CI: 1.7–3.0%) women were using implants and IUD respectively.

**Trends in LAPM contraceptive method use**

Long acting and permanent contraceptive method use increased significantly (Extended MH chi square for linear trend = 1421.15, $p < 0.01$) from 0.5% in 2000 to 11.6% in 2016. Implant use showed the highest change from 0.04% in 2000 to 8.8% in 2016 (Extended MH chi square for linear trend = 1231.41, $p < 0.01$) (Fig. 1). When analyzing the percent change in long acting and permanent contraceptive method use, the highest percentage of change was observed between 2005 and 2011. Both female sterilization and implant use showed the highest percentage increase at this period. But for IUD use, the highest increase was observed from 2011 to 2016 (Fig. 2).

**Factors associated with long acting and permanent contraceptive method use**

Multinomial logistic regression model was fitted to identify factors associated with long acting and permanent contraceptive method use. The analysis indicated that wealth index, occupation, sex of head of the household, history of abortion and ideal number of children were significantly associated with long acting and permanent contraceptive methods use (Table 4).

The odds of using long acting and permanent contraceptive methods compared to those not using any method for women in the richer wealth index was 2.6 (AOR 2.6; 95%CI 1.2–5.4) times higher compared to women in the poorest wealth quintile. Similarly, the odds of using long acting and permanent contraceptive methods compared to not using for women who were sales worker was 2.1 (AOR 2.1; 95%CI 1.1–3.9) times higher compared to women who were not working at the time of survey.

The odds of using long acting and permanent contraceptive methods compared to not using for women living in female headed households was 80% lower (AOR

**Table 2** Fertility and decision making characteristics of married or in union reproductive age women in Ethiopia, 2016

| Variable | Frequency | Percent |
|---|---|---|
| Knowledge of ovulatory period | | |
| During her period | 352 | 3.9 |
| After period ended | 2518 | 27.6 |
| Middle of the cycle | 2093 | 22.9 |
| Before period begins | 661 | 7.2 |
| At any time | 1894 | 20.7 |
| Do not know | 1610 | 17.6 |
| History of abortion | | |
| No | 8148 | 89.3 |
| Yes | 979 | 10.7 |
| Pregnancy can occur after birth and before period | | |
| No | 3349 | 36.7 |
| Yes | 5183 | 56.8 |
| Do not know | 595 | 6.5 |
| Fertility preference | | |
| Have another | 5084 | 55.7 |
| Undecided | 460 | 5.0 |
| No more | 3376 | 37.0 |
| Other | 206 | 2.3 |
| Ideal number of children | | |
| No child | 720 | 7.9 |
| 1–5 | 4327 | 47.4 |
| > 5 | 2926 | 32.1 |
| Non numeric | 1155 | 12.7 |
| Concordance on number of children | | |
| Both wants same | 3579 | 39.4 |
| Husband wants more | 2341 | 25.8 |
| Husband wants fewer | 662 | 7.3 |
| Do not know | 2503 | 27.6 |
| Number of children ever born | | |
| No child | 667 | 7.3 |
| 1–4 | 4688 | 51.4 |
| > 4 | 3771 | 41.3 |
| Number of living children | | |
| No living child | 709 | 7.8 |
| 1–3 children | 4031 | 44.2 |
| 4 or more children | 4387 | 48.1 |
| Age at first cohabitation | | |
| ≤ 19 years | 7224 | 79.1 |
| 20–24 years | 1476 | 16.2 |
| 25–29 | 330 | 3.6 |
| 30 or more | 97 | 1.1 |

**Table 2** Fertility and decision making characteristics of married or in union reproductive age women in Ethiopia, 2016 *(Continued)*

| Variable | Frequency | Percent |
|---|---|---|
| Decision maker on the respondent's health care | | |
| Respondent alone | 1434 | 15.7 |
| Respondent & partner | 6029 | 66.1 |
| Partner alone | 1623 | 17.8 |
| Other | 41 | 0.4 |
| Decision maker on large household purchase | | |
| Respondent alone | | |
| Respondent & partner | 993 | 10.9 |
| Partner alone | 6181 | 67.7 |
| Other | 1912 | 20.9 |
| | 40 | 0.4 |
| Decision maker to visit family or relatives | | |
| Respondent alone | 1670 | 18.3 |
| Respondent & partner | 6007 | 65.8 |
| Partner alone | 1422 | 15.6 |
| Other | 28 | 0.3 |
| Decision maker on what to do with husband money | | |
| Respondent alone | 636 | 7.0 |
| Respondent & partner | 6291 | 68.9 |
| Partner alone | 1998 | 21.9 |
| Other | 148 | 1.6 |
| Decision maker on respondent's first marriage | | |
| Self | 3215 | 35.2 |
| Parents | 5536 | 60.7 |
| Other | 376 | 4.1 |

0.2; 95%CI 0.1–0.5) compared to women living in male headed household. The odds of using long acting and permanent of contraceptive methods compared to not using for women who had history of abortion was 80% lower (AOR 0.5; 95%CI 0.1–0.5) compared to women who had no history of abortion. Similarly, The odds of using long acting and permanent method of contraceptive compared to not using for women whose ideal number of children is 1–5 was 4.2 (AOR; 4.2, 95%CI 1.4–13.0) times higher compared to women who desired no more children.

## Discussion

### Long acting and permanent contraceptive method use

This analysis identified that only 11.6% Ethiopian mothers were using long acting or permanent contraceptive methods. About 9 and 2% of mothers were using implants and IUD respectively. The proportion of women using female sterilization (0.4%) was almost negligible. Vasectomy was nil. The proportion of women using long acting and permanent

**Table 3** Exposure to mass media and family planning messages among married or in union reproductive age women in Ethiopia, 2016

| Exposure variable | Number | Percent |
|---|---|---|
| Frequency of reading newspaper | | |
| Not at all | 8371 | 91.7 |
| Less than once a week | 552 | 6.0 |
| At least once a week | 205 | 2.2 |
| Frequency of listening radio | | |
| Not at all | 6360 | 69.7 |
| Less than once a week | 1383 | 15.2 |
| At least once a week | 1384 | 15.2 |
| Frequency of watching TV | | |
| Not at all | 6996 | 76.7 |
| Less than once a week | 1013 | 11.1 |
| At least once a week | 1117 | 12.2 |
| Own mobile phone | | |
| No | 7192 | 78.8 |
| Yes | 1935 | 21.2 |
| Use of internet | | |
| Never | 8911 | 97.6 |
| Yes | 216 | 2.3 |
| Heard family planning message on radio on last few months | | |
| No | 7103 | 77.8 |
| Yes | 2024 | 22.2 |
| Heard family planning messages on TV on last few months | | |
| No | 7837 | 85.9 |
| Yes | 1290 | 14.1 |
| Read about family planning messages on newspaper/magazine last few months | | |
| No | 8827 | 96.7 |
| Yes | 300 | 3.3 |
| Received family planning text message on mobile phone | | |
| No | 8936 | 97.9 |
| Yes | 191 | 2.1 |
| Visited by field worker in the last 12 months | | |
| No | 6431 | 70.5 |
| Yes | 2696 | 29.5 |
| Field worker talk about family planning | | |
| No | 1068 | 39.6 |
| Yes | 1628 | 60.4 |
| Visited health facility in the last 12 months | | |
| No | 4682 | 51.3 |
| Yes | 4445 | 48.7 |
| Told about family planning in the health facility | | |
| No | 2669 | 60.0 |
| Yes | 1777 | 40.0 |

contraceptives methods was very low compared to the national family planning target of 2020 and the existing high demand for long acting and permanent contraceptive methods. The current practice was also low compared to the national health sector transformation plan and the family planning coasted implementation targets (to increase contraceptive prevalence rate to 55% at the end of 2020 by increasing the share of implant, IUD, female sterilization and vasectomy to 33, 15, 1.5 and 0.5% respectively in the method mix) [20]. In addition, the method mix was dominated by short acting contraceptive methods. Therefore, the government shall intensify task shifting activities launched on 2009. Awareness creation activities to avoid the prevailing myths and misconceptions are crucial.

The proportion of women using long acting and permanent contraceptive methods in this study (11.6%) was much lower than the level of use at global level (which accounted for 56%). In 2015, 19% of married or in-union women relied on female sterilization and 14% used the IUD [7]. The proportion of women using long acting and permanent contraceptive methods in Ethiopia was lower than a study conducted in Kampala, Uganda [21]. But it was similar with a study conducted in Rwanda (10.4%) [22].

The level of long acting and permanent contraceptive method use in this study was lower than meta-analysis done in Ethiopia [23]. The reason for this is that most of the studies included in the meta-analysis were facility based and based on urban settings both of which increase the proportion of women using long acting and permanent contraceptive methods [24–29].

#### Trends of long acting and permanent contraceptive method use

Long acting and permanent contraceptive methods use increased significantly (Extended MH Chi square for linear trend = 1421.15, $p < 0.01$) in the 16 years period although the level of use was still low compared to the national targets and the existing demand. This finding was similar with a study conducted in Lusaka Zambia which showed that long acting and reversible method use increased from less than 1 to 9% from 2004 to 2011 [30].

Implant use showed the highest change from 0.04% use in 2000 to 8.8% in 2016. This may be due to the task shift designed by the ministry of health. Health extension workers were trained to insert implants [31]. This made the implant accessible to the rural women. The highest percentage change in long acting and permanent contraceptive methods use was observed between 2005 and 2011. The percent change in long acting and permanent contraceptive use was lower from 2011 to 2016. The reason for this may be the presence of high demand for long acting and permanent contraceptive methods from 2005 to 2011. In addition, the government exerted significant effort to address that need at

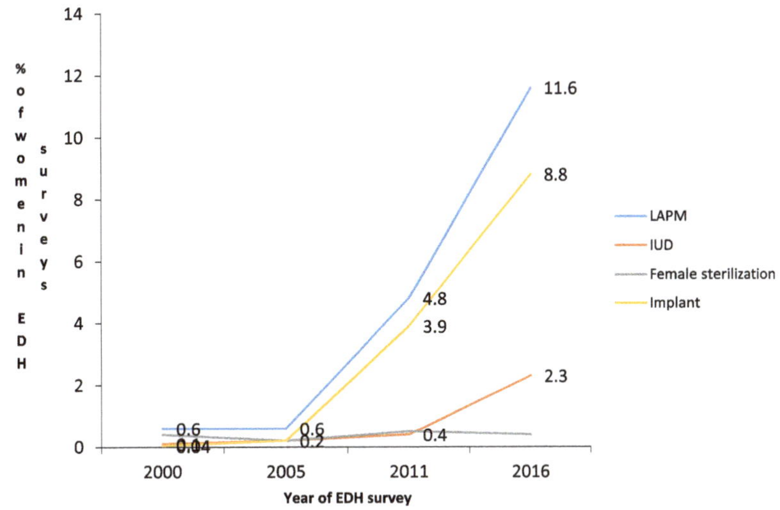


**Fig. 1** Trends in long acting and permanent contraceptive method use in Ethiopia, from 2000 to 2016

that time. Since that huge gap was addressed from 20,005 to 2011, the percent change from 2011 to 2016 seems lower. But this does not mean long acting and permanent contraceptive method use was lower. Both female sterilization and implant showed the highest percentage increase at this period. But for IUD use, the highest increase was observed from 2011 to 2016. Further qualitative study is needed to explore the reason and learn to increase long acting and permanent contraceptive methods use in Ethiopia.

### Factors associated with long acting and permanent contraceptive method use

The odds of using long acting and permanent contraceptive methods compared to non-use for women in the richer wealth index was higher compared to women in the poorest wealth quintile. This finding was similar with a multi country study conducted in developing countries based on DHS data and the 2011 EDHS data [32, 33]. This may be due to financial barriers to access long acting and permanent methods of contraceptives in Ethiopia. Except implants which are available in health posts, other long acting and permanent contraceptive methods are not easily accessible in Ethiopia. The users have to travel to access these methods of contraceptives. In addition, there is belief or misconception that long acting and permanent contraceptive methods are not convenient for working women [11, 34]. And the poorest are more likely to engage in activities which are more labor intensive. Because of this, the poor may refrain from using these methods.

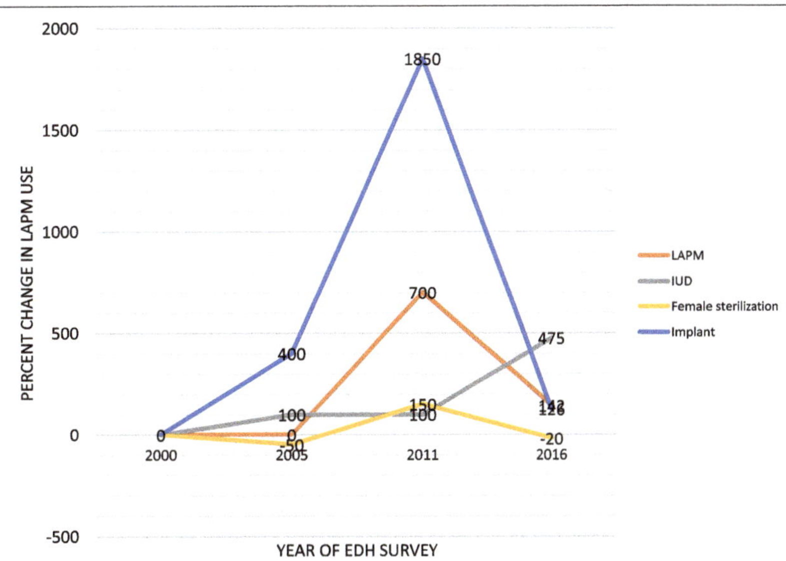


**Fig. 2** Percent change in long acting and permanent contraceptive method use among married or in union reproductive age women in Ethiopia, 2000–2016

**Table 4** Factors associated with long acting and permanent contraceptive methods use in Ethiopia, 2016

| Variable | LAPM use AOR(95%CI) |
|---|---|
| Region | |
| Tigray | 1.0 |
| Amhara | 1.3(0.4–4.4) |
| Oromia | 0.4(0.1–1.7) |
| SNNPR | 1.1(0.2–5.6) |
| Addis Ababa | 1.5(0.5–5.2) |
| Other regions | 0.4(0.1–1.4) |
| Highest education attended | |
| No education | 1.0 |
| Primary | 0.9(0.5–1.5) |
| Secondary | 0.8(0.3–1.9) |
| Higher | 1.4(0.5–3.7) |
| Religion | |
| Orthodox | 1.0 |
| Muslim | 0.9(0.4–2.0) |
| Protestant | 2.0(0.8–4.6) |
| Other | 0.03(0.005–0.2) |
| Ethnicity | |
| Amhara | 1.0 |
| Oromo | 1.4 (0.5–4.0) |
| Tigrie | 0.9(0.3–2.9) |
| Sidama | 0.7(0.1–3.4) |
| Welaita | 0. 3(0.04–2.8) |
| Other | 0.4(0.1–1.2) |
| Wealth index | |
| Poorest | 1.00 |
| Poorer | 1.5(0.7–3.3) |
| Middle | 1.8(0.9–3.8) |
| Richer | 2.6(1.2–5.4)** |
| Richest | 2.1(0.8–7.3) |
| Husband's/partner occupation | |
| Did not work | 1.0 |
| Sales worker | 2.0(0.6–6.5) |
| Skilled agriculture | 2.2(0.7–7.3) |
| Subsistence farming | 2.2(0.7–7.3) |
| Other | 2.4(0.8–7.3) |
| Women's occupation | |
| Not working | 1.0 |
| Agriculture | 1.7(0.9–2.9) |
| Sales | 2.1(1.1–3.9)* |
| Other | 1.7(1.0–3.1) |
| Sex of head of the household | |
| Female | 0.2(0.1–0.5)*** |
| Male | 1.00 |

**Table 4** Factors associated with long acting and permanent contraceptive methods use in Ethiopia, 2016 *(Continued)*

| Variable | LAPM use AOR(95%CI) |
|---|---|
| Use of internet | |
| Never | 1.0 |
| Yes | 1.6(0.7–4.1) |
| Time of ovulation | |
| Middle of the cycle | 1.0 |
| Other | 0.8(0.5–1.3) |
| History of abortion | |
| No | 1.0 |
| Yes | 0.2 (0.1–0.5)*** |
| Pregnancy can occur after birth and before period | |
| No | 1.0 |
| Yes | 1.0(0.7–1.5) |
| Ideal number of children | |
| No child | 1.0 |
| 1–5 children | 4.2(1.4–13.0)* |
| More than five | 2.1(0.7–6.1) |
| Non numeric | 2.2(0.6–7.8) |
| Concordance on number of children | |
| Husband wants more | 1.0 |
| Both wants same | 0.7(0.4–1.1) |
| Husband wants fewer | 0.7(0.4–1.1) |
| Do not know | 0.6(0.3–1.0) |
| Number of living children | 1.00(0.8–1.1) |
| Age at first cohabitation | 1.0(0.8–1.0) |
| Heard family planning on radio on last few months | |
| No | 1.0 |
| Yes | 0.9(0.7–1.3) |
| Hear family planning by text message on mobile phone | |
| No | 1.0 |
| Yes | 2.6(0.8–8.7) |
| Heard about family planning at community event/conversation | |
| No | 1.0 |
| Yes | 0.7(0.5–1.1) |
| Field worker talked about family planning | |
| No | 1.0 |
| Yes | 1.4(0.9–2.1) |
| Visited health facility in the last 12 months | |
| No | 1.0 |
| Yes | 0.8(0.5–1.3) |
| Decision on your first marriage | |
| Self | 1.0 |
| Parents | 0.7(0.4–1.1) |
| Other | 1.0(0.4–1.5) |

The odds of using long acting and permanent contraceptive methods compared to non-use for women who were sales worker was higher compared to women who were not working. Many studies in Ethiopia identified that occupation is associated with long acting and permanent contraceptive methods use. A study in Harar city indicated that daily laborers were less likely to use long acting reversible contraceptive methods compared to house wives [35]. A study conducted in Jigjiga showed that employee women were more likely to use long acting and permanent contraceptive methods compared to house wives [36]. Similar study in Areka town, Southern Ethiopia, indicated that government employees were more likely to use long acting and reversible methods [37]. The possible reason for this is that sales workers are better educated than others which improves their information processing skill. From the data, about 33% of nonworking women attended no education but only 6.2% of sales women did so. Sales workers had also better access to mass media which exposes them to family planning messages. There are evidences in Ethiopia that indicate educated women are more likely to use long acting and permanent contraceptive methods compared to women who did not attend formal education [35, 38, 39].

The odds of using long acting and permanent contraceptive methods compared to non-use for women living in female headed households was lower compared to women living in male headed household. This finding was similar with a study conducted in Lesotho [40]. The possible reason for this may be that female headed households do have less frequent sexual intercourse compared to male headed households. The husband may be away from home for different reasons. As a result the woman may not use contraceptives or may use short acting methods.

The odds of using long acting and permanent contraceptive methods compared to non-use for women who had history of abortion was lower compared to women who had no history of abortion. This finding contradicts a study in Luanda, Angola, which indicated that history of abortion was associated with contraceptive use [41]. The reason for this may be that women with abortion may have desire for other children. These women may not use contraceptives or will use short acting methods. Women who had abortion may also associate the abortion with long acting methods use and refrain from using.

The odds of using long acting and permanent methods of contraceptive compared to not using for women whose ideal number of children is 1–5 was higher compared to women who did not want any child. This finding contradict with a community based study conducted in Amhara region, Ethiopia which indicated that women with higher ideal number of children are less likely to use long acting methods [42]. The reason for this may be that women who desired no children are older women who are using short acting methods or not using any method thinking that they are approaching menopause.

The strength of this study is that it is based on nationally representative, large data. On the other hand, some factors are not included in the analysis as it is secondary data.

## Conclusion

Although increasing significantly, the current level of long acting and permanent contraceptive methods use was still low in Ethiopia compared to the national targets. The odds of long acting and permanent contraceptive methods use were high among women in the richer wealth index, among women who were sales workers and among women who desired more children. On the other hand, the odds of use were lower among women with female headed households and women with history of abortion.

Further research is needed to identify the different levels of change in long acting and contraceptive use in Ethiopia. Emphasis should be given to women in the lower wealth quintile and women who had history of abortion to improve long acting and permanent contraceptive method use.

### Abbreviations

AOR: Adjusted Odds Ratio; CSA: Central Statistical Agency; EDHS: Ethiopian Demographic and Health Survey; FMoH: Federal Ministry of Health; IUD: Intrauterine Device; LAPM: Long Acting and Permanent contraceptive method; MH: Mantel-Haenszel; SSA: Sub-Saharan Africa; TV: Television

### Acknowledgements

The authors would like to acknowledge Pan African University, Institute of Life and Earth Science (including health and agriculture) and University College Hospital, Ibadan University for all assistance to prepare this manuscript. The authors are grateful to the DHS programs for allowing the data to use.

### Authors' contribution

Mr. Gedefaw Abeje Fekadu initiated the study, analyzed the data and prepared the manuscript. Professor Akinyinka O. Omigbodun, Dr. Olumuyiwa A. Roberts and Professor Alemayehu Worku Yalew assisted the development of the research idea, the analysis, interpretation and preparation of the manuscript. All authors read and approved the final manuscript.

### Author's information

Mr. Gedefaw Abeje Fekadu is PhD candidate in Reproductive health sciences Pan African University, Institute of Life and Earth Science (including health and agriculture), University of Ibadan, Ibadan, Nigeria and assistant professor of reproductive health in Bahir Dar University, Bahir Dar, Ethiopia. Professor Akinyinka O. Omigbodun is senior gynecologist and obstetrician in University College Hospital, University of Ibadan, Ibadan, Nigeria. Dr. Olumuyiwa A. Roberts is also senior gynecologist and obstetrician in the same institute. Professor Alemayehu Worku Yalew is professor of public health in Addis Ababa University, School of Public Health.

### Author details

[1]Pan African University, Institute of Life and Earth Sciences (including health and Agriculture), University of Ibadan, Ibadan, Nigeria. [2]College of Medicine and Health Sciences, School of Public Health, Bahir Dar University, Bahir Dar,

Ethiopia. [3]University College Hospital, University of Ibadan, Ibadan, Nigeria. [4]School of Public health, College of Medicine, Addis Ababa University, Addis Ababa, Ethiopia.

**References**


1. Guttmacher Intitute. Adding it up: investing in contraception and maternal and newborn health, 2017. 2017.
2. Gipson JD, Koenig MA, Hindin MJ. The effects of unintended pregnancy on infant, child, and parental health: a review of the literature. Stud Fam Plan. 2008;39(1):18–38.
3. Sonfield A, Kost K, Gold RB, Finer LB. The public costs of births resulting from unintended pregnancies: national and state-level estimates. Perspect Sex Reprod Health. 2011;43(2):94–102.
4. Blumenthal P, Voedisch A, Gemzell-Danielsson K. Strategies to prevent unintended pregnancy: increasing use of long-acting reversible contraception. Hum Reprod Update. 2010;17(1):121–37.
5. Joshi R, Khadilkar S, Patel M. Global trends in use of long-acting reversible and permanent methods of contraception: seeking a balance. Int J Gynecol Obstet. 2015;131:S60–S3.
6. Winner B, Peipert JF, Zhao Q, Buckel C, Madden T, Allsworth JE, et al. Effectiveness of long-acting reversible contraception. N Engl J Med. 2012; 366(21):1998–2007.
7. United Nations Department of economic and social affairs population division. Trends in contraceptive use worldwide 2015. 2015.
8. Lotke PS. Increasing use of long-acting reversible contraception to decrease unplanned pregnancy. Obstet Gynecol Clin N Am. 2015;42(4):557–67.
9. Hubacher D, Mavranezouli I, McGinn E. Unintended pregnancy in sub-Saharan Africa: magnitude of the problem and potential role of contraceptive implants to alleviate it. Contraception. 2008;78(1):73–8.
10. Mengistu Meskele WM. Factors affecting women's intention to use long acting and permanent contraceptive methods in Wolaita zone, southern Ethiopia: a cross-sectional study. BMC women's health. 2014;14:109.
11. Gebremariam A, Addissie A. Knowledge and perception on long acting and permanent contraceptive methods in Adigrat town, Tigray, northern Ethiopia: a qualitative study. Int J Family Med. 2014;2014.
12. Abrham Jemberie Temach GAFaAAA. Educational status as determinant of men's knowledge about vasectomy in Dangila town administration, Amhara region, Northwest Ethiopia. Reprod Health. 2017;14(54).
13. Organization WH. Primary health care systems (PRIMASYS): case study from Ethiopia, abridged version. Geneva2017.
14. Federal Democratic Republic of Ethiopia Ministry of Health. National Guideline for family planning Services in Ethiopia. 2011.
15. Yewondwossen Tilahun CL, Belayihun B, Hagos KL, Asnake M. Improving contraceptive access, use, and method mix by task sharing Implanon insertion to frontline health workers: the experience of the integrated family health program in Ethiopia. Global Health: Science and Practice. 2017;5(4).
16. MoH E. In: Heae c, editor. Health extension program in Ethiopia; 2007.
17. Federal democratic republic of Ethiopia ministry of health. Health sector transformation plan. 2015.
18. Ministry of Health Ethiopia, PMNCH, WHO, World Bank, AHPSR, Participants in the Ethiopia multistakeholder policy review (2015). Success Factors for Women's and Children's Health: Ethiopia. 2015.
19. Federal Democratic Republic of Ethiopia Minstry of Health. Family Planning 2017 [updated August 27, 2017]. Available from: http://www.moh.gov.et/ejcc/en/mch.
20. Minstry of Health Ethiopia. Costed implementation plan for family planning in Ethiopia, 2015/16–2020. 2016.
21. Anguzu R, Tweheyo R, Sekandi JN, Zalwango V, Muhumuza C, Tusiime S, et al. Knowledge and attitudes towards use of long acting reversible contraceptives among women of reproductive age in Lubaga division, Kampala district, Uganda. BMC research notes. 2014;7(1):153.
22. Bikorimana E. Barriers to the use of long acting contraceptive methods among married women of reproductive age in Kicukiro District. Rwanda International Journal of Scientific and Research Publications. 2015:513.
23. Mesfin YM, Kibret KT. Practice and intention to use long acting and permanent contraceptive methods among married women in Ethiopia: systematic meta-analysis. Reprod Health. 2016;13(1):78.
24. Melka AS, Tekelab T, Wirtu D. Determinants of long acting and permanent contraceptive methods utilization among married women of reproductive age groups in western Ethiopia: a cross-sectional study. Pan African Medical Journal. 2015;22(1).
25. Takele A, Degu G, Yitayal M. Demand for long acting and permanent methods of contraceptives and factors for non-use among married women of Goba town, bale zone, south East Ethiopia. Reprod Health. 2012;9(1):26.
26. Bulto GA, Zewdie TA, Beyen TK. Demand for long acting and permanent contraceptive methods and associated factors among married women of reproductive age group in Debre Markos town, north West Ethiopia. BMC Womens Health. 2014;14(1):46.
27. Mekonnen G, Enquselassie F, Tesfaye G, Semahegn A. Prevalence and factors affecting use of long acting and permanent contraceptive methods in Jinka town, southern Ethiopia: a cross sectional study. Pan African Medical Journal. 2014;18(1).
28. Haile A, Fantahun M. Demand for long acting and permanent contraceptive methods and associated factors among family planning service users, Batu town, Central Ethiopia. Ethiop Med J. 2012;50(1):31–42.
29. Alemayehu M, Belachew T, Tilahun T. Factors associated with utilization of long acting and permanent contraceptive methods among married women of reproductive age in Mekelle town, Tigray region, North Ethiopia. BMC pregnancy childbirth. 2012;12(1):6.
30. Hancock NL, Chibwesha CJ, Stoner MC, Vwalika B, Rathod SD, Kasaro MP, et al. Temporal trends and predictors of modern contraceptive use in Lusaka, Zambia, 2004–2011. Biomed Res Int. 2015;2015.
31. International P. Scale-up of task-shifting for community-based provision of Implanon. 2009–2011.
32. Ugaz JI, Chatterji M, Gribble JN, Banke K. Is household wealth associated with use of long-acting reversible and permanent methods of contraception? A multi-country analysis. Global Health: Science and Practice. 2016;4(1):43–54.
33. Yigzaw M, Zakus D, Tadesse Y, Desalegn M, Fantahun M. Paving the way for universal family planning coverage in Ethiopia: an analysis of wealth related inequality. Int J Equity Health. 2015;14(1):77.
34. Tilahun Y, Mehta S, Zerihun H, Lew C, Brooks MI, Nigatu T, et al. Expanding access to the intrauterine device in public health facilities in Ethiopia: a mixed-methods study. Global Health: Science and Practice. 2016;4(1):16–28.
35. Shiferaw K, Musa A. Assessment of utilization of long acting reversible contraceptive and associated factors among women of reproductive age in Harar City. Ethiopia Pan African Medical Journal. 2017;28(1).
36. Abdisa B, Mideksa L. Factors associated with utilization of long acting and permanent contraceptive methods among women of reproductive age Group in Jigjiga Town. Anat Physiol. 2017;7(254).
37. Kabalo MY. Utilization of reversible long acting family planning methods among married 15-49 years women in Areka town, southern Ethiopia. International Journal of Scientific Reports. 2016;2(1):1–6.
38. Tekelab T, Sufa A, Wirtu D. Factors affecting intention to use long acting and permanent contraceptive methods among married women eproductive age groups in Western Ethiopia: a community based cross sectional study. Fam Med Med Sci Res. 2015;4(158):2.
39. Bayisa A, Lema M. Factors associated with utilization of long acting and permanent contraceptive methods among women of reproductive age Group in Jigjiga Town. Anat Physiol. 2017;7(256).
40. Makatjane T. Contraceptive prevalence in Lesotho: does the sex of the household head matter? Afr Popul Stud. 1997;12(2):1–11.
41. Morris N, Prata N. Abortion history and its association with current use of modern contraceptive methods in Luanda, Angola. Open Access J Contracept. 2018;9:45.
42. Nejimu Biza MA, Surender Reddy P. Long acting reversible contraceptive use and associated factors among contraceptive users in Amhara Region, Ethopia, a community based cross sectional study. Med Res Chron. 2017;4(5).

# 16

# Determinants of modern contraceptive use among postpartum women in two health facilities in urban Ghana

Jonathan Ian Coomson[1] and Abubakar Manu[2*]

**Abstract**

**Background:** Postpartum contraception is important for spacing and limiting childbirth. Although the use of modern contraception has been shown to reduce maternal and child morbidities and mortalities, postpartum women have one of the highest unmet needs for family planning. Inter-birth intervals less than 24 months have adverse effects on both the mother and the child, yet very limited empirical evidence exist on contraceptive use among postpartum women in Ghana. This study sought to determine the prevalence and determinants of modern contraceptive use among postpartum women in the Tema Metropolis, Ghana.

**Methods:** A facility-based cross-sectional survey was conducted among 320 postpartum women with babies aged between three and 15 months. Participants were recruited from child welfare clinics in two government health facilities in the Tema metropolitan area using a simple random sampling technique. Data were analyzed using STATA version 15. Chi-square and multiple logistic regressions techniques were used to examine associations between postpartum contraceptive use and key independent variables. Statistical significance was set at $p = 0.05$. Adjusted odds ratios and their 95% confidence intervals were used to assess the strength of association.

**Results:** The prevalence rate of modern contraceptive use among postpartum women was 26.3%. Postpartum contraceptive use was significantly associated with past contraceptive use [AOR = 7.7 (95%CI: 3.4–17.5)]; return of menses [AOR = 4.3 (95%CI: 1.7–11.3)]; resumption of sexual activity [AOR = 4.7 (95%CI: 1.4–15.4)]; discussion of family planning with male partner [AOR = 3.1 (95%CI: 1.03–9.2)]; male partners' approval of modern contraception [AOR = 18.1 (95%CI: 6.3–51.6)]; family planning counselling received during antenatal care [AOR = 3.5 (95%CI: 1.3–9.9)] and knowledge of at least one modern methods of contraception available at the health facility [AOR = 4.7 (95%CI: 1.9–11.5)].

**Conclusions:** Postpartum contraceptive uptake is low among women in the Tema area. Factors that influence modern contraceptive uptake among postpartum women include past modern contraceptive use, resumption of sexual activity and menstruation, male partner involvement in contraception, family planning counselling during antenatal care and knowledge of the modern methods of contraception available at the health facility. Strengthening family planning education and counselling during antenatal care and using a multi-prong strategy to engage men as partners in family planning will improve postpartum contraceptive uptake.

**Keywords:** Modern contraceptives, Postpartum, Family planning, Women, Ghana

* Correspondence: amanu@ug.edu.gh
[2]Department of Population, Family and Reproductive Health, School of Public Health, University of Ghana, Accra, Ghana

## Background

Postpartum contraception is one of the means to prevent rapid repeat pregnancies to ensure good health outcomes in both mother and baby. However, in developing countries, postpartum contraceptive uptake is low [1]. The World Health Organization estimates that about 830 women die daily from complications of pregnancy and childbirth worldwide, and nearly all (99%) of these maternal deaths occur in developing countries [2]. An overwhelming number of these deaths could be prevented through interventions such as the use of modern contraceptive methods. Evidence shows that an estimated 20% of obstetric deaths would be prevented if modern contraceptive methods were used [3].

Postpartum women have one of the greatest unmet need for family planning but most often than not, do not receive the services needed in ensuring longer birth intervals and reducing unintended pregnancies [4]. In Sub-Saharan Africa (SSA), the low use of modern contraceptives has led to high rates of unintended pregnancies, unsafe abortions and unplanned births [5]. About two-thirds of women would like to avoid pregnancy in the first year after delivery but are not on any postpartum contraceptive method [6, 7]. Evidence shows that nearly 95% of women who are 0 to 12 months postpartum desire to avoid pregnancy in the next 24 months, but 70% of them do not use contraception [8]. Short inter-birth intervals, that is, inter-birth intervals less than 24 months, are associated with maternal morbidities such as uterine rupture and uteroplacental bleeding disorders (abruptio placenta and placenta praevia) and infant morbidities such as prematurity, low birth weight and stunting [9]. Research indicates that in developing countries, the death rate of children under 5 years would reduce by 13% if women waited for at least 24 months after birth before conceiving, while a 25% decrease would be achieved if the waiting time was at least 36 months [10].

Although knowledge of contraceptives is relatively high among women of reproductive age in Ghana, its use remains low [11]. In Ghana, contraceptive prevalence rate among married women is only 27% for all methods, and 22% for modern methods [12]. Some studies have looked at the predictors of contraceptive use by postpartum women in developing countries of which Ghana is included. However, most of these studies used secondary data from the Ghana Demographic and Health Survey (GDHS) in 2008. Published research materials on postpartum contraceptives concerning Ghana are mostly those done on the global or regional scale using secondary data from demographic and health surveys [1, 13, 14]. Recently published research works which used primary data to study the factors that influence postpartum contraceptive use in Ghana are limited. This study, therefore, seeks to estimate the prevalence of postpartum modern contraceptive use and to assess the factors that influence modern contraceptive use among postpartum women in the Tema area of Ghana. In-depth knowledge of the factors that influence the use of postpartum modern contraceptives could be used to plan future educational programs on postpartum contraceptive, thereby reducing the maternal and child morbidities and mortalities associated with short inter-birth intervals. Results of this study could also be used for institutional assessment and implementing reforms at the facility level to increase the uptake of postpartum modern contraceptives.

## Methods

### Study design

This study employed a facility-based cross-sectional design using the quantitative method with structured questionnaires to obtain data from postpartum women with babies aged between three and 15 months.

### Study area, population and period

The study was conducted from May to June 2018, at the Tema General Hospital (TGH) and the Tema Polyclinic (TP). The facilities, located in the Tema Metropolis, about 30 km to the East of Accra, are the two main government facilities in the Tema District, both of which are operated under the Ghana Health Service (GHS) and offer various services including reproductive and child health services. The study population was all postpartum women attending the child welfare clinic of TGH and TP.

### Sample size determination and sampling procedure

The sample size was calculated based on Cochran's formula $n \geq [(Z_{\frac{\alpha}{2}})^{2} P (1-P)]/d^{2}$.

[15], with the following assumptions: Prevalence (P) of postpartum modern contraceptive use = 22.6% [16], margin of error (d) = 5%, $Z_{\frac{\alpha}{2}}$ = 1.96 at 95% confidence interval and a non-response rate of 10%. The total minimum sample size was 300 participants.

Proportion-to-size sampling was done to know the number of participants that was needed from each facility. Based on average monthly attendance at the two child welfare clinics, about 68% of the participants were recruited from TGH while the remaining 32% were recruited from TP.

At the facility level, a simple random sampling technique was used in selecting participants in the study. Postpartum women assessing the child welfare clinic of TGH and TP who met the criteria for the study were numbered from one till the last person. Pieces of papers with the corresponding numbers just like the numbering of the women were put in an opaque container, mixed thoroughly and blindly selected by a volunteer midwife.

Postpartum women who had their numbers selected were then invited to participate in the study for that particular day after informed consent had been sought from them. With the help of four research assistants, a maximum of 25 participants were interviewed per day in TGH whilst that of TP was a maximum of 10 interviews per day.

### Inclusion criteria

1. All women of reproductive age who delivered 3–15 months prior to the study, accessing the child welfare clinic of TGH and TP and who were willing to be participants in the study.
2. For postpartum women who were below 18 years at the time of data collection, written informed consent were sought from their guardian or parent who accompanied them to the hospital. Postpartum mothers below the age of 18 years who came to the health facility without a guardian or parent were excluded from the study.

### Exclusion criteria

1. Postpartum women who had had a hysterectomy (surgical removal of the uterus).
2. Postpartum women who did not speak and understand English, Twi or Ga were excluded from the study due to the language barrier.
3. Postpartum women who were pregnant at the time of accessing the Child Welfare Clinic of TGH and TP.

### Measures

Postpartum modern contraceptive use was the dependent variable; and was measured directly with a yes/no response (yes = 1 and no = 0). Postpartum women were asked to indicate whether they were currently using a modern contraceptive method.

The independent variables such as the use of modern contraceptives before last delivery, resumption of sexual activity, resumption of menstruation after delivery, discussion of family planning with male partner after delivery of last child, male partner's approval of modern contraceptives, antenatal and postnatal care attendance and whether family planning counselling occurred during these visits were measured directly with yes or no questions where yes = 1 and no = 0.

Regarding knowledge of modern contraceptive methods available at the health facility, women were asked a yes/no question on whether they knew the available contraceptive methods being offered at the health facility. Women who responded in the affirmative were asked to name the types of contraceptives being offered at the health facility. Women who correctly named at least one method were deemed to have knowledge of the available methods at the health facility. Women who said they knew the available methods but could not mention correctly any method as well as those who answered no were assumed to have no knowledge of the contraceptive methods available at the facility.

Knowledge of postpartum modern contraceptive side effects was computed by asking women to list the side effects of modern contraceptives they knew. Women who knew no side effect or correctly listed only one side effect were assumed to have a low knowledge of contraceptive side effects. Participants who correctly listed between two to three side effects were deemed to have moderate knowledge. Postpartum women who knew four or more side effects of modern contraceptives were assumed to have high knowledge of the side effects of modern contraceptives.

Knowledge of postpartum physiology was a created composite variable, where women were asked three yes/no questions where yes = 1 and no = 0. The questions included whether or not a postpartum woman can become pregnant when breastfeeding, can become pregnant when her menses has not returned and whether sexual activity had any effect on the time of the return of her menstrual cycle after delivery. A score of 0 or 1 was deemed as low knowledge, 2 as moderate knowledge and 3 as high knowledge.

### Data quality assurance

Four research assistants were recruited and trained. They were trained to ensure correct interpretation of the questionnaires. Research assistants were also trained on how to protect the confidentiality and privacy of participants. The principal investigator supervised and monitored the activities of the research assistants daily during data collection. Questionnaires were constructed in a lay-man's language so as to make it easily understandable and precise as much as possible after a pre-test was conducted on 30 individuals at both the Lekma Hospital and Polyclinic.

### Data processing and analysis

Data were entered into Microsoft Excel spreadsheet (Microsoft Office 2010) and cleaned to eliminate all irregularities. The data were then exported into STATA version 15, coded and cleaned for analysis. Univariate analysis was carried out using frequencies and percentages to describe the exposure and outcome variables independently. Bivariate analysis using the Pearson's Chi square was carried out to examine associations between postpartum modern contraceptive use and the various independent variables. All the independent variables which were found to be significantly associated with postpartum modern contraceptive use were fitted in a multivariate analysis using the binary logistic regression technique to determine predictors of postpartum contraceptive use. Odds ratios and their 95% confidence intervals were used to assess the strength of association. A $p$-value of 0.05 was used to determine statistical significance.

## Results

### Socio-demographic characteristics of respondents

Table 1 presents socio-demographic characteristics of study participants. The median age of participants was 29 years (IQR: 26–33.5). About half of the respondents 159 (49.7%) were between the ages of 20–29 years. Participants' age ranged between 17 and 47 years. Majority of the study participants 284 (88.7%) were married or cohabiting. Only 14 (4.4%) of respondents had no formal education with a vast majority 280 (87.6%) having at least secondary or vocational education. Nearly a quarter 77 (24.1%) of respondents were unemployed. Almost all women in the study (97.2%) had partners who had at least primary education.

**Table 1** Socio-demographic characteristics of respondents

| Characteristics | Frequency ($n = 320$) | Percent |
|---|---|---|
| Age of mother | | |
| ≤ 19 | 9 | 2.8 |
| 20–29 | 159 | 49.7 |
| 30–39 | 137 | 42.8 |
| 40–49 | 15 | 4.7 |
| Marital status | | |
| Single/divorced/widowed | 36 | 11.3 |
| Married/cohabiting | 284 | 88.7 |
| Education of mother | | |
| No formal education | 14 | 4.4 |
| Primary | 26 | 8.1 |
| Secondary/vocational | 204 | 63.8 |
| Tertiary | 76 | 23.8 |
| Occupation of mother | | |
| Public salaried worker | 32 | 10.0 |
| Private salaried worker | 66 | 20.6 |
| Trader | 113 | 35.3 |
| Unemployed | 77 | 24.1 |
| Other | 32 | 10.0 |
| Education of partner | | |
| No formal education | 9 | 2.8 |
| Primary | 3 | 0.9 |
| Secondary/vocational | 183 | 57.2 |
| Tertiary | 125 | 39.1 |

### Reproductive health characteristics of respondents

The median number of pregnancies of respondents was 2.5 (IQR: 2–3). About two out of every five women (42.8%) had only one child. Modal age group of the last child of participants was 6–8 months. The median age of the last child was 7 months [5–9]. Almost two thirds (63.7%) of respondents had the desire to have another child and of those who desired to have another child, about 84% (171) of them desired to have the next child after 21 months from the time of the study. About two in five (43%) of participants said the pregnancy which resulted in the birth of their last child was not planned or intended. Majority of participants 315 (98.4) had their last delivery in a health facility. Almost all the women 315 (97.5%) had at least one antenatal visit with nearly half (46.5%) meeting the current WHO's recommendation of at least eight antenatal care contacts before delivery [17]. Postnatal care attendance was almost universal 319 (99.7%) with nine in 10 women (90.9%) satisfying the WHO's recommendation of at least three visits [18] during the postnatal care period (Table 2).

### Postpartum contraceptive prevalence rate

Modern contraceptive prevalence among the postpartum women was 26.3 95% CI: 21.5–31.4%. Majority 177 (55.3%) of participants had never used any form of modern contraceptive method in their reproductive lives. Of the 143 participants who had used modern contraceptives in the past, a little over two-fifth (42.7%) obtained information about contraceptive use from health workers. Almost a third (29.8%) of postpartum women who were using modern contraceptives were using injectables (Fig. 1). Of the 284 (73.7%) postpartum women who were currently not using any modern method of contraception, more than one-third (36.9%) reported that fear of the side effects was the main problem for non-use of contraception (Fig. 2).

### Predictors of postpartum modern contraceptive use

Tables 3 and 4 summarize bivariate association between postpartum modern contraceptive use and socio-demographic and reproductive health characteristics respectively. Women's age ($p = 0.027$) was the only socio-demographic characteristic found to be associated with postpartum modern contraceptive use. The use of modern contraceptive in the past ($p < 0.001$), return of menstruation ($p = 0.049$), resumption of sexual activity ($p < 0.001$) and discussion of family planning among spouses ($p < 0.001$) were significantly associated with current modern contraceptive use postpartum women. Other variables significantly associated with modern contraceptive use were male partner approval of modern contraception ($p < 0.001$), whether family planning counselling was received during antenatal care ($p = 0.008$), family

**Table 2** Reproductive health characteristics of participants

| Variable | Frequency (n = 320) | Percent |
|---|---|---|
| Number of past pregnancies | | |
| 1 | 64 | 20.0 |
| 2 | 96 | 30.0 |
| 3 | 88 | 27.5 |
| 4 | 54 | 16.8 |
| More than 4 | 18 | 5.7 |
| Number of children | | |
| 1 | 137 | 42.8 |
| 2 | 101 | 31.6 |
| 3 | 50 | 15.6 |
| 4 | 26 | 8.1 |
| More than 4 | 6 | 1.9 |
| Age of child | | |
| 3–5 months | 98 | 30.6 |
| 6–8 months | 111 | 34.7 |
| 9–11 months | 75 | 23.4 |
| 12–15 months | 36 | 11.3 |
| Desires to have another child | | |
| No | 116 | 36.3 |
| Yes | 204 | 63.7 |
| When next child is wanted | *N* = 204 | |
| Within 21 months | 33 | 16.2 |
| After 21 months | 171 | 83.8 |
| Ever used modern contraceptive | | |
| No | 177 | 55.3 |
| Yes | 143 | 44.7 |
| Last pregnancy planned/intended | | |
| No | 138 | 43.1 |
| Yes | 183 | 56.9 |
| Menstruated after delivery | | |
| No | 124 | 38.7 |
| Yes | 196 | 61.3 |
| Resumed sexual activity | | |
| No | 110 | 34.4 |
| Yes | 210 | 65.6 |
| Current modern contraceptive use | | |
| No | 236 | 73.7 |
| Yes | 84 | 26.3 |
| Discussed family planning with partner | | |
| No | 156 | 48.8 |
| Yes | 164 | 51.2 |
| Partners' approval of modern contraception | | |
| No | 101 | 31.6 |
| Yes | 111 | 34.7 |
| I do not know | 108 | 33.7 |
| Place of delivery | | |
| Health facility | 315 | 98.4 |
| home | 5 | 1.6 |
| Antenatal attendance | | |
| No | 8 | 2.5 |
| Yes | 312 | 97.5 |
| Number of antenatal attendance | *N* = 312 | |
| Less than 8 visits | 167 | 53.5 |
| 8 or more visits | 145 | 46.5 |
| FP counselling at antenatal | *N* = 312 | |
| No | 80 | 25.6 |
| Yes | 232 | 74.4 |
| Postnatal attendance | | |
| No | 1 | 0.3 |
| Yes | 319 | 99.7 |
| Number of postnatal attendance | *N* = 319 | |
| Less than 3 visits | 29 | 9.1 |
| 3 or more visits | 290 | 90.9 |
| FP counselling at postnatal | *N* = 319 | |
| No | 200 | 62.7 |
| Yes | 119 | 37.3 |
| Knowledge of side effects | | |
| Low knowledge | 108 | 33.8 |
| Moderate knowledge | 155 | 48.4 |
| High knowledge | 57 | 17.8 |
| Knowledge of postpartum physiology | | |
| Low knowledge | 54 | 16.9 |
| Moderate knowledge | 131 | 41 |
| High knowledge | 135 | 42.1 |
| Knowledge of FP methods available at health facility | | |
| No | 184 | 57.5 |
| Yes | 136 | 42.5 |

planning counselling at postnatal care ($p < 0.001$) and knowing at least one modern contraceptive methods available at the health facility ($p < 0.001$).

#### Multivariate logistic regression

Table 5 presents results of multiple logistic regression of postpartum contraceptive use and selected independent variables. Postpartum women who had ever used a modern contraceptive were 7.7 times likely to be currently using a modern contraceptive compared to those who

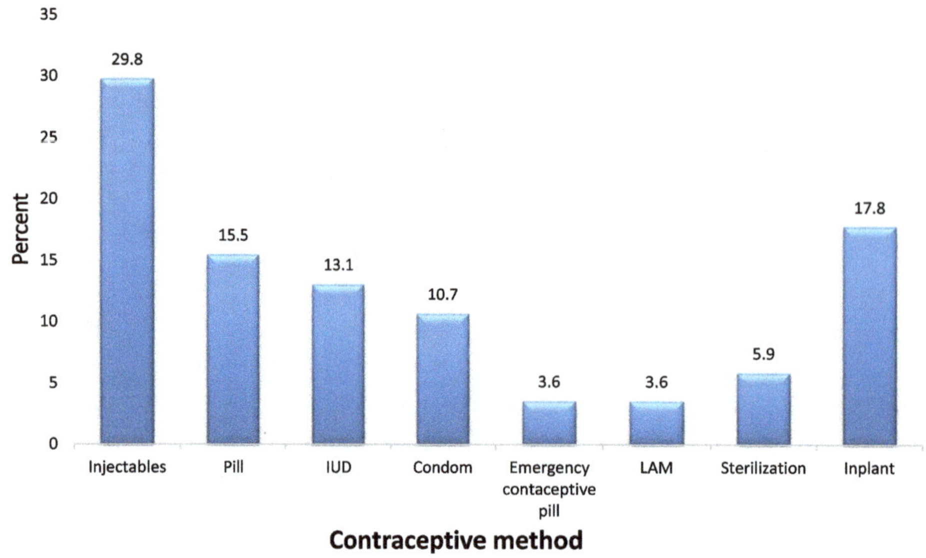


**Fig. 1** Preferred methods of postpartum modern contraception

had never used a modern contraceptive method [AOR = 7.7 (95% CI: 3.4–17.5)]. Postpartum women whose menses had returned compared to those who were yet to have a return of menstrual flow were 4.3 times likely to be using a modern contraceptive method [AOR = 4.3 (95% CI: 1.7–11.3)]. Likewise, women who have resumed sexual activity have 4.7 times increased odds of using a modern method of contraception compared to those who are yet to resume sexual activity after delivery [AOR = 4.7 (95% CI: 1.4–15.4)]. Spouses who have discussed family planning have 310% increased odds of using a postpartum modern contraceptive compared to spouses who have not had any discussion on family planning [AOR = 3.1 (95% CI: 1.03–9.2)]. There was an 18.1 higher odds of using modern contraceptives among postpartum women whose partners' approved of the use of modern contraceptives compared to women whose partners' did not [AOR = 18.1 (95% CI: 6.3–51.6)]. Postpartum women who received family planning counselling during antenatal care visits at health facilities were 3.5 times likely to be on modern contraceptives during the study than those who said they received no family planning counselling during antenatal care [AOR = 3.5 (95% CI: 1.3–9.9)]. Lastly, postpartum women who knew at least a modern contraceptive method

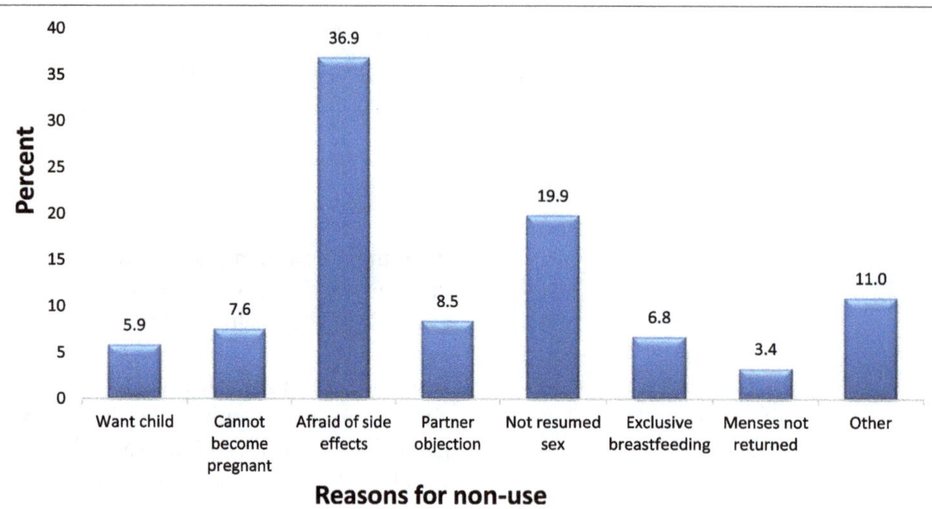


**Fig. 2** Reasons for non-use of postpartum modern contraception

**Table 3** Bivariate analysis of socio-demographic characteristics associated with current postpartum modern contraceptive use

| Characteristic | Contraceptive use, n (%) | | Chi square | P-value |
|---|---|---|---|---|
| | No | Yes | | |
| Age of mother | | | | |
| 10–19 | **7** (3.0) | 2 (2.4) | 9.20 | 0.027 |
| 20–29 | 126 (53.4) | 33 (39.3) | | |
| 30–39 | 96 (40.6) | 41 (48.8) | | |
| 40–49 | 7 (3.0) | 8 (9.5) | | |
| Marital status | | | | |
| Single/widow/divorced | 24 (10.2) | 12 (14.3) | 1.05 | 0.305 |
| Married/cohabiting | 212 (89.8) | 72 (85.7) | | |
| Education of mother | | | | |
| No formal education | 10 (4.3) | 4 (4.8) | | 0.298* |
| Primary | 22 (9.3) | 4 (4.8) | | |
| Secondary/vocational | 144 (61.0) | 60 (71.4) | | |
| Tertiary | 60 (25.4) | 16 (19.0) | | |
| Occupation of mother | | | | |
| Unemployed | 59 (25.0) | 18 (21.4) | 0.43 | 0.511 |
| Employed | 177 (75.0) | 66 (78.6) | | |
| Education of partner | | | | |
| No formal education | 8 (3.4) | 1 (1.2) | | 0.349* |
| Primary | 2 (0.9) | 1 (1.2) | | |
| Secondary/vocational | 129 (54.6) | 54 (64.3) | | |
| Tertiary | 97 (41.1) | 28 (33.3) | | |

*Fisher's exact

available at the health facility (Tema General Hospital and Tema Polyclinic) were 4.7 times likely to be currently using a modern method of contraception than women who had no idea of the contraceptive methods available at the health facility [AOR = 4.7 (95% CI: 1.9–11.5)].

## Discussion

This study sought to find the prevalence of modern contraceptive methods among postpartum women attending the child welfare clinic of Tema General Hospital and Tema polyclinic as well as assess the determinants of modern contraceptive use. Determinants of modern contraceptive uptake among postpartum women include past modern contraceptive use, resumption of sexual activity and menstruation, male partner involvement in contraception, family planning counselling during antenatal care and knowledge of the modern methods of contraception available at the health facility.

The prevalence of postpartum modern contraceptive use was 26.3% with the 95% confidence interval of 21.5 to 31.4%. This finding is in line with the modern contraceptive prevalence rate of 22% found during the GDHS of 2014 [12]. The low prevalence of modern contraceptive use among postpartum women in this study could result in rapid repeat pregnancies with the resultant short inter-birth interval, which have been shown by several studies [19–24] to be detrimental to the health of both the mother and the child. Past modern contraceptive use, return of menstrual cycle, resumption of sexual activity, discussion of family planning with male partner and male partners' approval of contraceptives were found to be associated with postpartum modern contraceptive use. Other factors significantly associated with modern contraceptive use among postpartum women were family planning counselling during antenatal care and knowledge of at least one modern contraceptive method available at the health facility.

The most preferred method of contraception was injectables (29.8%) which was consistent with several studies around the world [1, 12, 25–27]. All these studies showed a preference of women for short acting hormonal contraceptive methods such as injectables and the pill. However, long acting reversible methods such as IUDs and implants as well as permanent methods are known to be more effective in pregnancy prevention [28]. In this study, the commonest reason given by women for not being on any modern contraceptive method was the fear of side effects (36.9%). Non-use of modern contraceptive methods due to health concerns and fear of side effects are also common reasons given by women in Africa and other parts of the world [12, 14, 29].

Past modern contraceptive use prior to the last pregnancy increased the likelihood of current modern contraceptive use among postpartum women. This association is also seen in other studies across the world [30, 31]. This relationship may be due to the fact that women recognize the benefits of modern contraceptive use after initial use and continue to use them later on in life. Perhaps, they realize that the myths and side effects of contraceptives are over-exaggerated when they use it themselves and continue to use them in the postpartum period to space and limit childbirth.

Additionally, women whose menstrual cycle had returned after delivery were more likely to use modern contraception. This findings is in consonance with existing evidence indicating that most women prefer to use contraception when they had resumed menstruation [25, 32]. A survey of 17 low and middle income countries [33] using secondary data from their demographic and health surveys revealed a trend of postpartum women waiting for the return of their menses before the uptake of a modern method of contraception. The public health implication of this finding is that it can lead to a rise

**Table 4** Bivariate analysis of other factors associated with postpartum modern contraceptive use

| Characteristic | Contraceptive use, n (%) | | Chi square | p-value |
|---|---|---|---|---|
| | No | Yes | | |
| Number of past pregnancies | | | | |
| 1 | 53 (22.5) | 11 (13.1) | 7.87 | 0.096 |
| 2 | 75 (31.8) | 21 (25.0) | | |
| 3 | 62 (26.3) | 26 (31.0) | | |
| 4 | 35 (14.8) | 19 (22.6) | | |
| More than 4 | 11 (4.6) | 7 (8.3) | | |
| Number of children | | | | |
| 1 | 107 (45.3) | 30 (35.7) | 7.39 | 0.117 |
| 2 | 72 (30.5) | 29 (34.5) | | |
| 3 | 38 (16.1) | 12 (14.3) | | |
| 4 | 14 (5.9) | 12 (14.3) | | |
| More than 4 | 5 (2.2) | 1 (1.2) | | |
| Age of child | | | | |
| 3–5 months | 76 (32.2) | 22 (26.2) | 2.04 | 0.564 |
| 6–8 months | 82 (34.8) | 29 (34.5) | | |
| 9–11 months | 51 (21.6) | 24 (28.6) | | |
| 12–15 months | 27 (11.4) | 9 (10.7) | | |
| Desires another child | | | | |
| No | 84 (14.5) | 32 (21.2) | 0.17 | 0.682 |
| Yes | 152 (85.5) | 52 (78.8) | | |
| When next child is desired | | | | |
| Within 21 months | 22 (66.7) | 11 (33.3) | 1.28 | 0.259 |
| After 21 months | 130 (76.0) | 41 (24.0) | | |
| Ever used modern contraceptive | | | | |
| No | 154 (65.3) | 23 (27.4) | 35.95 | < 0.001 |
| Yes | 82 (34.7) | 61 (72.6) | | |
| Last pregnancy planned/intended | | | | |
| No | 101 (42.8) | 37 (44.0) | 0.04 | 0.842 |
| Yes | 135 (57.2) | 47 (56.0) | | |
| Menses returned | | | | |
| No | 99 (42.0) | 25 (29.8) | 3.88 | 0.049 |
| Yes | 137 (58.0) | 59 (70.2) | | |
| Resumed sexual activity | | | | |
| No | 103 (43.6) | 7 (8.3) | 34.24 | < 0.001 |
| Yes | 133 (56.4) | 77 (91.7) | | |
| Discussed FP with partner | | | | |
| No | 144 (61.0) | 12 (14.3) | 54.15 | < 0.001 |
| Yes | 92 (39.0) | 72 (85.7) | | |
| Partner approves modern contraception | | | | |
| No | 84 (35.6) | 17 (20.2) | 75.76 | < 0.001 |
| Yes | 50 (21.2) | 61 (72.6) | | |
| I do not know | 102 (43.2) | 6 (7.2) | | |

**Table 4** Bivariate analysis of other factors associated with postpartum modern contraceptive use *(Continued)*

| Characteristic | Contraceptive use, n (%) | | Chi square | p-value |
|---|---|---|---|---|
| | No | Yes | | |
| Place of delivery | | | | |
| Health facility | 232 (98.3) | 83 (98.8) | | 1.000* |
| home | 4 (1.7) | 1 (1.2) | | |
| ANC attendance | | | | |
| No | 6 (2.5) | 2 (2.4) | | 1.000* |
| yes | 230 (97.5) | 82 (97.6) | | |
| FP counselling at antenatal | | | | |
| No | 68 (29.6) | 12 (14.6) | 7.068 | 0.008 |
| Yes | 162 (70.4) | 70 (85.4) | | |
| PNC attendance | | | | |
| No | 0 (0.0) | 1 (1.2) | | 0.262* |
| Yes | 236 (100.0) | 83 (98.8) | | |
| FP counselling at PNC | | | | |
| No | 166 (70.3) | 34 (41.0) | 22.66 | < 0.001 |
| Yes | 70 (29.7) | 49 (59.0) | | |
| Knowledge of side effects | | | | |
| Low knowledge | 75 (31.8) | 33 (39.3) | 3.84 | 0.147 |
| Moderate knowledge | 122 (51.7) | 33 (39.3) | | |
| High knowledge | 39 (16.5) | 18 (21.4) | | |
| Knowledge of postpartum physiology | | | | |
| Low knowledge | 41 (17.4) | 13 (15.5) | 1.42 | 0.491 |
| Moderate knowledge | 92 (39.0) | 39 (46.4) | | |
| High knowledge | 103 (43.6) | 32 (38.1) | | |
| Knowledge of available FP methods | | | | |
| No | 163 (69.1) | 21 (25.0) | 49.23 | < 0.001 |
| Yes | 73 (30.9) | 63 (75.0) | | |

*Fishers' exact

in unplanned and unintended pregnancies because women mistakenly think postpartum amenorrhoea means they cannot become pregnant. Pregnancy is possible in postpartum women because ovulation, which is the releases of eggs by the ovary can occur before menstruation [34, 35].

As expected, women who had resumed sexual activity after delivery were more likely to use modern contraception. This finding is consistent with two studies from East Africa that found that resumption of sex predicts modern contraceptive use among postpartum women [32, 36].

It was also evident that family planning discussion among couples after last delivery increases postpartum contraceptive uptake. Hameed et al. [37] demonstrated in the Punjab Province of Pakistan, that when couples jointly make the decision to use contraceptives, its use was significant than

**Table 5** Logistic regression analysis of factors influencing postpartum modern contraceptive use

| Variable | COR (95% CI) | p-value | AOR (95% CI) | p-value |
|---|---|---|---|---|
| Age of mother | | | | |
| 10–19 | Ref | | Ref | |
| 20–29 | 0.9 (0.2–4.6) | 0.916 | 1.5 (0.2–9.3 | 0.683 |
| 30–39 | 1.5 (0.3–7.5) | 0.625 | 1.6 (0.3–10.5) | 0.610 |
| 40–49 | 4.0 (0.6–26.0) | 0.146 | 2.4 (0.2–30.7) | 0.490 |
| Ever used modern contraceptive | | | | |
| No | Ref | | Ref | < 0.001 |
| Yes | 5.0 (2.9–8.6) | < 0.001 | 7.7 (3.4–17.5) | |
| Menstruated after delivery | | | | 0.003 |
| No | Ref | | Ref | |
| Yes | 1.7 (1.0–2.9) | 0.050 | 4.3 (1.7–11.3) | |
| Resumed sexual activity | | | | 0.011 |
| No | Ref | | Ref | |
| Yes | 8.5 (3.7–19.3) | < 0.001 | 4.7 (1.4–15.4) | |
| Discussed family planning with partner | | | | |
| No | Ref | | Ref | 0.044 |
| Yes | 9.4 (4.8–18.3) | < 0.001 | 3.1 (1.03–9.2) | |
| Partners' approval of modern contraceptive use | | | | |
| No | Ref | | Ref | |
| Yes | 6.0 (3.2–11.4) | < 0.001 | 18.1 (6.3–51.6) | < 0.001 |
| I do not know | 0.3 (0.1–0.8) | 0.013 | 7.7 (1.6–38.1) | 0.012 |
| Family planning counselling at antenatal | | | | |
| No | Ref | | Ref | |
| Yes | 2.4 (1.2–4.8) | 0.009 | 3.5 (1.3–9.9) | 0.016 |
| Family planning counselling at postnatal | | | | |
| No | Ref | | Ref | 0.139 |
| Yes | 3.4 (2.0–5.7) | < 0.001 | 2.0 (0.8–5.3) | |
| Knowledge of available family planning methods at the health facility | | | | |
| No | ref | | Ref | 0.001 |
| Yes | 6.7 (3.8–11.8) | < 0.001 | 4.7 (1.9–11.5) | |

when the decision was made to use it only by the woman. This goes a long way to show the importance of involving the male partner in decisions regarding contraception. Likewise, male partners' approval of modern contraceptives increases its use. This association is not surprising because in many parts of the world especially SSA, husbands are the heads of families and major decisions such as fertility desires has to be approved by them.

Postpartum modern contraceptive use was significantly associated with family planning counselling during antenatal care as seen in several studies across the world [1, 30, 32, 38–41]. Appropriate family planning information and counselling at antenatal care visit allows women enough time to decide which method will be suitable for them in the postpartum period. Family planning counselling during antenatal care may motivate women who were otherwise indecisive to use modern contraceptive methods during the postpartum period.

Knowledge of at least one method of modern contraception available at the health facility increased modern contraceptive use by postpartum women. This relationship may be explained by the fact that in Ghana, health facilities are the major sources of some contraceptive methods [12] and therefore one is expected to know the available methods at the facility before choosing a suitable method.

The study is one of the few in the Tema area that seeks to determine the predictors of modern contraceptive use among postpartum women, thereby adding to the body of knowledge on postpartum contraception. Another strength of this study is that reliable data and appropriate methods were used, thereby ensuring that the findings reflect accurately on modern contraceptive use among postpartum women in the Tema area. A limitation of the study is in its design. The cross sectional study design made it impossible to establish causal relationships. Therefore, associations were the best ways to interpret results. Another limitation of the study was recall bias. Postpartum women had to recall certain reproductive health characteristics and behaviours that occurred in the past. Some of these behaviours were self-reported and there was practically no way to independently verify them. Sexual activity and contraceptive use are considered intimate issues in Ghana. This has a potential to lead to some reluctance in answering questions which bordered on those issues. However, this concern was addressed when the confidentiality and privacy of women were respected in the study. Again, this was a facility-based study in an urban setting, and therefore results can only be generalizable to similar urban settings.

## Conclusions

Postpartum modern contraceptive uptake is low among women in the Tema area. Injectables are the most preferred method of modern contraception while the fear of side effects is the major reason for modern contraceptive non-use. Modern contraceptive uptake among postpartum women in the Tema area is influenced by past modern contraceptive use, resumption of sexual activity and menstrual cycle after last delivery, the male partner's involvement in contraception, family planning counselling given by health care providers during antenatal care and postpartum women knowing at least one methods of modern contraception available at the health facility.

There should be an increased advocacy by the Tema Metropolitan Health Directorate to engage men as partners in family planning educational programs since their influence is huge in modern contraceptive uptake among postpartum women. Efforts should be made at the facility level by authorities and health managers to strengthen family planning counselling during antenatal care.

### Abbreviations

AOR: Adjusted Odds Ratio; CI: Confidence Interval; COR: Crude Odds Ratio; GDHS: Ghana Demographic and Health Survey; GHS: Ghana Health Service; IQR: Interquartile Range; SSA: Sub-Saharan Africa; TGH: Tema General Hospital; TP: Tema Polyclinic; WHO: World Health Organization.

### Acknowledgements

We wish to thank all postpartum women at the two health facilities, who spent their valuable time in answering questions during data collection. We also acknowledge our four research assistants, who worked diligently during the data collection process. Our sincere gratitude also goes to the management and staff of the two health facilities, who supported this study in diverse ways.

### Authors' contributions

JIC and AM conceptualized and designed the study. JIC was responsible for study implementation and acquisition of data, conducted data analysis and interpretation, and drafted the initial version of the manuscript. AM contributed to data interpretation, reviewed and revised the manuscript critically for important intellectual content. Both authors read and approved the final manuscript.

### Author details

[1]3M&C Health System, LG DTD 10081, East Legon, Accra, Ghana.
[2]Department of Population, Family and Reproductive Health, School of Public Health, University of Ghana, Accra, Ghana.

### References

1. Moore Z, Pfitzer A, Gubin R, Charurat E, Elliott L, Croft T. Missed opportunities for family planning: an analysis of pregnancy risk and contraceptive method use among postpartum women in 21 low- and middle-income countries. Contraception. 2015;92(1):31–9. https://doi.org/10.1016/j.contraception.2015.03.007.
2. Blencowe H, Cousens S, Jassir FB, Say L, Chou D, Mathers C, et al. National, regional, and worldwide estimates of stillbirth rates in 2015, with trends from 2000: a systematic analysis. Lancet Glob Heal. 2016;4(2):e98–108 Available from: http://linkinghub.elsevier.com/retrieve/pii/S2214109X15002752. [cited 2017 Oct 14].
3. Collumbien M, Gerressu M, Cleland J. Non-use and use of ineffective methods of contraception. In: Ezzati M, Lopez A, Anthony R, Murray C, editors. Comparative quantification of health risks; 2004. p. 1255–320. Available from: http://researchonline.lshtm.ac.uk/id/eprint/17866.
4. Winikoff B, Mensch B. Rethinking postpartum family planning. Stud Fam Plan. 2015;22(5):294–307.
5. Apanga PA, Adam MA. Factors influencing the uptake of family planning services in the Talensi district, Ghana. Pan Afr Med J. 2015;20:1–9.
6. Ross JA, Winfrey WL. Contraceptive use, intention to use and unmet need during the extended postpartum period. Int Fam Plan Perspect. 2001;27(1):20 Available from: http://www.jstor.org/stable/2673801?origin=crossref.
7. Rossier C, Bradley SEK, Ross J, Winfrey W. Reassessing unmet need for family planning in the postpartum period. Stud Fam Plan. 2015;46(4):355–67.
8. WHO | Postpartum family planning, editor. essential for ensuring health of women and their babies. World Health Organisation: World Health Organization; 2018. Available from: https://www.who.int/reproductivehealth/topics/family_planning/world-contraception-day-2018/en/. [cited 2019 May 25]
9. Conde-Agudelo A, Rosas-Bermúdez A, Castano F, Horton MH. Effects of birth spacing on maternal, perinatal, infant, and child health: a systematic review of causal mechanisms. Stud Fam Plan. 2012;43(2):93–114.
10. Rutstein SO. Effects of preceding birth intervals on neonatal, infant and under-five years mortality and nutritional status in developing countries: evidence from the demographic and health surveys. Int J Gynecol Obstet. 2005;89(Suppl 1):S7–S24.
11. Opoku B. Contraceptive Preferences of Post-Abortion Patients in Ghana. J Women's Heal Care. 2012;01(02) Available from: https://www.omicsgroup.org/journals/2167-0420/2167-0420-1-109.digital/2167-0420-1-109.html.
12. Ghana Statistical Service, Ghana Health Service, ICF Macro International. Ghana Demographic and Health Survey 2015;
13. Tsui AO, Brown W, Li Q. Contraceptive practice in sub Saharan Africa. HHS Public Access. 2017;43:166–91.
14. Sedgh G, Hussain R. Reasons for Contraceptive Nonuse among Women Having Unmet Need for Contraception in Developing Countries Reasons for Contraceptive Nonuse among Women Having Unmet Need for Contraception in Developing Countries For decades , the of unmet need for the contr 2017;45(2):151–169.
15. Cochran WG. Sampling Techniques. 3rd ed. Hoboken: Wiley; 1977.
16. Faabar A. Factors influencing postpartum contrceptive use in the Jirapa District. Legon: University of Ghana; 2014.
17. World Health Organization. WHO Recommendations on Antenatal care for positive pregnancy experience. WHO Recomm Antenatal care Posit pregnancy Exp. 2016;152 Available from: http://apps.who.int/iris/bitstream/10665/250796/1/9789241549912-eng.pdf.
18. World Health Organization. WHO recommendations on postnatal care of the mother and newborn. World heal organ; 2013. p. 1–72. Available from: http://apps.who.int/iris/bitstream/10665/97603/1/9789241506649_eng.pdf
19. Asgharpour M, Villarreal S, Schummers L, Hutcheon J, Shaw D, Norman WV. Inter-pregnancy interval and pregnancy outcomes among women with delayed childbearing: protocol for a systematic review. Syst Rev. 2017;6(1):75 Available from: http://systematicreviewsjournal.biomedcentral.com/articles/10.1186/s13643-017-0464-0.

20. Dim CC, Ugwu EO, Iloghalu EI. Duration and determinants of inter-birth interval among women in Enugu, South-Eastern Nigeria. J Obstet Gynaecol (Lahore). 2013;33(2):175–9. https://doi.org/10.3109/01443615.2012.747494.
21. Rodrigues T, Barros H. Short interpregnancy interval and risk of spontaneous preterm delivery. Eur J Obstet Gynecol Reprod Biol. 2008;136(2):184–8.
22. Stover J, Ross J. How increased contraceptive use has reduced maternal mortality. Matern Child Health J. 2010;14(5):687–95.
23. Van Eijsden M, Smits L, Van der Wal M, Bonsel G. Association between short interpregnancy intervals and term birth; 2008. p. 147–53.
24. Wendt A, Gibbs CM, Peters S, Hogue CJ. Impact of increasing inter-pregnancy interval on maternal and infant health. Paediatr Perinat Epidemiol. 2012;26(Suppl 1):239–58.
25. Abera Y, Mengesha ZB, Tessema GA. Postpartum contraceptive use in Gondar town, Northwest Ethiopia: a community based cross-sectional study. BMC Womens Health. 2015;15(1):19. https://doi.org/10.1186/s12905-015-0178-1.
26. Jalang' OR, Thuita F, Barasa SO, Njoroge P. Determinants of contraceptive use among postpartum women in a county hospital in rural Kenya. BMC Public Health. 2017;17(1):1–8.
27. Pasha O, Goudar SS, Patel A, Garces A, Esamai F, Chomba E, et al. Postpartum contraceptive use and unmet need for family planning in five low-income countries. Reprod Health. 2015;12(S2):S11. https://doi.org/10.1186/1742-4755-12-S2-S11.
28. World Health Organization. Family planning: a global handbook for providers: evidence-based guidance developed through worldwide collaboration. World Health Organization; 2011. p. 59–81. Available from: https://apps.who.int/iris/handle/10665/44028.
29. White K, Teal S, Potter J. Contraception after delivery and short interpregnancy intervals among women in the United States. Obstet Gynecol. 2015;125(6):1471–7.
30. Achyut P, Mishra A, Montana L, Sengupta R, Calhoun LM, Nanda P. Integration of family planning with maternal health services: an opportunity to increase postpartum modern contraceptive use in urban Uttar Pradesh, India. J Fam Plan Reprod Heal Care. 2016;42(2):107–15.
31. Gebremedhin AY, Kebede Y, Gelagay AA, Habitu YA. Family planning use and its associated factors among women in the extended postpartum period in Addis Ababa, Ethiopia. Contracept Reprod Med. 2018;3(1):1. https://doi.org/10.1186/s40834-017-0054-5.
32. Abraha TH, Teferra AS, Gelagay AA. Postpartum modern contraceptive use in northern Ethiopia: prevalence and associated factors. Epidemiol Health. 2017;39:e2017012. https://doi.org/10.4178/epih.e2017012.
33. Borda MR, Winfrey W, McKaig C. Return to sexual activity and modern family planning use in the extended postpartum period: an analysis of findings from seventeen countries. Afr J Reprod Health. 2010;14(4):72–9 Available from: http://www.ncbi.nlm.nih.gov/pubmed/21812200.
34. Borda M, Winfrey W. Postpartum fertility and contraception: an analysis of findings from 17 countries; 2010.
35. Bouchard T, Febring R, Schneider M. Efficacy of a new postpartum transition protocol for avoiding pregnancy. J Am Board Fam Med. 2013:35–44.
36. Bwazi C, Maluwa A, Chimwaza A, Pindani M. Utilization of postpartum family planning services between six and twelve months of delivery at Ntchisi District hospital , Malawi. Health (Irvine Calif). 2014;06(14):1724–37. https://doi.org/10.4236/health.2014.614205.
37. Hameed W, Azmat SK, Ali M, Sheikh MI, Abbas G, Temmerman M, et al. Women's empowerment and contraceptive use: the role of independent versus couples' decision-making, from a lower middle income country perspective. PLoS One. 2014;9(8):e104633.
38. Barber SL. Family planning advice and postpartum contraceptive use among low-income women in Mexico. Int Fam Plan Perspect. 2007;33(1):6–12.
39. Eluwa GI, Atamewalen R, Odogwu K, Ahonsi B. Success providing postpartum intrauterine devices in private-sector health care facilities in Nigeria: factors associated with uptake. Glob Heal Sci Pract. 2016;4(2):276–83.
40. Hernandez LE, Sappenfield WM, Goodman D, Pooler J. Is effective contraceptive use conceived prenatally in Florida? The association between prenatal contraceptive counseling and postpartum contraceptive use. Matern Child Health J. 2012;16(2):423–9.
41. Mengesha ZB, Worku AG, Feleke SA. Contraceptive adoption in the extended postpartum period is low in Northwest Ethiopia. BMC Pregnancy Childbirth. 2015;15(1):160. https://doi.org/10.1186/s12884-015-0598-9.

# 17

# Factors associated with early resumption of sexual intercourse among women during extended postpartum period in Northwest Ethiopia

Birye Dessalegn Mekonnen

**Abstract**

**Background:** Postpartum sexual health and practice need to be integrated in the current maternal healthcare services to address sexual health problems. However, postpartum sexual practice has received little attention, and was not often discussed by healthcare providers during prenatal and postnatal care. Thus, this study was aimed to assess early resumption of sexual intercourse and associated factors among postpartum women in Gondar city, Northwest Ethiopia.

**Methods:** A community based cross-sectional study was conducted from January 20 to February 20, 2020. A systematic random sampling technique was used to select 634 postpartum women. A pretested, structured and interviewer-administered questionnaire was used to collect data. Data were entered into Epi Info 7.2.2 and exported to SPSS version 20 for analysis. Bivariable and multivariable logistic regressions analysis were done. Variables with *p*- value of $\leq$ 0.05 were considered as statistically significant.

**Results:** The magnitude of early resumption of sexual intercourse after childbirth was found to be 26.9% (95% CI: 23.2, 30.8). Urban resident (AOR = 6.12, 95% CI: 2.41, 15.66), parity of one (AOR = 2.26, 95% CI: 1.66, 7.78), husband demand (AOR = 2.66, 95% CI: 1.72, 4.11), postnatal care (AOR = 1.45, 95% CI: 1.06, 2.18) and use of family planning (AOR = 2.72, 95% CI: 1.51, 3.43) were factors significantly associated with early resumption of sexual intercourse.

**Conclusion:** The study found that more than one fourth of women had resumed sexual intercourse within six weeks of following childbirth. The finding of this study suggests the need of integrating discussions of postpartum sexual activity into routine prenatal, intrapartum and postnatal care with collaborative effort of policy makers, program planners, health care providers and other stakeholders. Moreover, spousal communication on postpartum sexual activity should be encouraged.

**Keywords:** Early resumption of sexual intercourse, Postpartum women, Ethiopia

Correspondence: birye22@gmail.com
Department of Nursing, Teda health Science College, P.O.BOX: 790 Gondar, Ethiopia

## Background

During the first weeks after giving birth women face physical, psychological, social, and emotional challenges as well as changes in sexual function practices [1]. Postpartum period is the period beginning immediately after the birth of the child, and it is an ideal time to deliver interventions that improve the health and survival of both the newborn and the mother [2]. Although childbirth bring many changes to the postpartum sexual health and well-being of mothers, a period following childbirth has great expectation for parents as they look forward to getting new healthy baby [3].

Sexual practice during the postpartum period is an important element that has been identified in women's healthcare which needs increasing attention worldwide [4]. According to the World Health Organization (WHO) recommendations, as part of an overall assessment following childbirth all women should be assessed regarding resumption of sexual intercourse and possible dyspareunia [5]. However, in developing countries, health promotion and education on postpartum sexual health is limited in current maternal health care services [6, 7]. Thus, substantial proportion of postpartum women do not receive information or advice about when to resume sexual activity after birth [5].

Interest in sexual activity often decrease for the period of pregnancy, but eventually return to normal during postpartum period [8]. In many countries of sub-Saharan Africa, sexual intercourse after birth is sensitive issue and considered a taboo, and sexual abstinence after childbirth is a common cultural practice [9, 10].

Initiation of sexual intercourse early in the postpartum period may expose women at risk of getting pregnant, which is most likely unintended. Though more than 90% of women during the postpartum period want to either delay or avoid future pregnancies globally, women usually resume sexual activity without use of any modern contraceptives [11]. Though the resumption of sexual activity following childbirth varies from culture to culture, WHO recommends that women should wait till 24 months after childbirth, before becoming pregnant again [12].

Even though there is limited information on factors that affect women's early return to sexual activity during the postpartum period, biological, psychological, socio-logical and religious practice, educational status and parity of the women were identified factors that can affect women's decision on their sexual practice within the postpartum period [8, 13–15].

Women may have problems with sexual function and relationship in their postnatal period, for which they may require adequate information, counseling and support to be prepared for resumption of sexual intercourse in the postpartum, and to avoid complications such as puerperal infection and unwanted pregnancies [14]. Since, postpartum sexual health is inseparable from sexuality and sexual function, perceived sexual problems in the postpartum period need to be addressed [7, 16]. However, postpartum sexual practice has received little attention with policy makers, programmers and other stakeholders, and was not often discussed by health care providers during prenatal and postnatal care [17, 18]. For the effective intervention of postpartum sexual health, determine the magnitude of early sexual resumption and understanding the sexual experiences of women during the postpartum period is important. Therefore, the aim of this study was to assess the early resumption of sexual intercourse after childbirth and associated factors among women in the extended postpartum period in Gondar city, Northwest Ethiopia. This study can help policy makers, health care professionals and other stakeholders to provide information on postpartum sexual practice to women and their partners during antenatal care and after childbirth.

## Methods

### Study design, period and area

A community-based cross-sectional study was conducted from January 20, 2020 to February 20, 2020 at Gondar city. Gondar city is located 727 KM Northwest of Addis Ababa, capital of Ethiopia. It is divided in to seven sub cities and 25 kebeles. According to the 2013 population projection estimate, there were 258,178 residents and more than half of them were females [19]. The city has one comprehensive specialized hospital, eight governmental health centers and 14 rural health posts that are providing maternal and other health services to the population.

### Source and study population

The source population was all women of child bearing age who gave birth in the past 12 months prior to the study period in Gondar city, northwest Ethiopia. The study participants were women who gave birth in the past 12 months prior to the study and lived at least for 6 months in the selected Kebeles, but those who were sick and unable to respond during study period were excluded.

### Sample size determination and sampling procedure

The sample size was determined using single population proportion formula considering the following assumptions: expected proportion of women who resumed sexual intercourse within the six weeks postpartum of 50%; marginal error of 5, 95% confidence level, design effect 1.5 and estimated non response rate of 10%. Finally, the total sample size calculated was 634.

A multistage cluster sampling technique was used to identify the participants. First, out of the six sub-cities of

Gondar city, Maraki sub-city was chosen by the simple random sampling technique. From Maraki sub-city, four kebeles (College mazoria, Samuna ber, Shiro meda and Hidassie) were selected using the lottery method. Then, the total sample size was allocated proportionally to each selected kebeles. The study subjects were selected by systematic random sampling. The sampling interval was 2 obtained by dividing the study population to the sample size (1167/634 ≈ 2). The first household was chosen at the center of each Keble by lottery method as a starting point, and then the data collectors were going in the right direction until the required sample size was achieved. If there were more than one eligible woman in the selected household, one was considered by lottery method for the interview.

#### Data collection tool and procedure

Structured and pretested questionnaire adapted from related literatures [8, 13, 20–23] was used. Data were collected through face-to-face interview at the participant's home. The questionnaire was first developed in English, then translated into Amharic, and finally retranslated into English to check the consistency. Four diploma female midwives as data collectors and two supervisors were involved in the data collection process. Training was given to the data collectors and supervisor. The collected data were checked for completeness daily.

#### Variables of the study

In this study, the dependent variable was the early resumption of postpartum sexual intercourse (before or after six weeks postpartum), which is defined as having the first penetrative sexual intercourse after childbirth. The timing of sexual resumption was categorized into resumption before 6 weeks (early resumption) and after 6 weeks (recommended resumption). The independent variables include marital status; age, religion, use of contraceptive, place of residence, monthly income, woman's education, partner's education, mode of delivery, total child ever born, current working status of respondent, breastfeeding, menstrual resumption, family planning use, antenatal care (ANC), place of delivery and PNC.

#### Data quality control

Training was given to the data collectors and supervisor on general objective of the study, contents of the tool, how to approach the study participants and keep their confidentiality. The tool was pre-tested on 5% (32 women) of the sample in Debark town which was out of the study area before starting actual data collection.

#### Data processing and analysis

Data were entered using EPI-INFO version 7.2.2.2 and exported to Statistical Package for Social Sciences (SPSS) version 20 for further analysis. Descriptive statistics were computed to describe the study population in relation to relevant variables. For the wealth index, a principal component analysis was conducted. Both bivariable and multivariable logistic regression model were carried out to identify associated factors. Variables with *p*-values of $\leq$ 0.2 in the bivariate analysis were further fitted to multivariable logistic regression analysis. Adjusted Odds Ratio (AOR) with 95% confidence intervals (CI) was computed to determine the strength and presence of association. Variance inflation factors (VIF) was used to check assumptions regression model, and model goodness of fit was tested by the Hosmer–Lemeshow model goodness-of-fit test. Finally, variables with p- values of $\leq$ 0.05 were considered as statistically significant.

#### Ethical approval

Ethical clearance was obtained from the Institutional Review Board (IRB) of University of Gondar, College of Medicine and Health Sciences, Institute of Public Health. An official letter of cooperation was written to Gondar city administration. The benefit of the study was explained to the respondents, and then verbal informed consent was received from the participants before interviewing them. Confidentiality of the information was maintained by excluding personal identifiers in the questionnaire.

### Results

#### Socio-demographic characteristics of study participants

In this study, a total of 634 study participants were responded the interviewed with a response rate of 100%. The mean age of the respondents was 28.3 (SD ±5.5) with the minimum and the maximum age of 18 and 50 years respectively. Majority, 611(89.5%) of the participants were married and about, 546(86.6%) of women were urban residents. Five hundred forty-six (86.2%) of participants were followers of Orthodox Christian. Regarding to educational status, 224(35.3%) of women had completed secondary school while 267(43.7%) of their husband had completed higher education (Table 1).

#### Obstetrical and sexual history of participants

The median number of living children was 2 per women (IQR = 1.0 3.0) with nearly, 304(47.9%) of women had two to three living children. Majority, 389 (61.4%) of participants had vaginal delivery with no episiotomy/ tears, and 325 (51.2%) of their babies were aged between 6 and 24 weeks old.

Among the participants, 569 (89.7%) had already resumed sexual intercourse after delivery. Of the participants who had resumed sexual intercourse, 153(26.9%) with 95% CI (23.2, 30.8) resumed before 6 weeks after childbirth and 416 (73.1%) resumed after 6 weeks. The

**Table 1** Socio-demographic characteristics of mothers in the extended postpartum period, Gondar city, northwest Ethiopia, 2020 ($n = 634$)

| Variables | Number | Percent |
|---|---|---|
| Age | | |
| 18–24 | 205 | 32.3 |
| 25–34 | 331 | 52.2 |
| ≥ 35 | 98 | 15.5 |
| Marital status | | |
| Married | 611 | 96.4 |
| Unmarried (in union) | 23 | 3.6 |
| Religion | | |
| Orthodox | 546 | 86.2 |
| Muslim | 82 | 12.9 |
| Protestant | 6 | 0.9 |
| Residence | | |
| Urban | 546 | 86.2 |
| Rural | 88 | 13.8 |
| Educational level | | |
| No formal education | 116 | 18.3 |
| Primary school complete | 105 | 16.6 |
| Secondary school complete | 224 | 35.3 |
| Higher education complete | 189 | 29.8 |
| Occupation | | |
| Housewife | 416 | 65.6 |
| Government employee | 70 | 11.0 |
| Private employee | 112 | 17.7 |
| Merchant | 19 | 3.0 |
| Others (Daily laborer, student, Tella sellers) | 17 | 2.7 |
| Husband's education status ($N = 611$) | | |
| No formal education complete | 92 | 15.1 |
| Primary school complete | 88 | 14.4 |
| Secondary school complete | 164 | 26.8 |
| Higher education complete | 267 | 43.7 |
| Husband's occupation ($N = 611$) | | |
| Farmer | 41 | 6.7 |
| Government employee | 198 | 32.4 |
| Private employee | 165 | 27.0 |
| Merchant | 131 | 21.4 |
| Daily laborer | 59 | 9.7 |
| Others *(Driver, student, job seekers)* | 17 | 2.8 |
| Monthly income | | |
| Lowest | 64 | 10.1 |
| Second | 191 | 30.1 |
| Middle | 101 | 15.9 |
| Fourth | 142 | 22.4 |
| Highest | 136 | 21.5 |

timing of resumption of sexual intercourse ranged between 2 and 46 weeks with a median of 12 weeks. The major reason (76.1%) for resumed sexual intercourse after delivery were partner demand. In relation to problems noted after resuming sexual intercourse, about 394(69.2%) of participants had no problems experienced and 89(15.6%) had experienced pain during sexual intercourse.

Concerning maternal healthcare service utilization about 617(97.3%) of the respondents had antenatal attendance, about 577 (91.0%) of women delivered their last child at public health facilities and 347(54.7%) attended postnatal clinic after their last delivery. More than half, 329(51.9%) women were using a family planning method. Of the participants who use family planning method, only 56(17.1%) were initiated by 6 weeks following childbirth (Table 2).

### Factors associated with early resumption of sexual intercourse after delivery

Variables that had $p$ values $\leq 0.2$ in the bivariate analysis were included in the multivariable logistic regression model. In the multivariable logistic regression analysis, place of residence, parity, husband demand for sexual intercourse, use of family planning, and PNC visit were significantly associated with early resumption of sexual intercourse after childbirth. Women living in urban setting were 6.12 times (AOR = 6.12, 95% CI: 2.41, 15.66) more likely to initiate early sexual intercourse after childbirth than those who live in rural areas. The odds of early resumption of sexual intercourse after childbirth among women with one parity were about 2.26 times higher than women with five and above parity (AOR = 2.26, 95% CI: 1.66, 7.78). The odds of early sexual intercourse resumption after childbirth in husband demand for sexual intercourse were about 2.66 times higher than women's desire (AOR = 2.66, 95% CI: 1.72, 4.11). Women who obtained PNC were about 1.45 times higher odds to initiate early sexual intercourse than who did not (AOR = 1.45, 95% CI: 1.06, 2.18). Women who were using family planning were about 2.72 times higher odds to resume early sexual intercourse (AOR = 2.72, 95% CI: 1.51, 3.43) than those who did not use (Table 3).

## Discussion

The objectives of this study was to assess the timing of sexual intercourse resumption after childbirth and identify factors associated with early resumption of sexual intercourse among postnatal women. Accordingly, the finding shows that more than one fourth of women had resumed sexual intercourse by 6 weeks of postpartum. This implies that substantial proportion of women could be at risk of unintended pregnancy, especially when they delay to initiate postpartum contraceptive methods or

**Table 2** Reproductive and obstetric characteristics of mothers of extended postpartum period in Gondar city, northwest Ethiopia, 2020 ($n = 634$)

| Variables | Number | Percent |
|---|---|---|
| Parity | | |
| 1 | 227 | 35.8 |
| 2–4 | 373 | 58.8 |
| ≥ 5 | 34 | 5.4 |
| Alive children by now | | |
| 1 | 232 | 36.6 |
| 2–3 | 304 | 47.9 |
| ≥ 4 | 98 | 15.5 |
| Was the last pregnancy planned? | | |
| Yes | 593 | 93.5 |
| No | 41 | 6.5 |
| Mode of delivery for current child | | |
| Vaginal without episiotomy/tear | 389 | 61.4 |
| Vaginal with episiotomy/tear | 75 | 11.8 |
| Instrumental (Forceps and vacuumed delivery) | 41 | 6.5 |
| Emergency Cesarean section | 89 | 14.0 |
| Elective Cesarean section | 40 | 6.3 |
| Breastfeed currently | | |
| Yes | 614 | 96.8 |
| No | 20 | 3.2 |
| Sexual intercourse resumed after recent birth | | |
| Yes | 569 | 89.7 |
| No | 65 | 10.3 |
| Timing of resumption sexual intercourse ($n = 569$) | | |
| Before 6 weeks | 153 | 26.9 |
| After 6 weeks | 416 | 73.1 |
| Problems noted after resuming sexual intercourse ($n = 569$) | | |
| No problem | 394 | 69.2 |
| Pain during sex | 89 | 15.6 |
| Vaginal bleeding/discharge | 34 | 6.0 |
| Lack of desire | 29 | 5.1 |
| Vaginal dryness | 23 | 4.0 |
| Did you seek medical advice for sexual problem ($n = 175$)? | | |
| Yes | 52 | 29.7 |
| No | 123 | 70.3 |
| Reason for resuming sexual intercourse | | |
| I wanted sex | 136 | 23.9 |
| Partner demand | 433 | 76.1 |
| Ever advised about postpartum sexual activity | | |
| Yes | 181 | 28.5 |
| No | 453 | 71.5 |

**Table 2** Reproductive and obstetric characteristics of mothers of extended postpartum period in Gondar city, northwest Ethiopia, 2020 ($n = 634$) *(Continued)*

| Variables | Number | Percent |
|---|---|---|
| Time from childbirth | | |
| Less than 6 weeks | 36 | 5.7 |
| 6–24 weeks | 325 | 51.2 |
| 24–46 weeks | 273 | 43.1 |
| Using any family planning | | |
| Yes | 329 | 51.9 |
| No | 305 | 48.1 |
| Have ANC follow up | | |
| Yes | 617 | 97.3 |
| No | 17 | 2.7 |
| Place of delivery | | |
| Public health facility | 577 | 91.0 |
| Private clinics | 13 | 2.1 |
| Home | 44 | 6.9 |
| Postnatal care | | |
| Yes | 347 | 54.7 |
| No | 287 | 45.3 |

intensity of breastfeeding could not be guaranteed. Evidence revealed that short birth interval is relatively rare when sexual activity is delayed in the postpartum [9]. Furthermore, sexual abstinence is beneficial to the mother, for the body's recovery and the process of healing the birth injuries [24, 25].

In this study, the magnitude of early sexual intercourse resumption was found to be 26.9% (95% CI: 23.2, 30.8). This finding is consistent with similar studies done in Nigeria [26] and Ghana [15], which reported early sexual intercourse resumption as 29.7 and 23.9% respectively. However, this finding was higher than the findings of similar studies previously done in Uganda (21.9%) [21] and Northern Nigeria 21.7% [27]. However, this finding was found to be lower when compared with study done in United States (43%) [28], Nigeria (38.9%) [20], and Iban (37.4%) [8]. The possible explanation for these variations could be due to differences in socio-cultural, social beliefs and norms, religious practices, and sexual attitudes of women in different parts of the world. Early sexual resumption is influenced by subjective norms, social beliefs, and values held by society about postpartum sexual abstinence [29].

The present study revealed that women who live in urban setting were 6.12 times (AOR = 6.12, 95% CI: 2.41, 15.66) more likely to resume early sexual intercourse after childbirth than rural dwellers. This finding is consistent with other studies done in Nigeria [22] and Eswatini [24]. This could be due to the fact that women

**Table 3** Bivariable and multivariable analysis for early resumption of sexual intercourse among mothers of extended postpartum period in Gondar city, northwest Ethiopia, 2020

| Variables | Timing of resumption | | COR (95% CI) | AOR (95% CI) |
|---|---|---|---|---|
| | Before 6 weeks | After 6 weeks | | |
| Residence | | | | |
| Urban | 146 | 352 | 3.79(1.18, 5.89) | **6.12(2.41, 15.66)** |
| **Rural** | **7** | **64** | **1** | **1** |
| Age | | | | |
| 18–24 | 49 | 138 | 0.97(0.54, 1.72) | 0.92(0.43, 1.99) |
| 25–34 | 82 | 214 | 0.90(0.52, 1.55) | 0.99(0.52, 1.86) |
| ≥ 35 | 22 | 64 | 1 | 1 |
| Educational status | | | | |
| No formal education | 34 | 64 | 0.53(0.11, 0.92) | 0.54(0.29, 1.02) |
| Primary school complete | 30 | 57 | 0.54(0.31, 0.95) | 0.49(0.26, 1.94) |
| Secondary school complete | 49 | 154 | 0.89(0.55, 1.44) | 0.88(0.52, 1.48) |
| College/University complete | 40 | 141 | 1 | 1 |
| Parity | | | | |
| 1 | 46 | 153 | 1.57(0.64, 3.86) | **2.26(1.66, 7.78)** |
| 2–4 | 99 | 246 | 1.17(0.49, 2.80) | 1.81(0.59, 5.54) |
| ≥ 5 | 8 | 17 | 1 | 1 |
| Breastfeed currently | | | | |
| Yes | 149 | 404 | 0.91(0.29, 2.85) | 1.01(0.29, 3.48) |
| No | 4 | 12 | 1 | 1 |
| Reason for resuming sexual intercourse | | | | |
| I wanted sex | 59 | 77 | 1 | 1 |
| Partner demand | 94 | 339 | 2.76(1.82, 4.16) | **2.66(1.72, 4.11)** |
| Ever advised about postpartum sexual activity | | | | |
| Yes | 35 | 109 | 1.20(0.77, 1.85) | 1.32(0.79, 2.19) |
| No | 118 | 307 | 1 | 1 |
| Using any family planning | | | | |
| Yes | 65 | 250 | 2.04(1.40, 2.97) | **2.72(1.51, 3.43)** |
| No | 88 | 166 | 1 | 1 |
| Have postnatal care | | | | |
| Yes | 69 | 244 | 1.73(1.19, 2.51) | **1.45(1.06, 2.18)** |
| No | 84 | 172 | 1 | 1 |

living in rural area are more likely to adhere to traditional practices, and the cultural practice of sexual abstinence during the postpartum period. In addition, most women in rural residents separated from their spouses or partners and stayed with parents or relatives during the postpartum period [24, 30].

This study was also identified that husband demand for sexual intercourse were about 2.66 times higher than women's desire (AOR = 2.66 95% CI: 1.72, 4.11) to early resumption of sexual intercourse after childbirth. This finding is supported by other studies done in Eswatini [24] and Tanzania [30]. This attributed to the male partner's demand and pressure for sexual intercourse. In African, women usually initiate sexual intercourse against their will due to fear that the men will go elsewhere to have sex with other women [24, 27, 31]. Furthermore, the finding implies that the need of routine counseling and encouraging of couples, especially women, to voice out sexual concerns during the postpartum period. This could be achieved with the effort of health care providers through adopting existing guidelines to local cultural sensitivities and individual preferences [32].

Women with one parity were about 2.26 times higher (AOR = 2.26, 95% CI: 1.66, 7.78) to resume early sexual intercourse after childbirth than women with five and above parity. This finding is in agreement with a study conducted in Uganda [21]. The possible explanation for this might be that women might need another child within a short time interval, so that they couldn't assume that they are at risk of getting pregnancy.

Women who obtained PNC were about 1.45 times higher odds to initiate early sexual intercourse than who did not (AOR = 1.45, 95% CI: 1.06, 2.18). This might be due to that postnatal care visit could give the opportunity of getting more information and counselling from health professionals on exclusive breast feeding and postpartum contraceptive use, so that they can initiate postpartum contraception on recommended time. Studies reported contraceptive use as one of the factors associated with early postpartum resumption of sexual intercourse [21, 23, 33]. Furthermore, women who obtained PNC could get more information on sexual practice following delivery including misconceptions and can help women to practice sexual intercourse with no fear of physiological changes.

Women who were using family planning were about 2.72 times higher odds to resume early sexual intercourse (AOR = 2.72, 95% CI: 1.51, 3.43) than those who did not use. This finding is consistent with other previous studies done in rural Uganda [34], Iban [8] and Uganda [21]. This finding could be justified by the fact that women expected themselves as achieved the recommended birth spacing intervals and risk free of unintended pregnancy as well as its consequences.

### Limitations of the study

This study has some limitations: the study did not assessed factors related to the health system, service providers and sociocultural related misconception on postpartum sexual activity. Although community based study was conducted to minimize sampling bias, less attention was given for women with severe comorbidities, which may reduce generalizability of study results. In addition, respondents might have limited ability to remember exact time of sexual resumption; and the study lacked detailed information on sexual function and satisfaction. Moreover, evidence on the role of postpartum intercourse in the improvement of sexual health and intimacy between partners was not assessed.

## Conclusion

The study found that more than one fourth of women had resumed sexual intercourse within six weeks of following childbirth. Urban resident, one parity, husband demand for sexual intercourse, use of family planning, and having PNC visit were the significant factors of early resumption of sexual intercourse after childbirth. The finding of this study suggests that health care providers should give postpartum sexual health counseling and interactive health education, particularly for those women with few children and from urban areas. The finding also suggests the need of integrating discussions of postpartum sexual activity into routine prenatal, intrapartum and postnatal care with collaborative effort of policy makers, program planners, health care providers and other stakeholders. Moreover, spousal communication on postpartum sexual activity should be encouraged.

### Abbreviations

ANC: Antenatal care; AOR: Adjusted odd ratio; CI: Confidence intervals; OR: Odds ratio; PNC: Postnatal care; WHO: World Health Organization

### Acknowledgments

The author would like to thank University of Gondar for its technical support and ethical approval. The author is also grateful to the data collectors, supervisors and study participants for their cooperation and support during the study period.

### Author's contributions

BDM wrote the proposal, participated in data collection, analysis, report writing and drafted the manuscript. The author(s) read and approved the final manuscript.

### References

1. Lamont J. Female sexual health consensus clinical guidelines. J ObstetGynaecol Can. 2012;34:769–75..
2. WHO. WHO Technical Consultation on Postpartum and Postnatal Care. Geneva, Switzerland: World Health Organization; 2010 p 11–16 WHO/MPS/. 10.03. http://whqlibdoc.who.int/hq/2010/WHO_MPS_10.03_eng.pdf.
3. Organization WH. Postnatal Care for Mothers and Newborns: Highlights from the World Health Organization 2013 Guidelines. In. 2015; 25. 2019.
4. Radziah MSK, Jamsiah M, Normi M, MohdZahari TH, NurSyimah AT, Nor AM. Early resumption of sexual intercourse and its determinants among postpartum Iban mothers. International Journal of Reproduction, Contraception, Obstetrics and Gynecology Radziah M et al. Int J Reprod Contracept Obstet Gynecol. 2013;2(2):124–9.
5. Organization WH. Postnatal care for mothers and newborns: Highlights from the World Health Organization 2013 Guidelines. Avaible from: https://www.who.int.maternal.child.adolescent.publications/WHOMCA-PNC-2014-Briefer A. 2015;4.
6. Leeman L, Rogers R. Współżycie płciowe po porodzie. Aktywność seksualna kobiety po urodzeniu dziecka. Obstet Gynecol. 2012;119(3):647–55. https://doi.org/10.1097/AOG.0b013e3182479611.
7. O'Malley D, Higgins A, Smith V. Postpartum sexual health: a principle-based concept analysis. J Adv Nurs. 2015;71(10):2247–57. https://doi.org/10.1111/jan.12692.
8. Radziah M, Shamsuddin K, Jamsiah M, Normi M, Zahari T, Syimah A, et al. Early resumption of sexual intercourse and its determinants among postpartum Iban mothers. Int J Reprod Contracept Obstet Gynecol. 2013; 2(2):124–9. https://doi.org/10.5455/2320-1770.ijrcog20130603.
9. Borda M, Winfrey W. Postpartum fertility and contraception: an analysis of findings from 17 countries, Baltimore: Jhpiego. Afr J Reprod Health 2010; 14(4 Spec no): 72–79. 2010.
10. Woolhouse H, McDonald E, Brown SJ. Changes to sexual and intimate relationships in the postnatal period: women's experiences with health professionals. Aust J Prim Health. 2014;20(3):298–304. https://doi.org/10.1071/PY13001.
11. Organization. WH. Partner release programming strategies for postpartum family planning Global Health. Sci Pract. 2014;2(1):4–9.
12. Anzaku AMS. Postpartum resumption of sexual activity, Sexual Morbidity and Use of Modern Contraceptive Among Nigerian Women in Jos. Ann Med Health Sci Res. 2014;4(2):210–6.

13. Kola M, Owonikoko AGA, Aramide M, Tijani, et al. Determinants of resumption of vaginal intercourse in puerperium period in Ogbomoso: consideration for early use of contraceptives. Int J Reprod Contracept Obstet Gynecol. 2014;3(4):1061–6. https://doi.org/10.5455/2320-1770.ijrcog20141236.
14. Mbekenga CKOP, Pembe AB, Draj E, Christensson K. Prolonged sexual abstinence after childbirth: gendered norms and perceived family health risks. Focus group discussions in a Tanzanian suburb. BMC Int Health Hum Rights. 2013;13:4 https://www.biomedcentral.com/1472-698X/13/4.
15. Eliason SK, Bockarie AS, Eliason C. Postpartum fertility behaviours and contraceptive use among women in rural Ghana. Contracept Reprod Med. 2018;3(1):13 https://doi.org/0.1186/s40834-018-0066-9.
16. Organization WH. Consolidated guideline on sexual and reproductive health and rights of women living with HIV: World Health Organization; 2017.
17. Jonas K, Crutzen R, van den Borne B, Reddy P. Healthcare workers' behaviors and personal determinants associated with providing adequate sexual and reproductive healthcare services in sub-Saharan Africa: a systematic review. BMC Pregnancy Child. 2017;17(1):86. https://doi.org/10.1186/s12884-017-1268-x.
18. Olsson A, Robertson E, Falk K, Nissen E. Assessing women's sexual life after childbirth: the role of the postnatal check. Midwifery. 2011;27(2):195–202. https://doi.org/10.1016/j.midw.2009.04.003.
19. Bureau (ARHB): ARH. Wereda Based plan 2010. Bahir Dar, Ethiopia 2012.
20. Adenike O-BI, Oke OS, Kola OM, Akande R, Tolulope F, Oluwatosin D, et al. Post-partum resumption of sexual intercourse and the uptake of modern contraceptives among women attending a tertiary hospital in SOUTH West Nigeria. J Health Med Nurs 2017;1(1):65–80. ISSN 2520-4025.
21. Alum AC, Kizza IB, Osingada CP, Katende G, Kaye DK. Factors associated with early resumption of sexual intercourse among postnatal women in Uganda. Reprod Health. 2015;12(1):107. https://doi.org/10.1186/s12978-015-0089-5.
22. Fagbamigbe A, Awoyelu I, Akinwale O, Akinwande T, Enitilo B, Bankole O. Factors contributing to the duration of postpartum abstinence among Nigerian women: semi-parametric survival analysis. Heliyon. 2018;4(12): e01032 https://doi.org/10.1016/j.heliyon.2018.e.
23. Zhuang C, Li T, Li L. Resumption of sexual intercourse post partum and the utilisation of contraceptive methods in China: a cross-sectional study. BMJ Open. 2019;9(3):e026132. https://doi.org/10.1136/bmjopen-2018-.
24. Shabangu Z, Madiba S. The role of culture in maintaining post-partum sexual abstinence of Swazi women. Int J Environ Res Public Health. 2019; 16(14):2590. https://doi.org/10.3390/ijerph16142590.
25. Imo CK, Okoronkwo E, Ukoji V, Mbah C. Postpartum sexual abstinence and its implications for under-five health outcome among childbearing women in South-East Nigeria. Afr J Reprod Health. 2018;22(4):102–11.
26. Ezebialu I, Eke A. Resumption of vaginal intercourse in the early postpartum period: determinants and considerations for child spacing in a Nigerian population. J Obstet Gynaecol. 2012;32(4):353–6 https://doi.org/10.3109/01443615.2011.652701.
27. Iliyasu Z, Galadanci HS, Danlami KM, Salihu HM, Aliyu MH. Correlates of postpartum sexual activity and contraceptive use in Kano, northern Nigeria. Afr J Reprod Health. 2018;22(1):103–12. https://doi.org/10.29063/ajrh2018/v22i1.10.
28. Sok C, Sanders JN, Saltzman HM, Turok DK. Sexual behavior, satisfaction, and contraceptive use among postpartum women. J Midwifery Women's health. 2016;61(2):158–65. https://doi.org/10.1111/jmwh.12409.
29. Vaismoradi M, Turunen H, Bondas T. Content analysis and thematic analysis: implications for conducting a qualitative descriptive study. Nurs Health Sci. 2013;15(3):398–405.
30. Reuben Mahiti G, Mbekenga CK, Dennis Kiwara A, Hurtig A-K, Goicolea I. Perceptions about the cultural practices of male partners during postpartum care in rural Tanzania: a qualitative study. Glob Health Action. 2017;10(1):1361184.
31. Mbekenga CK, Christensson K, Lugina HI, Olsson P. Joy, struggle and support: postpartum experiences of first-time mothers in a Tanzanian suburb. Women Birth. 2011;24(1):24–31 https://doi.org/10.1016/j.wombi.2010.06.004.
32. Lamont J, Bajzak K, Bouchard C, Burnett M, Byers S, Cohen T, et al. Female sexual health consensus clinical guidelines. J Obstet Gynaecol Can. 2012; 34(8):769–75 https://doi.org/10.1016/S701-2163(16)35341-5.
33. Kitessa D, Rulisa S, Ntasumbumuyange D, Aimable M, Pritchett N, Ghebre R. Immediate Postpartum Family Planning Preferences Among Couples in Rwanda. Rwanda Med J. 2019;76(4):1–7.
34. Osinde MO, Kaye DK, Kakaire O. Influence of HIV infection on women's resumption of sexual intercourse and use of contraception in the postpartum period in rural Uganda. Int J Gynecol Obstet. 2012;116(2):171–2 https://doi.org/10.1016/j.ijgo.2011.09.018.

18

# A qualitative study exploring barriers to adequate uptake of antenatal care in pre-conflict Syria: Low cost interventions are needed to address disparities in antenatal care

Rima Mourtada[1,2*], Hyam Bashour[3] and Fiona Houben[4]

**Abstract**

**Background:** Syria has made progress in reducing maternal mortality and morbidity before the conflict in 2011. Despite the improvement in antenatal care (ANC) coverage and patterns of use, analyses of national surveys demonstrated wide regional variations in uptake, timing and number of visits even after controlling for women's socio-demographic characteristics. This study compares two governorates: Latakia, where uptake of ANC was high and Aleppo, where uptake of ANC was low to highlight the barriers to women's adequate uptake of ANC that existed in Syria pre-conflict.

**Methods:** This qualitative study carried out 30 semi-structured interviews with (18–45-year-old) pregnant women from Aleppo and Latakia (recruited purposively from different types of health facilities in rural and urban areas), and 15 observation sessions at health facilities. Transcripts and fieldnotes were analyzed using the Framework Method with attention to the dimensions of availability, accessibility and acceptability of services.

**Results:** Inadequate uptake of ANC in Aleppo included not attending ANC, seeking care with providers who are not trained to provide ANC or discontinuing care. Three themes explained the regional disparities in the uptake of ANC in Aleppo and Latakia: women's assessment of their health status and reasoning of causes of ill health in pregnancy; women's evaluation of the risks of seeking ANC; and women's appraisal of the value of different types of service providers. Poor experiences at public health facilities were reported by women in Aleppo but not by women in Latakia. Evaluations of ANC services were connected with the availability, accessibility (geographical and financial) and acceptability of ANC services, however, women's views were shaped by the knowledge and prevailing opinions in their families and community.

(Continued on next page)

* Correspondence: rima.mourtada@yahoo.co.uk
[1]Department of Epidemiology and Population Health, London School of Hygiene and Tropical Medicine, Keppel St, Bloomsbury, London WC1E 7HT, UK
[2]Faculty of Health Sciences, American University of Beirut, Bliss Street, Beirut, Lebanon

(Continued from previous page)

**Conclusions:** Findings are utilized to discuss low-cost interventions addressing the disparities in ANC uptake. Interventions should aim to enable vulnerable women to make informed decisions focusing on regions of low uptake. Women's groups that foster education and empowerment, which have been effective in other low resource settings, could be of value in Syria. Increased use of mobile phones and social media platforms suggests mobile health technologies (mHealth) may present efficient platforms to deliver these interventions.

**Keywords:** Antenatal care, Conflict, Interventions, Syria

## Background

The vast majority of pregnancy-related complications that cause maternal and neonatal morbidity and mortality take place in low and middle-income countries (LMICs) [1, 2]. Most interventions, often introduced during antenatal care (ANC), improve the health of the mothers and the neonates concurrently [3].

ANC is defined as the care provided by skilled healthcare providers to pregnant women and adolescent girls in order to ensure the best health conditions for both mother and baby during pregnancy [4]. It is recommended that ANC should be initiated in the first trimester of pregnancy because most interventions should be implemented early in order to be effective [5, 6]. A minimum number of visits is important. The World Health Organization (WHO) formerly recommended four focused ANC visits for low-risk pregnancies with additional visits for high risk women following the 1990 model [7], however, this model was found to be associated with higher perinatal deaths compared to the model advocating for 8 visits [8]. Consequently, WHO's updated model in 2016 recommended 8 ANC visits; one visit in the first trimester, 2 visits in the second trimester and 5 visits in the third trimester [8].

Given the prominent role of ANC in protecting the health of mothers and babies, understanding the factors that influence women's access to and uptake of ANC services is extremely important in order to address any barriers that prevent demand for or provision of such services. A number of health seeking behaviour models have been developed to map some factors that have shown to have an influence on patients' health seeking behaviour. The most commonly used models, which focus on utilisation of the health services are the Pathway Models, the Health Care Utilisation Model or the Andersen Model and the "Four As" Model [9].

The Pathways Models describe the sequence of events that patients follow starting with acknowledging the symptoms, and ending with the use of different types of health services (traditional and non-traditional) [10]. Good's model, one example of the Pathway Models, highlights the crucial role of family and friends in the management of illness and consequently the decision making process regarding different therapeutic choices [11].

The Andersen and Newman Health Care Utilisation Model [12, 13] groups in a logic sequence three categories of factors, which influence health behaviour or treatment actions: 1- Predisposing factors that include the socio-cultural characteristics of the individual that existed prior to their health condition such as age, education, parity, health awareness and previous use of the service; 2- enabling factors that include the means or logistics required to obtain the services, and 3- needs factors that include perception of health status of the individual and perception of usefulness of health services.

The "Four As" model assembles key factors for health-seeking behaviour into four dimensions of access that overlap with "the Right to Health" elements as well. "The Right to Health means that governments must generate conditions in which everyone can be as healthy as possible." Such conditions range from ensuring availability of health services, healthy and safe working conditions, adequate housing and nutritious food [14]. The "Right to Health" contains four elements: 1- availability: a sufficient quantity of functioning public health and health care facilities, goods and services, as well as programmes, 2-accessibility: health facilities, goods and services accessible to everyone and it has four overlapping dimensions (non-discrimination, physical accessibility, economical accessibility (affordability) and information accessibility). 3- acceptability: all health facilities, goods and services must be respectful of medical ethics and culturally appropriate as well as sensitive to gender and life-cycle requirements. 4- quality: health facilities, goods and services must be scientifically and medically appropriate and of good quality [15].

The health services "access" concept is also a function of demand and supply. Demand-side factors are defined as "those factors that affect demand and that operate at the individual, household or community level" whereas supply side factors are "factors derived from the health care production function, that interact to produce effective health care services" [10]. Access is hampered when individuals do not use services that could be beneficial to them on the demand side or when good quality effective care is not offered on the supply side, and both demand and supply sides are related [11]. Most studies that examine access to health care use frameworks that include the "4 As model" dimensions (that have supply and demand elements as described by Peters et al. [16]).

Individual and household factors that influence use of ANC include education, age, parity, socio-economic status, area of residence and knowledge about the characteristics of and need for medical treatment [13]. Cultural, religious and other social factors are among community factors that influence use of health services and these include autonomy, religion, social support and cultural beliefs [17–20].. A recent systematic review that examined provision and uptake of ANC emphasized the importance of traditional beliefs, which may consider pregnancy to be a normal event that does not require medical attention, in influencing women's health seeking behavior in LMICs. Cultural beliefs and the role of others that influence women's health seeking behavior in traditional societies are not captured with standard national household surveys.

Syria had made considerable progress in decreasing maternal and infant mortality before the conflict in 2011. Ninety six percent of women delivered with a skilled birth attendant, and 88% had at least one ANC with a skilled attendant. However, the number of women who had at least 4 ANC visits (according to the national guidelines following WHO recommendations at the time of the study) was much lower (64%) [21].

An earlier study by Mourtada et al. (2019) conducted secondary analyses of national health surveys which demonstrated wide regional variations in uptake, timing of first visit, number of visits to ANC and quality of ANC [22, 23]. Although women's socio-demographic characteristics are important determinants of service use, Mourtada et al' s analyses revealed that the regional disparities in ANC coverage and patterns of use remained even after controlling for women's main demographics [20], suggesting that there are additional factors contributing to the regional disparities in ANC coverage and use patterns, which are likely related to service provision on the supply side and socio-cultural and community factors on the demand side.

The Syrian conflict caused destruction to many health facilities in the country consequently interrupting maternal health care for many women [24] and likely deepening divisions in care quality. Post-conflict reconstruction of health services offers a unique opportunity to address the issues, which contributed to the regional disparities in ANC coverage and patterns of use that existed pre-conflict. Efforts to rebuild the health system in Syria are likely to focus on addressing supply side factors that are related to governance, infrastructure, rebuilding the destroyed health facilities and retaining the health workers [25] with the overall aim of achieving universal health coverage. However, high coverage does not always translate into positive health outcomes when health facilities are underutilized [26]. Therefore, it is important to address the demand-side barriers to adequate uptake of ANC that contributed to the regional variations in ANC coverage and patterns of use that were present before the conflict.

## Methods

### Aims of the study

The main aim of this qualitative study is to explore barriers to women's adequate uptake of ANC and regional differences in uptake. Findings are utilized to discuss potential low-cost interventions to increase women's uptake of ANC focusing on addressing the demand side barriers, which are discussed within three dimensions of the "Right to Health" model (availability, accessibility (geographical and financial) and acceptability).

### Study design

This qualitative study employed semi-structured interviews and observation to explore factors affecting utilization and quality of ANC in Syria. It was carried out in 2010, shortly before the eruption of the conflict and was part of a larger mixed-methods study that analyzed data from two national surveys (Pan Arab Project for Family Health (PAPFAM) (1996–2001) and Multiple Indicator Cluster Survey (MICS) (2004–2006). In this paper, we present the perspectives of women in two governorates in Syria; Latakia where uptake of ANC was high and Aleppo where uptake of ANC was low to explore barriers to adequate uptake of ANC [21]. Inadequate uptake of ANC in this study is defined as: not seeking ANC, seeking care with providers who are not trained to provide ANC or discontinuing care.

#### *Conceptual framework*

We have constructed a modified framework [23] (Fig. 1) that draws on a combination of two health care seeking behavior models: the Andersen and Newman Model that includes a wide range of women and health services related factors that demonstrate a strong influence on maternal health care service utilization in many settings; And Goods Pathway Model, which enables us to explore the role of the socio-cultural context, including the influence of significant others and the processes that guide women's selection of their ANC health sources. Three elements of the "Right to Health" Model constitute the main construct of the conceptual model. Women's choice of type of ANC service depends on the following dimensions of access: availability, accessibility (geographical and financial) and acceptability. We excluded quality as its definition (according to the "Rights to Health" framework focuses solely on the scientific and medical aspects of the service, which were examined in another study that focused on the provision of ANC content. In

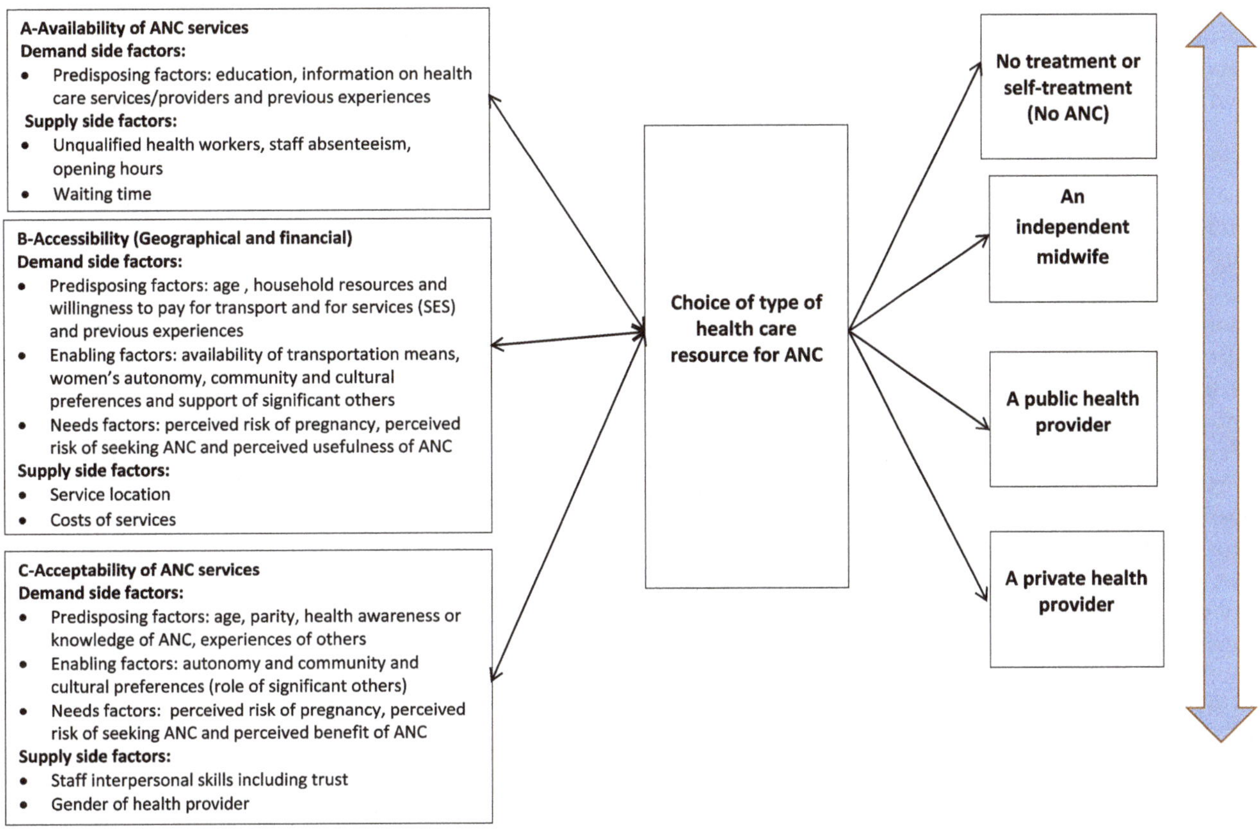


**Fig. 1** A modified conceptual framework based on three models for health care seeking behaviour

our model, we have classified the demand side and supply side factors that could be possible barriers to each dimension of access, following the classification suggested by Jacobs et al. [27]. For more details on the conceptual model, please refer to Appendix A (Additional File 1).

### *Study setting*

Table 1 provides an overview of Aleppo and Latakia governorates (referred to as Aleppo and Latakia in the paper) including the population size in each governorate in 2010 at the time of the study. Aleppo is the largest and most densely inhabited Syrian governorate. Latakia is much smaller and its capital, Latakia city, is the main port city of Syria on the Mediterranean Sea.

### *Study participants*

Participants included pregnant women aged 18–45 years living in Aleppo and Latakia attending ANC at different types of health facilities that provide ANC in Syria (private clinics/hospitals, public health centers/hospitals in urban and rural areas). We also included women who attended ANC with midwives who provided ANC independently at their own clinics in Aleppo (which was considered illegal as reported by health officials, as midwives in Syria are not trained to provide ANC

**Table 1** The general characteristics of Aleppo and Latakia governorates

| | Aleppo | Latakia |
|---|---|---|
| **Location** | Northern Syria | Western Syria |
| **Land area** | 1,850,000 ha | 230,000 ha |
| **Population** | 5,927,000 | 1,229,000 |
| **Number of districts** | 8 | 4 |
| **Number of villages** | 1453 | 432 |
| **Religion** | 90% are Muslims; the majority are Sunnis, mostly Arabs, followed by Kurds. The rest (10%) are Christians and Armenians | Mostly Alawites with some Sunni Muslims and Greek Orthodox Christians |

independently, especially examining women using an ultrasound and prescribing ANC tests, without the supervision of a doctor) as well as women who did not attend ANC (Table 2).

#### Sampling and recruitment

In each governorate, we employed purposive sampling to recruit the women from four randomly selected private clinics (from the list of private practices issued in 2009 by the Syrian Society of Obstetrics and Gynecology) and four randomly selected Public Health Centers (PHCs) (from the list issued in 2009 by the Ministry of Health). Please refer to Appendix B (Additional File 1) for a detailed description of the sampling process).

We contacted the doctor working at each health facility, explained the study and if they consented, we arranged to approach women at their health facilities. If doctors declined, we selected an alternative clinic/health center below them on the list. We approached pregnant women in the waiting areas at the health facilities independently of the health providers and emphasized that their decision to participate would not affect the health care they were receiving at this health facility. We gave them the option to be interviewed at a private room at the health facility after their appointment or at their homes at a time that is convenient for them. Women who preferred to be interviewed at their home shared their contact details. We contacted them the second day to arrange for their interview at home. None of the women we approached refused to participate.

To recruit women attending ANC with midwives who provide ANC independently, we obtained the phone numbers of midwives from the health officials in Aleppo who worked at the health directorate. We contacted the midwives, explained the study and approached women at the clinics of those who agreed to participate using the same method of recruitment as the other facilities. No midwives provided ANC independently in Latakia.

Women who did not attend ANC were recruited using the snowball technique of purposive sampling, with the help of women participating in our study. It was reflective of the regional differences in the pattern of ANC use that we were unable to locate and recruit women who did not attend ANC in Latakia. Our experience was confirmed by doctors and women in Latakia who confirmed that almost all women in Latakia attended ANC at least once. MICS survey data in 2006 shows that 97% of women in Latakia attended ANC and this percentage may have increased by the time we conducted our interviews in 2010 [21, 22].

We recruited 13 women attending ANC and 5 women not attending ANC in Aleppo, and 12 women attending ANC in Latakia (Table 2).

#### Data collection

Semi-structured audio-recorded interviews with pregnant women were carried out in both governorates. Semi-structured interviews allow the interviewees to talk more freely about their personal experiences and perceptions while also remaining focused on the topic [28].

The interviews were carried out in Arabic by the lead author as part of her PhD research. The interview guide covered the following topics: women's practices regarding their current pregnancies (and the reasons for these practices); places where they sought care, frequency of care; women's perceptions of the importance of ANC and certain elements of ANC. The guide was piloted with three women in each governorate and reviewed by the research panel.

We interviewed twelve women in Aleppo twice mainly because during the first interview these women were shy, and not always alone, which might have influenced their willingness to share information about their health seeking behavior. The interviews lasted between 30 and 45 min.

The lead author also conducted fifteen observation sessions, lasting approximately two hours each and recorded in fieldnotes at a range of health facilities in Aleppo and Latakia to validate the content of the interviews. The lead author observed the physical settings of the health facilities and the participants including women, doctors, staff and how they interacted in different settings.

The role of the researcher was known and agreed upon prior to the observations taking place [29, 30].

#### Data management and analysis

Interviews were transcribed verbatim and relevant quotes were translated into English. Data were analyzed by the lead author and codes were checked by a co-

**Table 2** An overview of the interviewed women in Aleppo and Latakia governorates

| | Women in Aleppo | Women in Latakia | Total |
|---|---|---|---|
| **Private clinics/hospitals** | 4 | 7 | 11 |
| **Public health centres/hospitals** | 4 | 5 | 9 |
| **Midwives clinics** | 5 | NA | 5 |
| **No ANC** | 5 | NA | 5 |
| **Total** | 18 | 12 | 30 |

author using the Framework Method for health research, a modified version of content analysis developed for policy relevant research [31, 32]. Familiarization with the data and the identification of persistent and contrasting themes led to the construction of a detailed index where all data were annotated according to the thematic framework and charted. In the final stage (mapping and interpretation), charts were reviewed carefully, examining different perceptions and experiences looking for similarities and differences and attempting to find associations between themes to provide an explanation for the findings. The refined themes were discussed in relation to the three dimensions of access under the "Right to Health" framework (discussed earlier) (Availability, accessibility (geographical and financial) and acceptability) of ANC services focusing on the demand side barriers under each dimension.

## Results

### Characteristics of study participants

Demographic characteristics of participants are in (Additional File 2).

### Barriers to adequate uptake of ANC

Three dominant themes emerged throughout the semi-structured interviews that explained barriers to adequate uptake of ANC, particularly in Aleppo. These were related to women's assessment of their own health status in pregnancy and reasoning about causes of ill health, women's perception of risks of seeking ANC, and women's appraisal of the value of different services and their treatment by providers.

#### *Theme 1: Women's assessment of their own health status in pregnancy and reasoning about the causes of ill health*

Women in Aleppo who never attended ANC and those who attended ANC but did not follow up regularly assessed their own health status and the risks during pregnancy differently to women in Latakia. Interviews indicated that some women in Aleppo associated seeking care with being ill or experiencing complications during pregnancy or even with being infertile: *"We do not have the habit of seeking ANC here. I will go to the doctor only if I feel sick or if I bleed." She added, "Some women in the village visit the doctor but those have fertility problems." (Participant 4, rural Aleppo, never used ANC, first interview).*

While some women did seek ANC during their first pregnancy, those who had successful pregnancy and childbirth with no complications felt that there was little value in seeking care in subsequent pregnancies: *"I did not want to follow this pregnancy up, I tried the first pregnancy, and everything was normal." (Participant 6, rural Aleppo, currently not attending ANC, first interview);* or chose to undertake a single visit during the pregnancy: *"I will visit the doctor but maybe I won't register to follow up like the first time. The first baby is different. You are scared because you know nothing, this is why you follow up..." (Participant 18, Aleppo City, attended ANC, private clinic, second interview).*

By contrast, all interviewed multiparous women in Latakia reported attending ANC regularly, either with private or public doctors (Additional File 2).

Some of the interviewed women who experienced complications and miscarriages did not perceive ANC to be protective. Their explanations for their losses included having had a shock, a nightmare, or the evil eye: *"People in the village told me that it is the evil eye that caused my miscarriage, so my mother and my husband advised me to go to the sheikh to disable the evil eye." (Participant 2, rural Aleppo, attended ANC, private clinic, one interview).*

It is notable that women living in rural Aleppo did describe the value of visiting the local health center to get vaccinated against tetanus (free at point of access) in their interviews. Observations undertaken in the accessible rural Aleppo health centers showed however, that the doctor was not available on a regular basis and that the doctors practicing were mostly males which could have discouraged some women from seeking ANC given the traditional beliefs in those communities.

#### *Theme 2: Women's evaluation of the risks associated with seeking ANC services*

Some women in Aleppo, mostly those living in rural areas, with little formal education and low-socioeconomic status, not only perceived there to be few benefits to attending ANC regularly, but further reported that seeking ANC might put their pregnancies at risk through the following: fear of hearing false bad news and fear of being asked to undergo a caesarean section. These perceptions were often founded on and expressed through stories from their immediate community (family members, friends and neighbors): *"I worry that the doctor might tell me some bad news that will stress me out. My cousin, who was nine months pregnant, was told by her doctor that the baby's position was not right and she would need a caesarean. She was stressed out, and at the end, she had a normal delivery. This affected her and she was stressed out for a whole month (Participant 3, rural Aleppo, not attending ANC, second interview)."* Similarly, participant 1 explained: *"The doctor reassured me .... If he told me that there is something wrong, I would have been scared and I would have followed up with another doctor." (Participant 1, Aleppo city, attending ANC, private clinic, second interview).*

Although some women in Latakia reported doubts about the usefulness of ANC or confidence in a doctor, they did not express similar fears that attending ANC could be the cause of harm: *"I monitored my previous pregnancy from the beginning and they did not discover that my baby was malformed until the end. Sometimes monitoring the pregnancy is useless unless both the doctor and the ultrasound are good." (Participant 27, Latakia city, attended ANC, private clinic, one interview).*

Some women avoided seeking ANC with doctors due to the belief that most doctors performed unnecessary caesarean sections or hurried the 'natural course' of birth: *"The midwife does not deliver you unless you are totally ready whereas the doctor gives you needles or operates on you when your delivery is delayed" (Participant 5, rural Aleppo, did not attend ANC, first interview); "Midwives have more patience, the doctor will not wait. I heard several stories where doctors did not wait, they ask for a caesarean right away (Participant 16, Aleppo city, attended ANC with a midwife, first interview)."* Not only had these women avoided ANC because they did not perceive any benefits, these women perceived seeking care as a risky venture and avoided seeking ANC with certain providers such as doctors or avoided seeking ANC altogether to 'protect' their pregnancies.

Our observations confirmed that the roads to the health facilities in some of the areas in rural Aleppo and poor urban Aleppo were in a poor condition, public transport was irregular and the distances were greater compared to the journeys described by women in Latakia. This may have contributed to women's perceptions of seeking ANC as risky.

#### *Theme 3: Women's appraisal of the value of different services and their treatment by providers*

A central theme that emerged from the accounts of women who attended ANC was their preference for private care, which included care with a private doctor or a private independent midwife, over public health centers. This was due to the following reasons: lack of knowledge about services offered by public health centers (PHCs), lack of trust in PHC services and poor experiences of provider-patient interaction at PHCs.

Some women in Aleppo and in Latakia were not well informed about the services offered at PHCs by clinicians: *"The staff did not mention that I could do the tests at the health center" explained Participant 8 (Aleppo city, attended ANC, PHC, first interview).* Participant 21 who lived in Latakia city and attended ANC at a PHC explained: *"The service here is good. I have never heard of this health center before. My sister told me about it. I did not even know that they have a gynecologist and an ultrasound." (one interview).*

Some women who were more familiar with the ANC services offered at PHCs however did not trust their quality, particularly, their ability to deal with or identify complications and preferred to visit a private doctor at the beginning of their pregnancy, only later following up the pregnancy at a PHC: *"I visited a private doctor at the beginning of my pregnancy. She reassured me that my pregnancy was fine. Therefore, I have decided to follow up at this health center [PHC]." (Participant 9, Aleppo city, attending ANC, second interview).*

A frequently reported experience in both governorates, but more commonly reported in Aleppo, was being mistreated by doctors and staff at PHC: *"they are cold, they do not make you feel comfortable, they do not understand what you want to tell them" (Participant 9, Aleppo city, attended ANC, PHC, first interview) and "I once visited a PHC but I lost my card and they did not agree to see me again, they refused to give me another card. They told me this is a lesson for you although I did not lose it on purpose." (Participant 7, Aleppo city, not currently attending ANC, second interview).* Impolite treatment of women by doctors and staff working in PHC in Aleppo was confirmed in observation sessions' fieldnotes. For example, a doctor scolded a woman for not being able to tell them how severe her headache was saying: *"How difficult could it be to tell me?"* On another occasion, a woman was rudely scolded by a nurse at the health center for mistakenly entering the wrong room.

By contrast, women who attended care with independent midwives described their relationship with their midwives more positively: *"Although it takes half an hour to get here, I prefer to seek care with her. I like her as she makes me feel good every visit. Good attitude is the most important thing...especially during the last month of pregnancy." (Participant 12, Aleppo city, attended ANC with a midwife, one interview); and "My midwife does not intimidate me and she never makes me feel I know nothing like doctors do." (Participant 14, Aleppo city, attended ANC with a midwife, one interview).*

The majority of women in Latakia were generally satisfied with how the doctors and staff treated them: *"The doctor here is so nice and has sense of humor (she smiles). She makes me feel at ease. It is all about attitude...I have decided to follow-up here." (Participant 29, rural Latakia, attends ANC, PHC, one interview).*

Although women in Aleppo expressed a preference for private clinics, their incapability to afford care limited their ability to attend ANC with a private doctor so women either discontinued ANC: *"The private doctor is too expensive, and the treatment at the health center is really bad, so we have to depend on God now, that's all we have" (Participant 8, Aleppo city, attended ANC, PHC, second interview),* or attended care with independent midwives who charged lower fees: *"She is not expensive, I pay only 200 SP for a visit, and sometimes she does not take money, and when she refuses to take money I give her a present." (Participant 15, Aleppo city, attended ANC with a midwife, second interview).*

## Discussion

The patterns of inadequate uptake of ANC as defined in this study (not seeking ANC, seeking care with providers who are not trained to provide ANC or discontinuing care) were prominent in Aleppo and the results generated insights into regional differences in ANC uptake. Overall, three dominant themes emerged, which explained different patterns of ANC seeking behavior among women in Aleppo and Latakia. The first theme focused on women's assessment of their health status in pregnancy and reasoning about the causes of ill health. Such perceptions were related to experiencing complications, women's parity level and their perception of the usefulness of ANC, and these were different for women in Latakia who described ANC as important regardless of their health status or parity level. The second theme described women's evaluation of the potential risks associated with seeking ANC services, which included fear of hearing bad news and fear of being asked to undergo a cesarean section. Women in Latakia were less likely to have such concerns or weighed these up differently to women in Aleppo. The third theme examined women's appraisal of the value of different services and their treatment by providers. Private providers were preferred to public services in both governorates and this was connected to the lack of knowledge about services provided at PHCs, lack of trust in services provided at PHCs and poor experiences of patient-provider interactions at PHCs. However, poor experiences with seeking ANC at PHCs were not reported to the same degree by women in Latakia.

We discuss our findings against the conceptual framework constructed for this study (Fig. 1) and under the three selected dimensions of access: availability, accessibility (geographical and financial) and acceptability focusing on the demand side barriers to accessing adequate ANC.

### Availability

Our results indicated that even when services were available, such as in the villages, where interviewed women did not seek ANC at all, there was low demand for them. A potential explanation for it could be that such women were often uneducated (Additional File 2) and consequently did not attempt to obtain information on such health facilities and the services they provide and were not empowered to do so (predisposing characteristics). On the other hand, the limited hours where doctors were present at such health facilities could also discourage women from attending ANC and may have contributed to the lower demand for such services.

### Accessibility (geographical and financial)

Our observations of the general settings confirmed that PHCs were often available and free of charge, however, geographical accessibility may have been an issue in some areas where road conditions were bad or regular transportation means were not available. As a result, accessibility (geographical and financial) of services could have been a challenge for vulnerable women in Aleppo with low autonomy, restricted access to financial resources and consequently limited mobility (enabling factors). Additionally, although it was not brought up during the interviews, women in traditional societies such as in Aleppo, are not allowed to leave the house unaccompanied (enabling factors), which makes seeking care even harder when services are not easily accessible. Therefore, even when women wanted to seek care despite their communities' traditional norms that did not perceive ANC as important, they may have been faced with other traditional norms that did not favor women going out alone (enabling factors). Accessing ANC becomes even more challenging when women are obliged to pay for transportation to go to a PHC or pay for ANC at private clinics that are closer to where they live. Moreover, women often evaluated the risks entailed in accessing ANC services (perceived risks of ANC). The poor road conditions in Aleppo and the potential negative implications of travel on pregnancy could have discouraged women from seeking care. Travel related risks resulting from inadequate infrastructure, distance to health facilities and lack of transportation were also brought up as barriers to ANC uptake in several studies included in a review that looked at reasons why women do not use ANC in LMICs [20].

### Acceptability of ANC services

Several issues were raised by interviewed women, which may have influenced their acceptability of ANC services. These were mainly related to perceived risks of pregnancy, perceived benefits of ANC and perceived risks of ANC (needs factors). The majority of women who did not seek ANC were from rural Aleppo where services were often available and accessible but those women were willing to seek care only when they perceived their case as risky or when they had problems conceiving (perceived risks of pregnancy and perceived benefits of ANC). Women's emic definitions of risk, which affected their perception of ANC benefits, differ from the etic or medical definitions which consider any pregnant woman at risk of developing complications. Whereas in those communities, pregnancy continues to be seen as a normal event that does not require regular medical follow-up, especially among multiparous women and women who did not experience any health complications or had a normal previous delivery.

Generally, women in traditional communities worry about the harmful effect of the evil eye on the unborn baby, which obliges many women to remain discrete about their pregnancy until their baby is born [33]. A number of women in rural and poor urban areas in Aleppo brought up the concept of "evil eye," and a few were convinced that it was responsible for their previous miscarriages reflecting their lack of trust in ANC benefits (perceived benefits of ANC), possibly because they were given no alternative explanations incorporating biomedical explanation of illness (low awareness of ANC). Additionally, women's fear of the harmful effect of the "evil eye" in these communities could have discouraged them or delayed them from seeking care, as seeking ANC would have been a clear announcement of their pregnancy (perceived risks of ANC). These beliefs did not disappear with time, possibly due to the isolation of these communities as well as the lack of interaction with other communities or the medical system, which may have contributed to increasing those women's vulnerability. This was unlikely the case for Latakia, as its smaller size and its geographical location on the Mediterranean Sea may have permitted additional exposure to the outer world and consequently resulted in a wider exposure to endorsed information.

Women's acceptability of ANC services affected their choice of type of ANC provider. For instance, women brought up issues such as fear of hearing false bad news and fear of undergoing a cesarean section when seeking care with doctors (perceived risks of ANC). Such fears clearly suggest the women's lack of trust in biomedical care. Preferences for normal vaginal childbirth were brought by women in rural Bangladesh in a study that examined women and obstetricians' attitudes towards cesarean delivery [34], however, the study revealed that women trusted their doctors' decisions performing cesarean sections unlike the women in this study who decided to discontinue ANC or seek care with independent midwives.

Lack of trust in public health care providers and being maltreated at PHCs were two main reasons when why women decided to go to a private doctor, an independent midwife or discontinue ANC when they could not afford private care. Another potential explanation of why many women preferred care with midwives, which was not brought up by women, is the preference for female health providers, which is particularly important for traditional women in Aleppo (enabling factors). A previous study that included 500 women in Damascus, Syria, confirmed women's preferences for females as birth attendants [35], so we assume that this might have been the case for women in Aleppo.

Poor staff attitude was among the main factors that prevent women from seeking ANC as demonstrated by a review that examined reasons why women seek ANC in LMICs [20]. Similarly, a recent study in Saudi Arabia demonstrated that the negative attitude of the staff and poor communication prevented women from attending ANC despite their awareness of its importance [36]. The same study also demonstrated the importance of the beliefs of others including family and community members and how they impaired women's access to ANC [34].

These perceptions of ANC and acceptability of certain types of services were related to prevailing cultural norms and the influence of others (enabling factors), which resulted in not perceiving ANC as being beneficial and which could have prevented vulnerable women with low autonomy from adequate uptake of ANC. These findings are in line with findings from other studies included in a recent review of factors influencing women's uptake of ANC [19]. Fourteen studies in the review confirmed the influence of traditional beliefs on shaping women's ANC seeking behavior, which translated into avoiding biomedical care [19]. Additionally, 16 studies that were included in the review established that for many women, pregnancy is still considered as a normal event that does not require medical attention, especially in LMICs [19].

The results of the current study have important implications for consideration of introducing low-cost interventions that address the demand side barriers to adequate uptake of ANC. Although universal health coverage is important to achieve positive health outcomes, its effectiveness becomes limited when services are not used or under-used. Our study demonstrated that vulnerable women, such as women in Aleppo were less likely to demand for ANC services even when they were available and accessible. Future interventions intending to increase adequate uptake of ANC should aim at addressing the needs of vulnerable women and strengthening their capacity and capabilities to enable them to make their own decisions without having to depend on the opinions of others [26]. We recommend 3 promising and inter-related approaches to strengthen women's competencies and eventually improve their uptake of ANC: education, empowerment using women's groups and Mobile Health Technologies (mHealth) as potential platforms to deliver education and empowerment interventions (Table 3).

Increasing women's access to education improves their status in the household and the community, improves their knowledge of ANC benefits and their knowledge about existing services and appropriate types of providers, thus increasing the likelihood of their adequate uptake of ANC. Another effective strategy in poor settings is empowerment using community mobilization through women's groups that encourage women to discuss their needs and the barriers they face when seeking care and encourage them to seek care at health facilities consequently improving maternal and birth outcomes [26, 37–41]. When education is coupled with

**Table 3** Potential low-cost interventions to address the demand-side barriers to adequate uptake of antenatal care

| | Dimensions of access | | |
|---|---|---|---|
| | **Availability** | **Accessibility (geographical and financial)** | **Acceptability** |
| **Education** | Improves knowledge about available ANC services and type of services provided by different types of providers (private, public). | Improves knowledge about available health services that are closest to where women live and types of services provided at such health facilities. | Increases knowledge about benefits of ANC improving trust in biomedical care and reducing reliance on unreliable sources of information. |
| **Empowerment** | Encourages women to be more proactive and obtain information on health services. | Increases women's autonomy to improve their access to resources that impact on their geographical and financial access to services. | Increases women's autonomy to enable them to communicate more effectively with health providers, improving the patient-provider relationship and the acceptability of services. |
| **mHealth tools** | **A platform to deliver messages to promote behavior change and improve uptake of ANC** | | |

empowerment, it improves women's accessibility to health services especially when women have an increased mobility as well as an increased access to financial resources. Additionally, education and empowerment improve women's ability to communicate effectively with health care providers thus enabling them to raise their concerns regarding any negative news they may receive hence reducing the likelihood of being mistreated by health providers, and consequently improving their acceptability of ANC services.

The use of mobile phones was not widespread around the time of the study, especially among rural and poor women. Additionally, social platforms such as WhatsApp, which permit the free exchange of text and audio messages, were also not available. Given the high prevalence of mobile phones use these days [42], using Mobile Health technologies (mHealth) offers an effective and a low cost platform to promote behavior change and increase vulnerable women's uptake of ANC. A systematic review on the effectiveness of using mHealth in improving usage of ANC demonstrated that there is a strong evidence that delivering text messages reminders and education to the phones of pregnant women can improve their uptake of ANC [43].

When designing interventions for vulnerable women with limited mobility and reduced access to financial resources, it is important to consider interventions with a delivery mechanism that meets their needs. In the context of Syria, mHealth could be an effective platform to deliver such interventions without the need for women to leave their homes or use transportation, which is particularly important in settings where insecurity remains to be a major concern. Such platforms can be used to send reminders thorough text messages and deliver educational text and audio recorded messages on the importance of seeking ANC, risks of not seeking care and on available PHCs that provide ANC that are close to where women live. Also, mHealth can be an effective platform to deliver empowerment interventions. Such low-cost interventions using existing resources are worth exploring in a low-resource setting such as in Syria.

One of the main strengths of this study is that, unlike many studies, it chose not to present a generalized picture of 'Syrian women', their health care seeking behavior and their choice of different types of ANC providers but examined regional differences and patterns of ANC use and beliefs. This approach was grounded in the use of quantitative data to inform the study design [22] and was particularly relevant for patterns of ANC use, which differed substantially by region. The study also employed observation sessions, which helped triangulate the findings of the interviews.

The sample included in this study is relatively small and not representative of all women in both governorates, but as in any qualitative research, the sample is not usually selected for statistical representativeness, as the main objective of the study is to understand social processes. We could have missed important information by not including more women who did not use ANC at all in Aleppo, women who did not seek ANC in Latakia and by not including more women in rural Latakia. However, quantitative analyses of earlier surveys demonstrated that both rural and urban women in Latakia seek adequate ANC.

Interviewing women at home made them feel more at ease, since they were at a familiar setting. However, since many of them lived in households with many family members, interviews were often interrupted, and other family members like mothers and mothers in –law who participated occasionally. The presence of other family members might have made women feel less comfortable discussing their health seeking behaviour and biased their answers. Thus, to avoid such bias, we interviewed women in Aleppo for a second time and for a longer period, which helped to build rapport, encouraging the women to feel more comfortable sharing information about their ANC practices.

Courtesy bias, where women tried to give answers in favour of their doctors might have occurred with women in Latakia, as most participants preferred to be interviewed at health facilitates. Consequently, being interviewed at health facilities where those women received

ANC might have biased their answers towards favouring the services they have received at these particular health facilities and might have discouraged them from discussing the issues that they were not entirely satisfied with.

## Conclusions

We believe that our proposed interventions are likely to be effective in addressing the demand-side barriers to adequate uptake of ANC that existed pre-conflict and which were likely to have persisted post-conflict. Such interventions could be also explored to increase women's uptake of other maternal health care services including family planning and use of modern contraception methods. Furthermore, given the physical destruction caused by the conflict, which led to a decrease in the number of health facilities and which instigated the internal displacement of a large number of people, future research is needed to explore the additional demand side barriers that internally displaced women are currently experiencing when seeking ANC in their new host communities and as a result of using new and probably strained health facilities. Crafting appropriate interventions to increase women's uptake of ANC is likely to be more effective when it is contextual, pays attention to regional disparities in access and when it addresses the barriers that women are presently facing.

#### Abbreviations

ANC: Antenatal Care; LMICs: Lower and Middle-Income Countries; MICS: Multiple Indicator Cluster Survey; PAPFAM: Pan Arab Project for Family Health; PHCs: Public Health Centers; WHO: World Health Organization

#### Acknowledgements

We would like to thank the Syrian Ministry of Health and the Health directorates in Aleppo and Latakia. We would like to thank Dr. Oona Campbell (London School of Hygiene and Tropical Medicine) for her great contribution in conceptualizing the study. We also thank all women who participated in this study.

#### Authors' contributions

RM conceptualized the study and collected the data. RM analysed the data with FH's input. RM wrote the paper. FH commented on several drafts of the paper. HB commented on the final draft of the paper.

#### Author details

[1]Department of Epidemiology and Population Health, London School of Hygiene and Tropical Medicine, Keppel St, Bloomsbury, London WC1E 7HT, UK. [2]Faculty of Health Sciences, American University of Beirut, Bliss Street, Beirut, Lebanon. [3]Faculty of Medicine, University of Damascus, Damascus, Syria. [4]Faculty of Health and Wellbeing, Canterbury Christ Church University, North Holmes Road, Canterbury, Kent CT1 1QU, UK.

#### References

1. Alkema L, Chou D, Hogan D, Zhang S, Moller AB, Gemmill A, Fat DM, Boerma T, Temmerman M, Mathers C, Say L. Global, regional, and national levels and trends in maternal mortality between 1990 and 2015, with scenario-based projections to 2030: a systematic analysis by the UN. Maternal mortality estimation inter-agency group. Lancet. 2016;387(10017):462–74.
2. Cousens S, Blencowe H, Stanton C, Chou D, Ahmed S, Steinhardt L, Creanga AA, Tunçalp Ö, Balsara ZP, Gupta S, Say L. National, regional, and worldwide estimates of stillbirth rates in 2009 with trends since 1995: a systematic analysis. Lancet. 2011;377(9774):1319–30.
3. World Health Organization. WHO Recommended interventions for improving maternal and newborn health. WHO/MPS/07.05. Geneva: WHO; 2007.
4. Tunçalp Ö, Pena-Rosas JP, Lawrie T, Bucagu M, Oladapo OT, Portela A, Gülmezoglu AM. WHO recommendations on antenatal care for a positive pregnancy experience-going beyond survival. Bjog. 2017;124(6):860–2.
5. Kolsteren PW, De Souza S. Micronutrients and pregnancy outcome. Safe motherhood strategies: a review of the evidence; 2001.
6. Carroli G, Villar J, Piaggio G, Khan-Neelofur D, Gülmezoglu M, Mugford M, Lumbiganon P, Farnot U, Bersgjø P. WHO antenatal care trial research group. WHO systematic review of randomised controlled trials of routine antenatal care. Lancet. 2001;357(9268):1565–70.
7. AbouZahr C, Wardlaw T. Antenatal care in developing countries: promises, achievements and missed opportunities-an analysis of trends, levels and differentials, 1990–2001. Geneva: WHO; 2003.
8. World Health Organization. WHO recommendations on antenatal care for a positive pregnancy experience: summary: highlights and key messages from the World Health Organization's 2016 global recommendations for routine antenatal care. Geneva: WHO; 2018.
9. Sert G, Narman İ, Erkan O, Emre Ö, Özden, E, Tursun N, Başar Yunu. General Comment No. 22 (2016) on the Right to Sexual and Reproductive Health. Türkiye Biyoetik Dergisi. 2020;6(2):65-81.
10. Mackian S, Bedri N, Lovel H. Up the garden path and over the edge: where might health-seeking behaviour take us? Health Policy Plan. 2004;19(3):137–46.
11. Hausmann-Muela S, Ribera JM, Nyamongo I. Health-seeking behaviour and the health system response. Disease Control Piroirities Project working paper No14; 2003.
12. Andersen RM. Revisiting the behavioral model and access to medical care: does it matter? J Health Soc Behav. 1995;36(1):1–10.
13. Andersen R, Newman JF. Societal and individual determinants of medical care utilization in the United States. Milbank Q. 2005;83(4):1–28.
14. World Health Organization. The right to health. Fact Sheet N. 31. World Health Organization; 2002. https://www.who.int/gender-equity-rights/knowledge/right-to-health-factsheet31.pdf?ua=1. Accessed 20 Dec 2020.
15. Choi Y, Fabic MS, Adetunji J. Measuring access to family planning: conceptual frameworks and DHS data. Stud Fam Plan. 2016;47(2):145–61.
16. Peters DH, Garg A, Bloom G, Walker DG, Brieger WR, Hafizur RM. Poverty and access to health care in developing countries. Ann N Y Acad Sci. 2008; 1136(1):161–71.
17. Ensor T, Cooper S. Overcoming barriers to health service access: influencing the demand side. Health Policy Plan. 2004;19(2):69–79.
18. Simkhada B, Teijlingen ER, Porter M, Simkhada P. Factors affecting the utilization of antenatal care in developing countries: systematic review of the literature. J Adv Nurs. 2008;61(3):244–60.
19. Downe S, Finlayson K, Tunçalp Ö, Gülmezoglu AM. Provision and uptake of routine antenatal services: a qualitative evidence synthesis. Cochrane Database Syst Rev. 2019;6:CD012392.
20. Finlayson K, Downe S. Why do women not use antenatal services in low- and middle-income countries? A meta-synthesis of qualitative studies. PLoS Med. 2013;10(1):e1001373.
21. Syrian Central Bureau of Statistics, League of Arab States. Family Health Survey in Syrian Arab Republic; 2009.
22. Mourtada R, et al. London School of Hygiene and Tropical Medicine. 2014; PhD thesis.
23. Mourtada R, Bottomley C, Houben F, Bashour H, Campbell OM. A mixed methods analysis of factors affecting antenatal care content: a Syrian case study. PLoS One. 2019;14(3):e0214375.
24. DeJong J, Ghattas H, Bashour H, Mourtada R, Akik C, Reese-Masterson A. Reproductive, maternal, neonatal and child health in conflict: a case study on Syria using countdown indicators. BMJ Glob Health. 2017;1:2(3).
25. Abbara A, Blanchet K, Sahloul Z, Fouad F, Coutts A, Wasim M. The effect of the conflict on Syria's health system and human resources for health. World health & population. 2015;16(1):87–95.
26. Elmusharaf K, Byrne E, O'Donovan D. Strategies to increase demand for maternal health services in resource-limited settings: challenges to be addressed. BMC Public Health 2015;15(1):1–0.

27. Jacobs B, Ir P, Bigdeli M, Annear PL, Van Damme W. Addressing access barriers to health services: an analytical framework for selecting appropriate interventions in low-income Asian countries. Health Policy Plan. 2012;27(4): 288–300.
28. Pope C, Mays N. Qualitative methods in health research. Qualitative research in health care. 2006;3:1–1.
29. Mays N, Pope C. Qualitative research: observational methods in health care settings. Bmj. 1995;311(6998):182–4.
30. Mulhall A. In the field: notes on observation in qualitative research. J Adv Nurs. 2003;41(3):306–13.
31. Ritchie J, Spencer L. Qualitative data analysis for applied policy research. The qualitative researcher's companion. 2002;573(2002):305–29.
32. Pope C, Ziebland S, Mays N. Analysing qualitative data. Bmj. 2000;320(7227): 114–6.
33. Kridli SA. Health beliefs and practices among Arab women. MCN Am J Matern Child Nurs. 2002;27(3):178–82.
34. Begum T, Ellis C, Sarker M, Rostoker JF, Rahman A, Anwar I, Reichenbach L. A qualitative study to explore the attitudes of women and obstetricians towards caesarean delivery in rural Bangladesh. BMC pregnancy and childbirth. 2018;18(1):368.
35. Bashour H, Abdulsalam A. Syrian women's preferences for birth attendant and birth place. Birth. 2005;32(1):20–6.
36. Alanazy W, Rance J, Brown A. Exploring maternal and health professional beliefs about the factors that affect whether women in Saudi Arabia attend antenatal care clinic appointments. Midwifery. 2019;76:36–44.
37. Manandhar DS, Osrin D, Shrestha BP, Mesko N, Morrison J, Tumbahangphe KM, Tamang S, Thapa S, Shrestha D, Thapa B, Shrestha JR. Effect of a participatory intervention with women's groups on birth outcomes in Nepal: cluster-randomised controlled trial. Lancet. 2004;364(9438):970–9.
38. Prost A, Colbourn T, Seward N, Azad K, Coomarasamy A, Copas A, Houweling TA, Fottrell E, Kuddus A, Lewycka S, MacArthur C. Women's groups practising participatory learning and action to improve maternal and newborn health in low-resource settings: a systematic review and meta-analysis. Lancet. 2013;381(9879):1736–46.
39. World Health Organization. WHO recommendation on facilitated participatory learning and action cycles with women's groups during pregnancy. 2018. Accessed via: https://extranet.who.int/rhl/topics/improving-health-system-performance/implementation-strategies/who-recommendation-facilitated-participatory-learning-and-action-cycles-womens-groups-during. Accessed 15 Jun 2020.
40. Ishaku, Salisu Mohammed. "Engaging community women's groups for improved uptake of antenatal care services in Cross River State, Nigeria: An analysis of post-intervention findings," Ending Eclampsia Research Brief. 2018. Abuja: Population Council
41. Kearns AD, Caglia JM, ten Hoope-Bender P, Langer A. Antenatal and postnatal care: a review of innovative models for improving availability, accessibility, acceptability and quality of services in low-resource settings. BJOG Int J Obstet Gynaecol. 2016;123(4):540–8.
42. UKaid. The use of Mobile Technology for humanitarian Programming in syria Potential and Constraints. 2017. Accessed via: https://assets.publishing.service.gov.uk/media/58e273b040f0b606e70000a1/Research_Report_-_Mobile_Technology_in_Syria__Potential_and_Constraints___March_2017.pdf. Accessed 27 Dec 2020.
43. Watterson JL, Walsh J, Madeka I. Using mHealth to improve usage of antenatal care, postnatal care, and immunization: a systematic review of the literature. Biomed Res Int. 2015;1:2015.

# 19

# Are higher unintended pregnancy rates among minorities a result of disparate access to contraception?

Michele Troutman[1], Saima Rafique[2] and Torie Comeaux Plowden[3*]

**Abstract:** Unintended pregnancy is a major global issue. Women who experience an unintended pregnancy have a significant risk of morbidity and mortality. Additionally, these women also experience substantial financial hardships. Many women, particularly women of color, do not have adequate access to reliable and affordable contraception resulting in major health disparities among this group. This review explores the relationship between unintended pregnancy and inadequate access to contraception and is divided into 5 sections: addressing problems associated with unintended pregnancies, unintended pregnancy rate in the US, disparities of unintended pregnancy rates and access to care, addressing potential solutions, and finally conclusions.

**Keyterms:** unintended pregnancy, healthcare disparities, contraception, access to care.

## Introduction

An unintended pregnancy is any unplanned, mistimed or unwanted pregnancy at the time of conception [1]. In 2011, 48% of all pregnancies in the United States were unintended [2]. Similarly, women worldwide have high unintended pregnancy rates. In 2010–2014, 44% of all pregnancies worldwide were unintended [3]. Although we've begun to see a slow decline in these numbers with the aid of education, LARC methods, and access to family planning services, unintended pregnancy rates remain a major public health problem.

Unintended pregnancies have a substantial impact on public health. Women with unintended pregnancies have a higher percentage of late entry to care, alcohol and drugs use during pregnancy and higher rates of preterm birth [4]. Unintended pregnancies are often higher among adolescents, lower income, minority, and single women who have poverty rates twice that of other groups, making the financial impact of an unplanned conception even greater [5]. Improved access to contraception by age 20 has been shown to decrease the likelihood that a woman will subsequently live in poverty and thus increase one's quality of life [6]. With the onset of coronavirus disease 2019 (COVID-19) and the resurface of a national economic depression, it is important that now more than ever we consider the economic burden of these unintended pregnancies and the strain on national resources. Many organizations are significantly decreasing in-person and telehealth visits and reproductive access organizations have been forced to innovate in a more thoughtful way to reach those most at risk. There are slated state and national healthcare budget cuts although it remains unclear the long-term effects it will have on unintended pregnancies. While it is possible to increase clinic show rates with the use of technology and decreasing economic barriers, what remains is the constant gaping disparities in digital equity and patient perception regarding the care, or lack thereof, that they're receiving.

Unintended pregnancy is a public health emergency. The U.S. Department of Health and Human Services has identified reducing unintended pregnancy as a significant

* Correspondence: torie.c.plowden.mil@mail.mil
The views expressed herein are those of the authors and do not reflect the official policy or position of the US Army Medical Department, Department of the Army, Department of Defense, or the US Government.
[3]Department of Obstetrics and Gynecology, Womack Army Medical Center, Ft Bragg, NC, USA

goal in the Healthy People 2020 family planning objectives. The initiative focuses on improving pregnancy planning, spacing and prevention as a way to improve health outcomes while decreasing the economic burden. In order to accomplish the goal, barriers such as limited access to publicly funded services, limited transportation, lack of youth-friendly services, and inadequate services for men are identified as some of the issues to be addressed [7].

Although women of reproductive age of all races and ethnicities are at risk of unintended pregnancy, Hispanic and Black women are disproportionally at risk [8]. Globally, the at-risk population numbers are in the millions, making this a critical issue worldwide. Contributions to this disparity include income, insurance status, relationship status, and education level. Our objective was to examine the contributors to high rates of unintended pregnancies and to identify potential strategies to address this critical issue.

## Unintended pregnancy rates in America

In 2011, the rates of unintended pregnancy among African-American, Hispanic and Caucasian women that ended in birth were 33, 31, and 17% respectively in the United States [2]. Using data from the National Survey of Family Growth from 2006 to 2010, Kim et al. observed 50% of the 3577 pregnancies were unintended [9]. The study notes that women of color, particularly black women had higher rates than whites; 63% (Black women), 48% (Hispanic women) and 42% (Caucasian women). Although the rates were higher among black and Hispanic women, the difference was not statistically significant (Fig. 1). However, even the lowest rate of unintended pregnancy, 42%, would be considered unacceptable high by most healthcare providers. This number is particularly alarming given the failure rate of less than 1% for highly effective contraceptives [10].

## Disparities in unintended pregnancy and access to care

The medical literature has documented racial and ethnic disparities in access to healthcare, as well the quality of that care for more than a decade. In 2003, the Institute of Medicine determined "research suggests that healthcare providers' diagnostic and treatment decisions, as well as their feelings about patients, are influenced by patients' race or ethnicity and that these differences may contribute to disparities in health outcomes" [11]. Multiple studies have unfortunately demonstrated that African-American and Latina women from low socioeconomic backgrounds have been strongly encouraged to limit their family sizes and have been pressured to start contraception or proceed with tubal sterilization [12, 13].

Historically, the United States has had a shameful history regarding forced sterilizations and reproductive injustices which may lead minority women to be distrustful of contraception [14, 15]. There are also racial differences in contraceptive preferences. Because it is important to many African American women to avoid the use of hormones, they may be less likely to choose highly effective contraception such as implants, injectable contraception or levonorgestrel containing intrauterine devices (IUDs) [15]. Outside of preferences

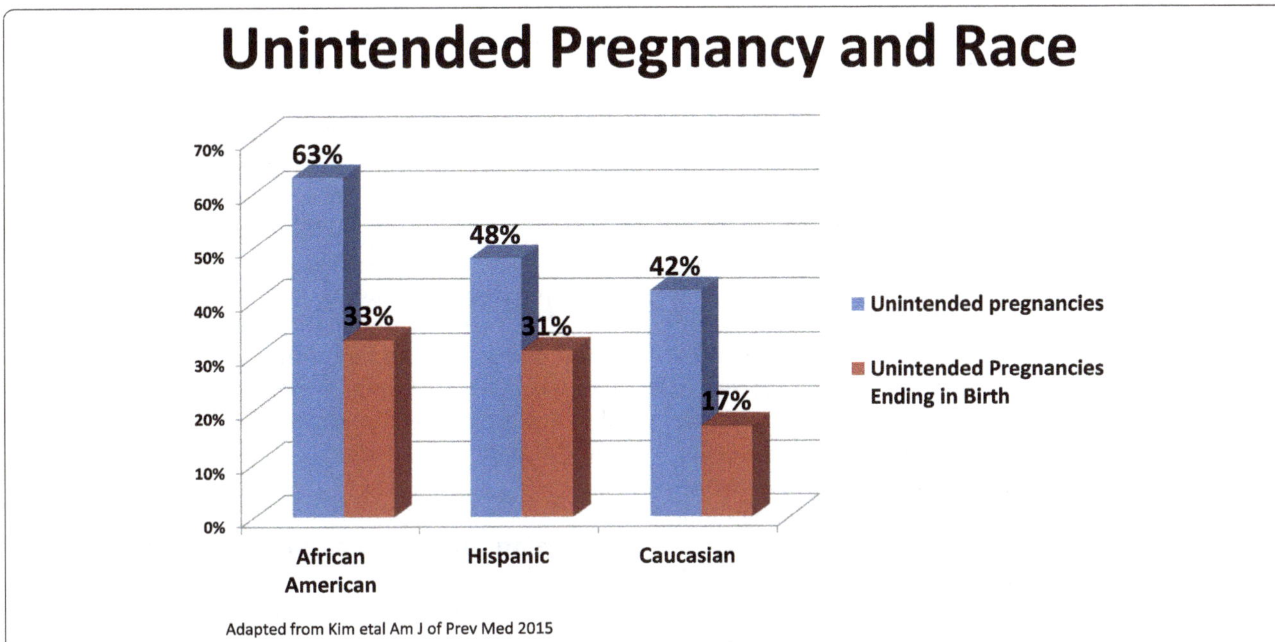


**Fig. 1** Unintended pregnancy and race

guided by historical weight, there are also distinctive barriers to reproductive access.

This idea of disparity in contraceptive access is echoed in the discordance between desired fertility and chosen method of contraception. A study of 110 (48 African-Americans, 43 Hispanics, 19 Caucasians) low-income women who lived in an underserved area found that 40% of women who did not desire pregnancy had unprotected intercourse within the last 12 months [16]. Similarly, a study examining contraception trends found that 16% of African-American women who were at risk of unintended pregnancy were not using contraception compared to about 9% of Hispanic, white and Asian women [8].

Attitudes and norms regarding contraception in minority groups are often different than those of Caucasian women. Frequently, when African-American and Latina women choose contraception, they choose less effective contraception options (i.e. condoms) compared to white women [12–14]. Interestingly, data from the contraceptive CHOICE project revealed that prior to enrollment in the study, African-American women who have had a history of discrimination were more likely to choose less efficacious contraceptive measures (specifically barrier methods, natural family planning and withdrawal) but after enrollment, 67% of these women elected to use long-acting reversible contraception (LARC) [16]. The script that was used in the CHOICE study provided important information about the effectiveness of various contraceptive methods, and patients were free to choose whatever method they desired. Patient education played a pivotal role in the success of the CHOICE project, but it is imperative that other contraceptive programs provide education and not coercion.

High unintended pregnancy rates, particularly among low-income women and women of color, have persisted despite the expanded options for highly efficacious contraceptives. LARC, which includes IUDs and subdermal contraceptive implants, are cost-effective and highly efficacious, with an annual failure rate of 0.05% (implants) and 0.2–0.8% (IUDs) [17]. Despite the efficacy of these methods, they are often associated with up-front out-of-pocket costs which may be prohibitive to poorer women [10, 17]. When women were given multiple options for contraception, and cost was not a consideration, 67% elected to use long-acting reversible contraceptive (LARC) [18]. In comparison, non-LARC contraceptive options were 20 times more likely to have an unintended pregnancy, demonstrating how much effective contraception is of paramount importance for preventing unintended pregnancy [19].

Any efforts to decrease unintended pregnancy will need to include elimination of barriers such as a lack of insurance, inadequate coverage that requires large out of pocket expenses, or extremely high premiums. One potential strategy is to educate third party payers about the cost savings associated with widely available contraception. One study estimated that the direct medical cost of unintended pregnancy in the United States was more than $4.6 billion annually [20]. Women ages 18–24 have the highest risk of unintended pregnancy. Using cost models, one review found that if 10% of women ages 20–29 who used oral contraception changed to LARC, the total costs associated with unintended pregnancy would decrease by $288 million per year [20]. Third party payers should consider access to contraception as effective preventive health care that will decrease medical costs.

Although decisions regarding contraception are often left up to the female partner, the role of the male partner must be examined as part of the strategy to decrease unintended pregnancy. Utilizing data from the 2006–2010 National Survey of Family Growth, one study attempted to better understand knowledge of contraception among young men [21]. Researchers found that although 96.6% of men reported formal sex education, Black men were less likely to receive contraceptive education [21]. Another study examining contraceptive knowledge found that men were more likely to "display serious gaps in objective knowledge about the major contraceptive options" [22]. Despite men often being left out of conversations involving contraception, counseling that reflects a couple's culture and values may help increase compliance especially amongst minority groups [23].

Age plays a significant role in the likelihood of having an unintended pregnancy. Young women who become sexually active at an early age are particularly at risk for an unplanned conception. Data from Demographic and Health Surveys revealed that a significant proportion of adolescents in 16 countries reported sexual activity. In 9 of these 16 countries, approximately 40% of women reported sexual activity before age 18 while men engaging in intercourse before age 18 ranged from 25 to 75% [24]. There is a clear need for access to contraception among adolescents in many of these countries. However, adolescents in low and middle-income countries face additional barriers regarding contraception. These include poor understanding of how to use various methods correctly and law or policies preventing young unmarried women from accessing contraception [24]. The following recommendations are potential solutions to the disparities of contraception access facing minority population.

## Addressing the problem: potential solutions [Table 1]

The Centers for Disease Control (CDC) recommends that "every woman, man and couple should be encouraged to have a reproductive life plan" [25].

**Table 1** Strategies to Decrease Unintended Pregnancy

**Strategies to Decrease Unintended Pregnancy**

| Strategy | Example |
|---|---|
| Increase Access | Universal Health Coverage |
| Decrease Cost | Negotiation by large health care organizations for lower prescription costs<br>Use of generic prescriptions |
| Increase Cultural Sensitivity | Education of Health Care Providers and Patients |
| Education of Providers | Incorporation of contraceptive education in medical school, nursing school , pharmacy school and residency curriculum |
| Education of Patients | Professional organizations such as ACOG, development of educational materials such as those used in CHOICE project |
| Education of third party payers | Use of published data to highlight cost savings of contraceptive use |

### Access/cost

Although multiple factors affect the unintended pregnancy rate, access to reliable and safe contraception can certainly positively impact this problem. Universal coverage of all contraceptive methods has been shown to decrease unintended pregnancy rates [12]. Negotiation with pharmaceutical companies by large health care organizations, such as HMOs, is also a potential strategy to decrease cost. On a global level, organizations like the Gates Foundation are investing in reasons for non-use, distribution and development for contraceptive technology [26].

### Culturally sensitive approach

African-American and Latina women suffer from misconceptions surrounding contraception, its use and efficacy [14]. The CHOICE project serves an example of using patient education to effectively overcome cultural beliefs that pose a barrier to the use of highly efficacious contraception. Access to care limitations based upon race, ethnicity and income is well documented and poses one of the most significant impediments to contraceptive access. Incorporation of contraceptive education as well as culturally sensitivity training into the curriculum of medical, nursing, and pharmacy schools and residency training programs are a tool that can be used to address these important issues.

### Appropriate physician education

Like patients, health care professionals often have limited knowledge about the availability and appropriate use of contraceptive methods. IUD use, one type of LARC, has been hampered by the persistence of incorrect myths including that they are contraindicated in young/adolescent nulliparous women, they lead to infertility and women will experience high rates of infection [17]. Residency programs in obstetrics/gynecology, family practice and pediatrics along with nurse practitioners and physician assistants should ensure that providers are aware and well-educated about LARC methods and its contraindications. Appropriate counseling by providers "not only promotes effective methods but also directly translates to increased use" [14]. Use of published materials by organizations such as the American College of Obstetricians and Gynecologists (ACOG), Society of Family Planning (SFP), and the use of apps such as Medical Eligibility Criteria app produced by the CDC (https://www.cdc.gov/reproductivehealth/contraception/usmec.htm) facilitate the appropriate selection of contraceptives for women with medical conditions such as hypertension. These tools aid women in locating effective contraception that they otherwise could have been denied as a result of a provider's fears about medical complications.

### Maximizing opportunities to educate patients

The ACOG strongly advocates for reproductive planning. In a recent committee opinion, the College emphasized that physicians should take every contact with their patients as a teachable moment [27]. Rather than limiting the discussion of contraceptive management to well women or contraceptive visits, every visit should be considered as a unique opportunity to address patient's reproductive plan and offer counseling, education and correct any misconceptions on available contraceptive options. Initiatives like "One Key Question" and "Providing Quality Family Planning Services" aim to enhance effective communication and improve understanding of a woman's reproductive health plan [28]. Adopting these strategies in day-to-day interactions will efficiently utilize available resources and further achieve the goal of preventing unintended pregnancies [29].

#### Empowering other health care providers

Emergency contraceptives is another excellent option geared towards decreasing the unintended pregnancy rates [30]. Now that these methods are available over the counter, many patients may seek advice from pharmacists [31]. Pharmacists can advise patients of emergency contraception, but, additionally can provide information regarding LARC and refer to an appropriate provider [31]. Nurse practitioners are becoming the primary providers of contraception for some women. Training these healthcare providers to provide not only counseling about LARC, but also placement of IUD and implants will help women access these methods more easily [31].

#### Using community resources

Disseminating information through various avenues including schools, health centers, the media, and peer education has been shown to improve uptake of LARC use [31]. Additionally, other resources that should be considered when targeting minority groups may include churches, community center, and salons. One limitation of LARC use is a lack of appropriately trained personnel. Charyeva et al. in their study in Northern Nigeria showed increased utilization of LARCS by training community health extension workers in their insertion and removal [32]. In Ethiopia, similar results were noted in the utilization of implants with the help of health extension workers [33]. These studies suggest that optimizing human resources and training ancillary staff to deliver these services could be another option in increasing the utilization of contraceptives and eventually decreasing unintended pregnancies in at risk communities worldwide.

#### Title X and reproductive access

Title X is a federal grant program through the US Department of Health and Human Services that provides comprehensive family planning and preventative health services, prioritizing low income families [34]. Recent proposed revisions to Title X will negatively impact access to legal abortion services and impede the provider's ability to discuss family planning options at federally funded centers. The regulations would most affect low income and minority women. Organizations like Planned Parenthood who serve 41% of Title X recipients, use funding to provide preventative services and prevent 1 million unintended pregnancies a year [35]. If these regulations are enacted, low income and minority women who rely on Title X centers for their reproductive needs will be much more vulnerable to unintended pregnancies.

## Conclusion

Unintended pregnancy continues to be a critical global issue, particularly among certain ethnic and racial groups as well as low income women. These unintended pregnancies can negatively impact women physically, emotionally, and financially. Easier access to effective contraception methods, particularly long-acting reversible contraception, can certainly help to address this public health issue. Physicians and other health-care providers need to ensure they are providing comprehensive care and have received appropriate contraceptive education as well as culturally sensitive training. Although access to contraception plays a large role in unintended pregnancy, the added impact of less efficacious contraceptive methods use, lack of patient and provider education and understanding are additional contributors. Contraceptive programs must utilize multiple wide ranging strategies to achieve success in decreasing unintended pregnancies and its surrounding disparities.

#### Abbreviations

COVID-19: Coronavirus disease 2019; IUD: Intrauterine device; LARC: Long acting reversible contraception; CDC: Centers for disease control; ACOG: American college of obstetricians and gynecologists; SFP: Society of family planning

#### Acknowledgements

The authors would like to acknowledge Dr. Alicia Christy for her feedback and critique of this manuscript.

#### Authors' contributions

MT, SR and TCP contributed to the writing of this manuscript. All authors read and approved the final manuscript.

#### Author details

[1]Department of Obstetrics and Gynecology, Beth Israel Deaconess Medical Center, Boston, MA, USA. [2]Advantia Ob/Gyn Shady Grove, Rockville, MD, USA. [3]Department of Obstetrics and Gynecology, Womack Army Medical Center, Ft Bragg, NC, USA.

#### References

1. Brown SS, Eisenberg L, Institute of Medicine (U.S.). Committee on Unintended Pregnancy. The best intentions: unintended pregnancy and the well-being of children and families. Washington, D.C.: National Academy Press; 1995. ix, 380 p. p.
2. Finer LB, Zolna MR. New England journal of medicine 2016; 374:843-852 March 3, 2016. DOI: https://doi.org/10.1056/NEJMsa1506575.
3. Bearak J, Popinchalk A, Alkema L, Sedgh G. Global, regional, and subregional trends in unintended pregnancy and its outcomes from 1990 to 2014: estimates from a Bayesian hierarchical model. Lancet Glob Health. 2018;6(4): e380–9. https://doi.org/10.1016/S2214-109X(18)30029-9.

4. Haider S, Stoffel C, Donenberg G, Geller S. Reproductive health disparities: a focus on family planning and prevention among minority women and adolescents. Glob Adv Health Med: Improving Healthc Outcomes Worldwide. 2013;2(5):94–9 PubMed PMID: 24416701. Pubmed Central PMCI D: 3833575.
5. Census Bureau US. Income, poverty, and health insurance coverage in the United States. In: Current population reports Consumer income P60. Washington, D.C.: Bureau of the Census.
6. Browne SP, LaLumia S. The effects of contraception on female poverty. J Policy Anal Manage: [the J Assoc Public Policy Anal Manage]. 2014;33(3): 602–22 Summer. PubMed PMID: 24988652.
7. U.S. Department of Health and Human Services. Healthy People 2020 topics and objectives Washington, DC.2010 [March 14, 2016]. Available from: https://www.healthypeople.gov/2020/topicsobjectives2020/objectivelist.aspx?topicid=13.
8. Mosher WD, Jones J, Abma JC. Intended and unintended births in the United States: 1982-2010. Natl Health Stat Rep. 2012;24(55):1–28 PubMed PMID: 23115878.
9. Kim TY, Dagher RK, Chen J. Racial/ethnic differences in unintended pregnancy: evidence from a national sample of U.S. women. Am J Prev Med. 2016;50(4):427–35.
10. Wilder V, Bromfield G, de Fiebre G, Prine L. Disparities in contraceptive care. J Health Care Poor Underserved. 2014;25(2):451–9 PubMed PMID: 24858860.
11. Smedley BD, Stith AY, Nelson AR, Institute of Medicine (U.S.). Committee on Understanding and Eliminating Racial and Ethnic Disparities in Health Care. Unequal treatment: confronting racial and ethnic disparities in health care. Washington, D.C.: National Academy Press; 2003. xvi, 764 p.
12. Dehlendorf C, Rodriguez MI, Levy K, Borrero S, Steinauer J. Disparities in family planning. Am J Obstet Gynecol. 2010;202(3):214–20 PubMed PMID: 20207237. Pubmed Central PMCID: 2835625.
13. Ayoola AB, Zandee GL, Johnson E, Pennings K. Contraceptive use among low-income women living in medically underserved neighborhoods. J Obstet Gynecol Neonatal Nurs. 2014;43(4):455–64 PubMed PMID: 24958447.
14. Casey F, Gomez-Lobo V. Disparities in contraceptive access and provision. Semin Reprod Med. 2013;31(5):347–59 PubMed PMID: 23934695.
15. Borrero S, Schwarz EB, Creinin M, Ibrahim S. The impact of race and ethnicity on receipt of family planning services in the United States. J Women's Health. 2009;18(1):91–6 PubMed PMID: 19072728. Pubmed Central PMCID: 2743980.
16. Kossler K, Kuroki LM, Allsworth JE, Secura GM, Roehl KA, Peipert JF. Perceived racial, socioeconomic and gender discrimination and its impact on contraceptive choice. Contraception. 2011;84(3):273–9 PubMed PMID: 21843693. Pubmed Central PMCID: 3539813.
17. Parks C, Peipert JF. Eliminating health disparities in unintended pregnancy with long-acting reversible contraception (LARC). Am J Obstet Gynecol. 2016;214(6):681–8.
18. Secura GM, Allsworth JE, Madden T, Mullersman JL, Peipert JF. The contraceptive CHOICE project: reducing barriers to long-acting reversible contraception. Am J Obstet Gynecol. 2010;203(2):115 e1–7 PubMed PMID: 20541171. Pubmed Central PMCID: 2910826.
19. McNicholas C, Madden T, Secura G, Peipert JF. The contraceptive CHOICE project round up: what we did and what we learned. Clin Obstet Gynecol. 2014;57(4):635–43 PubMed PMID: 25286295. Pubmed Central PMCID: 4216614.
20. Trussell J, Henry N, Hassan F, Prezioso A, Law A, Filonenko A. Burden of unintended pregnancy in the United States: potential savings with increased use of long-acting reversible contraception. Contraception. 2013; 87(2):154–61 PubMed PMID: 22959904. Pubmed Central PMCID: 3659779.
21. Farkas AH, Vanderberg R, Sucato GS, Miller E, Akers AY, Borrero S. Racial and ethnic differences in young men's sex and contraceptive education. J Adolesc Health. 2015;56(4):464–7 PubMed PMID: 25797633. Pubmed Central PMCID: 4371132.
22. Frost JJ, Lindberg LD, Finer LB. Young adults' contraceptive knowledge, norms and attitudes: associations with risk of unintended pregnancy. Perspect Sex Reprod Health. 2012;44(2):107–16 PubMed PMID: 22681426.
23. Warren JT, Harvey SM, Bovbjerg ML. Characteristics related to effective contraceptive use among a sample of nonurban Latinos. Perspect Sex Reprod Health. 2011;43(4):255–62.
24. Chandra-Mouli V, McCarraher DR, Phillips SJ, Williamson NE, Hainsworth G. Contraception for adolescents in low and middle income countries: needs, barriers, and access. Reprod Health. 2014;11(1):1 PubMed PMID: 24383405. Pubmed Central PMCID: 3882494.
25. Johnson K, Posner SF, Biermann J, Cordero JF, Atrash HK, Parker CS, et al. Recommendations to improve preconception health and health care--United States. A report of the CDC/atsdr preconception care work group and the select panel on preconception care. MMWR Recomm Rep. 2006; 55(RR-6):1–23 PubMed PMID: 16617292.
26. Family Planning: Strategy overview. Gates Foundation 2020. Retrieved from www.gatesfoundation.org.
27. Committee Opinion No. 654: Reproductive life Planning to reduce unintended pregnancy. Obstet Gynecol 2016;127(2):e66–9. PubMed PMID: 26942389.
28. Bellanca HK, Hunter MS. ONE KEY QUESTION(R): preventive reproductive health is part of high quality primary care. Contraception. 2013;88(1):3–6 PubMed PMID: 23773527.
29. Gavin L, Moskosky S, Carter M, Curtis K, Glass E, Godfrey E, et al. Providing quality family planning services: recommendations of CDC and the U.S. office of population affairs. MMWR Recomm Rep. 2014;63(RR-04):1–54 PubMed PMID: 24759690.
30. Devine KS. The underutilization of emergency contraception. Am J Nurs. 2012;112(4):44–50 quiz 1-2. PubMed PMID: 22421320.
31. Shoupe D. LARC methods: entering a new age of contraception and reproductive health. Contracept Reprod Med. 2016;2(4).
32. Charyeva Z, Oguntunde O, Orobaton N, Otolorin E, Inuwa F, Alalade O, et al. Task shifting provision of contraceptive implants to community health extension workers: results of operations research in northern Nigeria. Glob Health Sci Pract. 2015;3(3):382–94 PubMed PMID: 26374800. Pubmed Central PMCID: 4570013.
33. Asnake M, Henry EG, Tilahun Y, Oliveras E. Addressing unmet need for long-acting family planning in Ethiopia: uptake of single-rod progestogen contraceptive implants (Implanon) and characteristics of users. Int J Gynecol Obstet. 2013;123(Suppl 1):e29–32 PubMed PMID: 24035007.
34. HHS.gov. (2019). Funding History. Available at: https://www.hhs.gov/opa/title-x-family-planning/about-title-x-grants/funding-history/index.html.
35. Planned Parenthood Action Fund. Title X: Affordable Birth Control and Reproductive Health Care. Retrieved from http://www.plannedparenthoodaction.org/issues/health-care-equity/title-x.

# The role of pregnancy intendedness and prenatal contraceptive counseling on postpartum contraceptive use

Karina M. Shreffler[1*], Stacy Tiemeyer[1], Jameca R. Price[2] and Lance T. Frye[3]

**Abstract**

**Background:** The study was conducted to prospectively examine how pregnancy intendedness and prenatal provider counseling about postpartum contraceptive options are associated with lack of contraception use at 6 months post-birth (e.g., increased risk for a short interpregnancy interval).

**Methods:** Logistic regression models were used to examine risk for no postpartum contraception use among a sample of low-income and racially/ethnically diverse women recruited from two metropolitan perinatal clinics in Tulsa, OK.

**Results:** Women who reported that they were trying to get pregnant or "okay either way" about getting pregnant had significantly lower odds of using contraception at 6 months post childbirth than those who had unintended pregnancies. Having providers who discussed postpartum contraceptive options during pregnancy significantly increased the odds of contraceptive uptake among those who were planning or ambivalent about their pregnancies.

**Conclusions:** Intentions of a current pregnancy and provider contraceptive counseling matter for postpartum contraceptive use and the associated risk for a short interval subsequent pregnancy. Provider contraceptive counseling that accounts for the intendedness of a current pregnancy may offer a more targeted approach to prevent a short interval subsequent pregnancy.

**Keywords:** Family planning, Contraception, Counseling, LARC, Unintended pregnancy, Ambivalence

* Correspondence: karina.shreffler@okstate.edu

*This research was supported in part by the National Institute of General Medical Sciences of the National Institutes of Health (P20GM109097; Jennifer Hays-Grudo, PI). The content is solely the responsibility of the authors and does not necessarily represent the official views of the National Institutes of Health. For more information, contact: Karina M. Shreffler, Department of Human Development and Family Science, Oklahoma State University, 700 N. Greenwood Ave., Tulsa, OK, 74106. Phone: 918-594-8389. Email: karina.shreffler@okstate.edu.

[1]Oklahoma State University, 700 N. Greenwood Ave, Tulsa, OK 74106, USA

## Background

Nearly half (45%) of the 6.1 million pregnancies in the US each year are unintended [1]. The public health impact of unintended pregnancy is considerable: women who carry an unintended pregnancy to term are more likely to delay prenatal care, use alcohol and tobacco, and experience low infant birth weight, preterm birth, and maternal morbidity and mortality [2–6]. Most unintended pregnancies in the US occur because women and their partners do not use contraception consistently and effectively [7].

The most effective form of female contraception is tubal ligation [8]. Though so-called "short-term" contraceptive methods (e.g., oral and barrier methods of contraception) tend to be quite effective if used correctly [9], long-acting reversible contraception (LARC)--such an intra-uterine device (IUD) or implant—are highly effective at preventing first-time [10], rapid repeat [11], and unintended pregnancy [12]. ACOG and the American Academy of Pediatrics (AAP) recommend LARC methods as the best option for adolescents and women [13, 14]. Despite the proven effectiveness of LARC methods, their use in 2013 was not as widespread as condoms (32%) or birth control pills (27%) [12]. Approximately 14% of reproductive-aged women (ages 15–44) used an IUD or implant in 2013, though that is nearly a five-fold increase since 2002 [12, 15].

Promoting postpartum contraception such as LARC insertion has been identified as an effective and timely strategy to reduce inadequate birth spacing and unintended pregnancy [16]. Lack of knowledge about contraception, both perceived and actual, has been identified as the primary barrier to contraceptive uptake [17]. Women who discussed LARC methods with their providers are more than 13 times more likely to adopt intrauterine contraception than those who did not discuss the method with their providers [18]. Prenatal facilities differ considerably on practices regarding postpartum LARC insertion and communication with patients [19], but even within the same prenatal clinic, uptake of postpartum contraception can differ by patient characteristics. For example, women who have public (e.g., Medicaid) insurance as compared to private insurance are more likely to receive postpartum LARC insertion [20]. Yet it is unclear how characteristics of a prior pregnancy predict postpartum contraceptive use. Identifying circumstances that predict or disrupt postpartum uptake of effective contraception is therefore a critical need. Prior qualitative research with a non-pregnant sample of reproductive-age women found that ambivalence about getting pregnant is associated with being less receptive to LARC methods [21]. In the current prospective study of a sample of pregnant women ages 15–39, we examine how the intendedness of a pregnancy predicts risk for a subsequent pregnancy at 6 months postpartum as measured by contraceptive non-use and whether provider recommendations moderate the impact of intendedness.

## Methods

### Sample

We conducted enrollment for the longitudinal clinic-based cohort study between October 2016 and May 2017. After securing Institutional Review Board approval at the participating authors' institution, pregnant women were recruited from the two university-affiliated perinatal clinics in a city in the South-Central U.S. The participating clinics were purposively selected because they serve racially diverse, but socioeconomically disadvantaged and medically underserved patient populations. Recruitment of study participants took place in the obstetric practices of the participating centers during prenatal visits. Research and clinical partners worked together to develop a screening, recruitment and participant transfer protocol. All pregnant patients seen by providers during the designated recruitment times were screened for study eligibility. A screen to determine eligibility was completed by nursing staff and provided to the research staff. A patient was eligible for participation if she was 15+ years old and less than 28 weeks pregnant. The sample for this paper comes from the 177 patients who agreed to participate. The sample size at recruitment was determined by a power calculation for a study of rapid repeat pregnancy.

### Patient and public involvement

Neither patients nor the public were involved in the design, conduct, reporting, or dissemination plans of the research study.

### Measures

The measures used in this study come from longitudinal data collected during pregnancy and within the first 6 months postpartum. Most women completed the first survey during their first trimester (72%), and 90% of the women were less than 20 weeks pregnant. The first survey asked demographic, medical and pregnancy history, as well as a number of psychosocial measures. Additional survey assessments were sent to participants via text and email during their second and third trimesters, 2 months postpartum, 6 months postpartum, and 1 year postpartum.

#### *Dependent variable*

Our outcome variable, *contraceptive use* was assessed using post-birth survey data. From the six-month post-birth survey, we created a dichotomous variable indicating contraceptive use; respondents who indicated that they were not consistently using any form of contraception despite having regular heterosexual intercourse were coded as 0, with respondents either using contraception or not having sexual intercourse coded as 1. For descriptive purposes, we also created dummy variables for methods of contraception, though small cell sizes within the different methods prevented multivariate analysis.

#### *Independent variables*

To measure *pregnancy intendedness*, we used a question from the National Survey of Fertility Barriers that asked women about their reproductive behaviors at the time of their pregnancy: "Right before you got pregnant, would you say you were trying to get pregnant, trying NOT to get pregnant, or okay either way?" Responses were coded as dummy variables for "intended" (e.g., trying to get pregnant) and "ambivalent" (e.g., okay either way), as compared to those who were "unintended" (e.g., avoiding pregnancy) as the reference group.

We measured *contraceptive counseling* at the two-week post-birth survey with a question asking women, "Did your doctor, or any healthcare provider, discuss long-acting birth control options with you?" Response options were coded as yes (=1), no (=0), and don't know (=0).

#### *Control variables*

Our controls for the following sociodemographic variables collected at the first assessment include no desire for more children, race/ethnicity, parity, age, relationship status, economic hardship, and clinic where recruitment occurred. *No desire for more children* was measured with a question asking women if they wanted more children at any point after giving birth; no was coded as 1 with yes or unsure coded as 0. *Race/Ethnicity* was measured using Census coding recommendations with four categories: non-Hispanic white, non-Hispanic black, Hispanic, and Native American. *Parity* was calculated from reported live births as a continuous variable. *Age* was measured in years. We included a dummy variable indicating the respondent was in a *union* if she was married or cohabitating with a partner. *Economic hardship* was measured with seven items and included, "In the past year, did any of the following happen to you or members of your household because of a shortage of money" .... "went without meals;" "could not pay the mortgage or rent on time;" and "asked for financial help from friends or family." "Yes" responses were coded as 1 and summed to create an index of economic hardship. Additionally, although both medical practices served disadvantaged populations, there were a few differences between the obstetric practices. First, one practice served a slightly more urban population, and we observed differences in racial/ethnic distributions. Second, there were differences in institutional structures and affiliations. *Clinic 1* has the ability to do LARC placement at the time of delivery, whereas the other practice is affiliated with a religious-based institution that does not allow placement of LARC at delivery, though they can offer it at the post-birth clinic visit. Both clinics offer LARC at no charge to patients on public insurance. Due to these differences, we controlled for the location participants were recruited from in our analysis. Finally, we also controlled for whether the participants reported *prior unintended pregnancies* (1 = yes; 0 = no).

#### Analytic plan

We conducted logistic regression analyses to examine how pregnancy intendedness and provider contraceptive counseling predicted contraceptive non-use at 6 months. We ran all analyses in Stata. All variables in our analysis had fewer than 5% missing values. We used Stata's mi package to impute missing values on variables using chained equations in Stata to fit five imputation models.

## Results

### Sample characteristics

The analytical sample for the study included the approximately 71% of respondents who completed the survey assessments during pregnancy through the six-month post-birth follow up. This resulted in a final sample of 125 participants. Table 1 shows the descriptive statistics for the full sample as well as split into pregnancy intendedness groups. There was a fairly even split between pregnancy intendedness, with the largest group (40%) of the sample reporting that they were ambivalent about getting pregnant, 34% reporting that their pregnancies were intended, and 26% reporting that they were avoiding pregnancy (e.g., unintended) when it occurred. Two-thirds (66%) of participants reported that their providers discussed post-birth contraceptive options during pregnancy with them. The majority of the sample (56%) were at risk for a subsequent pregnancy at 6 months post-birth, meaning that they were sexually active and not using any form of contraception. The "unintended" group was the only one in which the majority of the women (69%) were using contraception 6 months after giving birth. Post-birth contraceptive methods by pregnancy intendedness status are depicted visually in Fig. 1. LARC methods were most popular among those with an unintended pregnancy, and among those who were ambivalent about getting pregnant, LARC was the most common contraceptive method used among those using contraception. More than half of those who had intended or were ambivalent about their pregnancies reported that they were sexually active and not using contraception 6 months after giving birth.

The logistic regression results are presented in Table 2. With all control variables included in the analysis (Model 1), women who reported their pregnancies were intended and those who were ambivalent about getting pregnant had significantly lower odds of using contraception at six-

**Table 1** Contraceptive Use and Contraceptive Counseling by Pregnancy Intention Status

| Characteristics | Total (*n* = 125) | Intended (*n* = 42) | Ambivalent (*n* = 50) | Unintended (*n* = 33) |
|---|---|---|---|---|
| | %/M (SD) | %/M (SD) | %/M (SD) | %/M (SD) |
| Contraceptive use at 6 months postpartum | 44% | 32% | 38% | 69% |
| Contraceptive counseling during pregnancy | 66% | 55% | 76% | 66% |
| Control variables | | | | |
| Desires no more births | 37% | 24% | 40% | 50% |
| Race/Ethnicity | | | | |
| White | 41% | 46% | 44% | 28% |
| Black | 28% | 27% | 22% | 41% |
| Hispanic | 14% | 15% | 12% | 16% |
| Native American | 17% | 12% | 22% | 16% |
| Parity | 1.27 (1.31) | 1.29 (1.45) | 1.08 (1.24) | 1.56 (1.21) |
| Age (years) | 25.84 (5.47) | 26.73 (5.82) | 25.86 (5.76) | 24.66 (4.87) |
| Residential partner | 65% | 76% | 71% | 41% |
| Economic hardship | 1.56 (1.82) | 1.71 (1.92) | 1.55 (1.91) | 1.34 (1.92) |
| Clinic 1 | 67% | 66% | 66% | 72% |
| Ever had unintended pregnancy | 57% | 48% | 55% | 70% |

months post birth than those who reported unintended pregnancies (OR = .19, $p < .01$ and OR = .30, $p < 05$, respectively). Latina and Native American women had lower odds of using contraception at 6 months postpartum than white women (OR = .23, $p < .05$; OR = .19, $p < .05$, respectively).

In Model 2, interactions between pregnancy intendedness and provider contraceptive counseling were added to the analysis. Findings indicate greater odds of contraceptive use among those who were ambivalent about their pregnancies when providers counseled them about post-.

birth contraception options during their pregnancy. To ease readability of the interaction findings, Fig. 2 presents the predicted probabilities of contraceptive use by pregnancy intention and provider counseling. Results indicate that among those who were ambivalent about their pregnancies, lack of provider contraceptive counseling was associated with significantly lower odds of contraceptive use at 6 months postpartum despite being

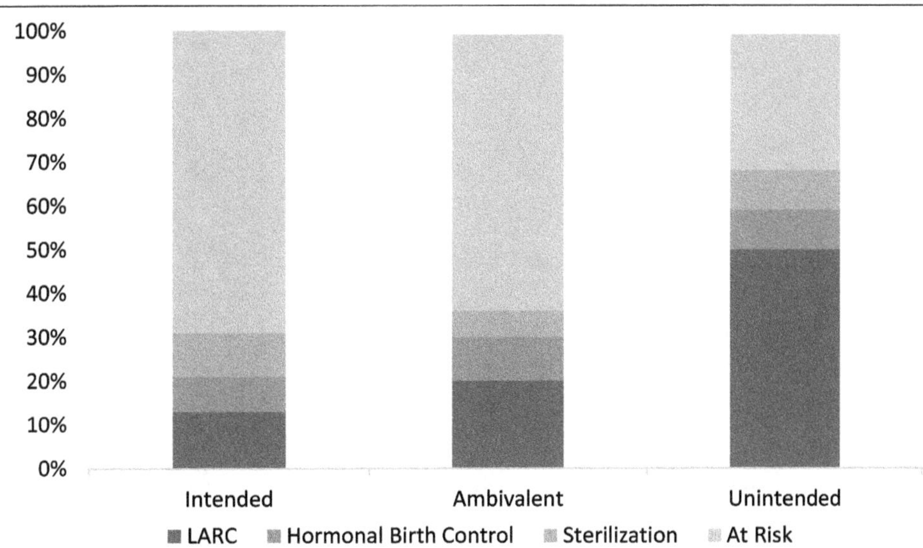


**Fig. 1** Contraception Use at 6 Months Postpartum by Pregnancy Intendedness

**Table 2** Logistic Regression Analysis Predicting Contraceptive Use at 6 Months Postpartum, with 95% CI ($N = 125$)

| | M1 | | M2 | |
|---|---|---|---|---|
| | aOR[a] | *p*-value | aOR[a] | *p*-value |
| Pregnancy intendedness | | | | |
| Unintended (reference) | | | | |
| Intended | .19 [.06,.65] | <.01 | .03 [.00,.33] | <.01 |
| Ambivalent | .30 [.10,.88] | <.05 | .02 [.00,.35] | <.01 |
| LARC counseling during pregnancy | .99 [.38,2.62] | | .10 [.01,1.09] | |
| Control variables | | | | |
| Desires no more children | 1.44 [.52,3.98] | | 1.50 [.52,4.31] | |
| Race | | | | |
| White (reference) | | | | |
| Black | .47 [.15,1.48] | | .39 [.12,1.26] | |
| Hispanic | .23 [.05,.1.00] | <.05 | .27 [.06,1.18] | |
| Native American | .19 [.05,.71] | <.05 | .18 [.04,.77] | <.05 |
| Parity | 1.82 [1.09,3.04] | <.05 | 1.79 [1.06,3.01] | <.05 |
| Age (years) | .91 [.82,1.02] | | .91 [.82,1.02] | |
| Residential partner | .79 [.31,2.05] | | .75 [.27,2.07] | |
| Economic hardship | 1.02 [.81,1.28] | | 1.03 [.81,1.31] | |
| Clinic 1 | 2.36 [.80,7.01] | | 2.40 [.75,7.63] | |
| Ever had unintended pregnancy | .48 [.15,1.51] | | .52 [.17,1.75] | |
| Pregnancy intention X contraceptive counseling | | | | |
| Intended X Counseling | | | 15.87 [.98,255.87] | |
| Ambivalent X Counseling | | | 32.53 [1.56,586.32] | <.05 |

[a] *aOR* Adjusted odds ratio

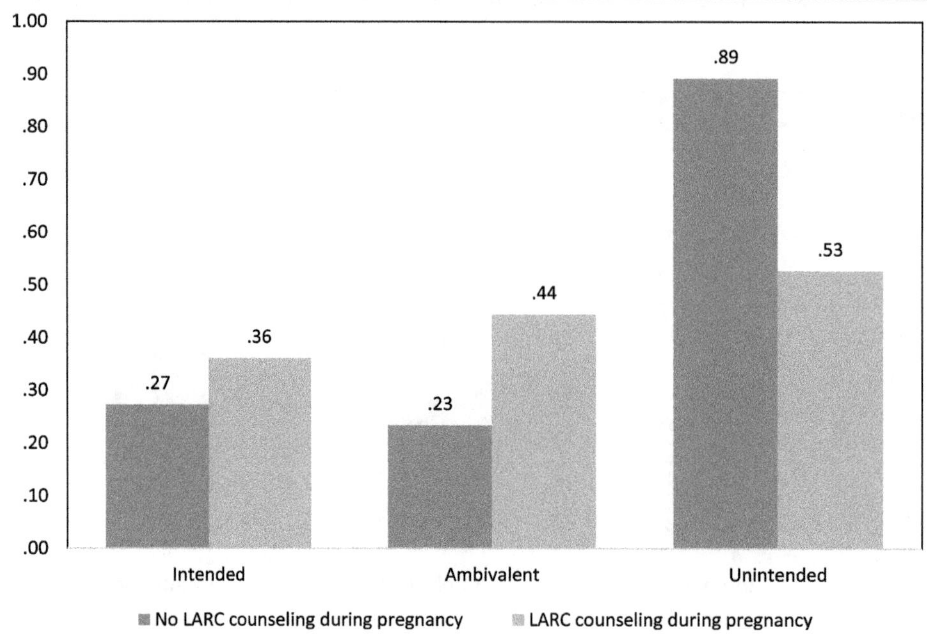


**Fig. 2** Predicted Probabilities of Contraceptive Use at 6 Months Postpartum by Pregnancy Intendedness

sexually active. The findings for those with unintended pregnancies were not in the expected direction, so we also created Fig. 3 to better understand how pregnancy intentions and provider counseling were associated with pregnancy risk at 6 months postpartum. Results suggest that those who were ambivalent about their pregnancies received the most counseling, and that women with unintended pregnancies were more likely to opt for postpartum contraception, even without discussions with their provider about post-birth contraception options.

## Discussion

Using a prospective, clinic-based sample of low-income pregnant women, we examined whether pregnancy intendedness and provider postpartum contraceptive counseling predicted risk for contraceptive non-use 6 months after giving birth. The findings from this study were consistent with prior findings that women interested in avoiding a subsequent pregnancy are most likely to opt for postpartum contraception [22]. Our findings highlighted that women who reported their pregnancy was intended or that they were ambivalent about getting pregnant were significantly less likely to use contraception following birth. The significant moderation between pregnancy intendedness and provider contraceptive counseling revealed that among pregnant women who were ambivalent about getting pregnant, receiving counseling about contraceptive options available after birth significantly increased the odds of using contraception at 6 months post birth.

This finding has critical implications for practitioners who provide contraceptive counseling. Ambivalence about getting pregnant is common; women often perceive both positive and negative consequences if they become pregnant [23], and those who report ambivalence tend to overestimate the risks associated with more effective contraceptive methods (e.g., LARC methods) and overestimate the effectiveness of oral contraception [24]. Providers who identify their patients as ambivalent have the opportunity to ask their patients about perceived benefits and adverse consequences if they become pregnant and to inform their patients about different contraceptive methods and their effectiveness. Our results suggest that this is a particularly receptive group for contraceptive counseling that can reduce the risk of a short inter-pregnancy interval.

This analysis has several limitations. Due to the nature of the sample being recruited from clinics serving primarily patients receiving public healthcare coverage, we were unable to examine insurance differences in post-birth contraceptive coverage. All participants had the option for free LARC insertion post-birth, however, which may explain why economic hardship did not significantly predict post-birth contraceptive use. Additionally, due to the small sample size, we were not able to empirically examine different methods of contraception. Future research should include a larger sample to allow for analysis of a wider array of methods to gain insight into those choices and consequences for short interpregnancy intervals. Still, a substantial proportion of our participants (56%) are at risk for a subsequent pregnancy (e.g., not using any form of contraception despite engaging in regular, heterosexual intercourse) only 6 months following a birth. Nonetheless, these limitations are offset by the strengths of this analysis, which include the prospective nature of the study and a predominately low-income and diverse sample. Future research is needed to further explore the findings about pregnancy intendedness and provider contraceptive counseling. For example, were women with intended pregnancies less likely to receive provider counseling because they were

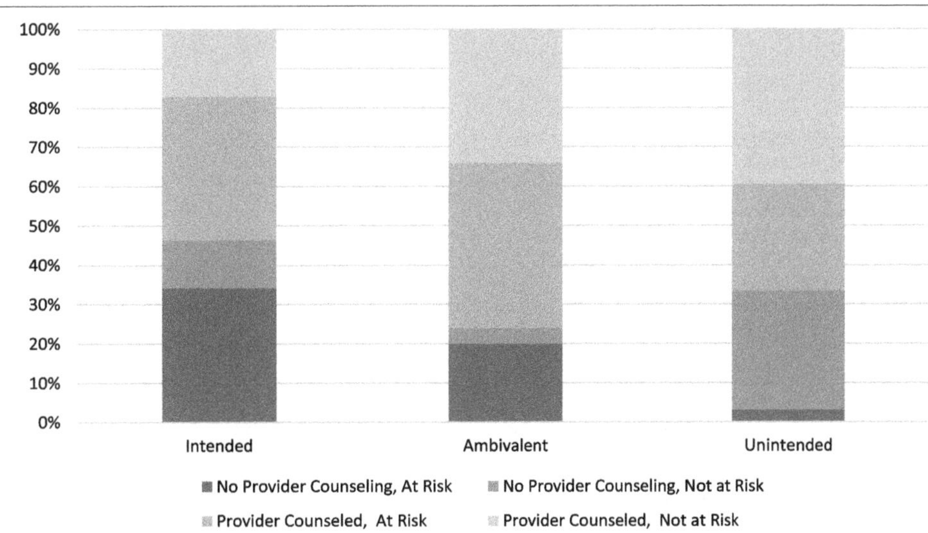


**Fig. 3** Provider Counseling and Risk for Short Interpregnancy Interval at 6 Months Postpartum by Pregnancy Intendedness

worried that a long-acting method may prevent them from having more children? Did women with unintended pregnancies report that they did not discuss contraception with providers because they had already decided to pursue contraception following birth, thus making contraceptive counseling unnecessary for those highly motivated to seek it?

## Conclusion

Our study highlighted the role that healthcare providers can play in encouraging women to uptake highly effective forms of contraception to delay a subsequent birth—particularly among women who expressed ambivalence about pregnancy. In conversations with pregnant women about post-birth contraception, providers should consider asking women about the intendedness of their current pregnancy. Women who are highly motivated to avoid pregnancy are most likely to opt for LARC or another contraceptive method after a birth, but those who are interested in giving birth again in the future should be informed about the risks for short interpregnancy intervals and the effectiveness of different forms of contraception.

#### Abbreviation

LARC: Long-acting reversible contraception

#### Acknowledgements

The authors would like to thank the HATCH participating clinics, and particularly Dr. Karen Gold, for their support.

#### Authors' contributions

KS and ST: Developed study, analyzed data, and wrote manuscript. JP, and LF: Coordinated data collection process and consulted on study design and analysis. All authors read and approved the final manuscript.

#### Author details

[1]Oklahoma State University, 700 N. Greenwood Ave, Tulsa, OK 74106, USA. [2]University of Oklahoma Health Sciences Center, 4502 E. 41st St, Tulsa, OK 74135, USA. [3]Oklahoma State University Center for Health Sciences, 1111 W. 17th St, Tulsa, OK 74107, USA.

#### References

1. Finer LB, Zolna MR. Declines in unintended pregnancy in the United States, 2008–2011. N Engl J Med. 2016;374(9):843–52.
2. Brown SS, Eisenberg L. The best intentions: unintended pregnancy and the well-being of children and families: National Academies Press; 1995.
3. Shah PS, Balkhair T, Ohlsson A, Beyene J, Scott F, Frick C. Intention to become pregnant and low birth weight and preterm birth: a systematic review. Matern Child Health J. 2011;15:205–16.
4. Kost K, Lindberg L. Pregnancy intentions, maternal behaviors, and infant health: investigating relationships with new measures and propensity score analysis. Demography. 2015;52:83–111.
5. Barber JS, Axinn WG, Thornton A. Unwanted childbearing, health, and mother-child relationships. J Health Soc Behav. 1999;40(3):231–57.
6. Orr ST, Miller CA, James SA, Babones S. Unintended pregnancy and preterm birth. Paediatr Perinat Epidemiol. 2000;14(4):309–13.
7. Gold RB, Sonfield A, Richards CL, Frost JJ. Next steps for America's family planning program. Leveraging the potential of Medicaid and title X in an evolving health care system. Guttmacher Institute: New York; 2009.
8. Chiou CF, Trussell J, Reyes E, Knight K, Wallace J, Udani J, et al. Economic analysis of contraceptives for women. Contraception. 2003;68(1):3–10.
9. Hatcher RA, Trussell J, Nelson AL, Cates W, Stewart FH, Kowal D. Contraceptive technology. Ardent Media: New York; 2007.
10. American College of Obstetricians and Gynecologists. Adolescents and long-acting reversible contraception: Implants and intrauterine devices. Committee opinion no. 539. Obstet Gynecol. 2012;120:983–8. https://doi.org/10.1097/AOG.0b013e3182723b7d.
11. Baldwin MK, Edelman AB. The effect of long-acting reversible contraception on rapid repeat pregnancy in adolescents: a review. J Adolesc Health. 2013;52(4):S47–53.
12. Finer LB, Lindberg LD, Desai S. A prospective measure of unintended pregnancy in the United States. Contraception. 2018;98(6):522–7.
13. American College of Obstetricians and Gynecologists. Increasing access to contraceptive implants and intrauterine devices to reduce unintended pregnancy. Committee opinion no. 642. Obstet Gynecol. 2015;126:e44–8. https://doi.org/10.1097/AOG.0000000000001106.
14. American Academy of Pediatrics. Contraception for adolescents: committee on adolescence. Pediatrics 2014;134(4):e1244-e1256. doi:https://doi.org/10.1542/peds.2014-2299.
15. Branum AM, Jones J. Trends in long-acting reversible contraception use among US women aged 15–44. Centers for Disease Control and Prevention, National Center for Health Statistics: US Department of Health and Human Services; 2015.
16. Moniz M, Chang T, Heisler M, Dalton VK. Immediate postpartum long acting reversible contraception: the time is now. Contraception. 2017;95(4):335.
17. Hall KS, Ela E, Zochowski MK, Caldwell A, Moniz M, McAndrew L, Steel M, Challa S, Dalton VK, Ernst S. "I don't know enough to feel comfortable using them:" Women's knowledge of and perceived barriers to long-acting reversible contraceptives on a college campus. Contraception. 2016;93(6):556–64.
18. Hladky KJ, Allsworth JE, Madden T, Secura GM, Peipert JF. Women's knowledge about intrauterine contraception. Obstet Gynecol. 2011;117(1):48.
19. Okoroh EM, Kane DJ, Gee RE, Kieltyka L, Frederiksen BN, Baca KM, Rankin KM, Goodman DA, Kroelinger CD, Barfield WD. Policy change is not enough: engaging provider champions on immediate postpartum contraception. Am J Obstet Gynecol. 2018;218(6):590–e1.
20. White K, Potter JE, Hopkins K, Grossman D. Variation in postpartum contraceptive method use: results from the pregnancy risk assessment monitoring system (PRAMS). Contraception. 2014;89(1):57–62.
21. Higgins JA. Pregnancy ambivalence and long-acting reversible contraceptive (LARC) use among young adult women: a qualitative study. Perspect Sex Reprod Health. 2017;49(3):149–56.
22. Guzzo KB, Eickmeyer K, Hayford SR. Does postpartum contraceptive use vary by birth intendedness? Perspect Sex Reprod Health. 2018;50(3):129–38.
23. Campo S, Askelson NM, Spies EL, Losch M. Ambivalence, communication and past use: understanding what influences women's intentions to use contraceptives. Psychol Health Med. 2012;17(3):356–65.
24. Sundstrom B, Ferrara M, DeMaria AL, Baker-Whitcomb A, Payne JB. Integrating pregnancy ambivalence and effectiveness in contraceptive choice. Health Commun. 2017;32(7):820–7.

# 21

# Discontinuation of implants use and associated factors among women attending health facility clinics in Hawassa City, Southern Ethiopia, 2019

Belay Amare Abebe[1*] and Mulu Reda Terefe[2]

**Abstract**

**Background:** Despite improving the availability and use of Implants, discontinuation is becoming a public health concern. A significant proportion of women discontinuing the service before its due date, which is of concern in the health system and its consequence may lead to a program failure. This might have also social and economic consequences for users. Only 8% of married women in Ethiopia use implants. Apart from its low utilization, premature removal is common for unknown reasons. However, there is paucity of information on discontinuation of implants use and associated factors in the study area.

**Objective:** The study was aimed to assess discontinuation of implants use and associated factors among women attending health facility clinics in Hawassa city, southern Ethiopia, from March, 01-April, 01/2019.

**Methods:** Facility based cross sectional study design was used. Out of 16 health facilities, 9 of them were selected for this study using simple random sampling. Total sample size of this study was determined to be 351. Data were collected from study subjects using pretested, structured questionnaire through a face-to-face interview. Data was analyzed using descriptive statistics and logistic regression. The result is presented using the Crude Odds ratio as well as Adjusted Odds Ratio with the corresponding 95% confidence level.

**Result:** Out of 351 study participants, the overall proportion of implants discontinuation was 49.3%(95% CI: 44.2–55.0). Lack of counseling about side effects (AOR = 2.394; 95% CI: 1.422–4.030), developing side effects (AOR = 6.325; 95% CI: 3.719–10.757) and lack of post insertion follow-up (AOR = 2.241; 95% CI: 1.186–4.234) the major factors associated with discontinuation of Implants.

**Conclusion and recommendation:** In this study, the overall proportion of discontinuation of Implants among women who were using Implants was high. Health professionals could give pre-insertion counseling about side effects and post insertion dates for follow-up to improve of utilization of implants.

**Keywords:** Associative factors, Discontinuation, Implants

* Correspondence: gideteb60@gmail.com
[1]Department of Midwifery, College Medicine and Health Sciences, University of Hawassa, PO Box-1560, Hawassa, Ethiopia

## Backround

Modern contraception is highly effective in preventing unintended pregnancy and reducing maternal mortality. Family planning (FP) is a process that usually involves a discussion between a woman, a man, and a trained family planning service provider focusing on family health and the desires of the couple to either limit or space their family size [1]. Contraceptives discontinuation is removal of the methods by the women due to any reason. Implants are long-acting and extremely effective at preventing pregnancy, with a clinical failure rate less than 1% [19].

Discontinuation of effective methods of contraception is a universal problem, though rates vary widely by population and country [8]. Every year, about one-third of the 182 million pregnancies occurring worldwide are unplanned [7, 21]. Globally, 33 million accidental pregnancies are estimated to occur among women reportedly using a contraceptive method, either traditional or modern [25].

Evidence from 60 demographic and health surveys conducted on causes and consequences of contraceptive discontinuation; on average, 38% of women discontinue using reversible methods by the 12th month and 64% by the 36th month in 19 countries [25].

According to a report based on developing countries, Implanon discontinuation within the first year ranges from 2% in Nigeria to 23% in UK [2, 3].

Contraceptive discontinuation contributes to unplanned pregnancies, unwanted births and termination of pregnancies that expose a risk to the health of women. This unplanned pregnancy has impacts on larger family size and ultimately contributes to higher overall fertility rates which may result social, economic and physical health disabilities [18, 23].

According to [11], contraceptive discontinuation in the 5 years preceding the survey were > 35% within 12 months' use [11].

Only 8% of married women in Ethiopia use implants [12, 26]. Apart from its low utilization, premature removal is common for unknown reasons. In addition, there is limited information on discontinuation of implants use and associated factors in the study area. Therefore, this study was aimed to assess discontinuation of implants use and associated factors among women attending health facility clinics in Hawassa city, Southern Ethiopia, from March, 01 to April, 01/2019.

The findings of this study will enhance the planning and decision-making capacity of health professionals to seek possible solutions to the problems of the community in collaboration with the stake holders concerned. In addition, the findings will help local programmer managers, planners and other concerning organizations working in the field of family planning and maternal health to plan new strategies and prepare training programs based on the identified factors to enhance retention of utilization in the community. Finally, this study will provide baseline data for other researchers to investigate a prospective future study in the field.

### Conceptual framework (Fig. 1)

## Methods and materials

### Study area and period

Hawassa City Administration, is the capital city of Southern nation nationality people, and Sidama Zonal administration, located 275 km to the south of the capital city of Ethiopia, Addis Ababa. The city administration is divided in 8 sub cities, of which 7 are urban having 21 kebeles and one peri-urban with 12 kebeles with a total population of 387,087 in 2017 (CSA, 2017). The study was conducted in nine health facilities, i.e. HURH, AGH, Hawassa family guidance association, Hawassa Merry stop international clinic, Millinium HC, Alamura HC, Adare HC, Tulla HC and Tilite HC of Hawassa City, Southern Ethiopia, from March, 01 to April 01/2019.

### Study design

Facility based cross-sectional study was used.

### Study population

All reproductive age women who were using Implants and came to the selected health institutions for contraceptives related reasons during the actual data collection period.

### Inclusion and exclusion criterias

All reproductive age women who were using Implants and came to the selected health institutions for contraceptives related reasons during the actual data collection period were included in the study. Women who were unable to communicate and respond like hearing loss were excluded from the study.

### Sample size determination

Outcome variable and various factors significantly associated with the outcome variable in previous studies were considered to determine the sample size. Accordingly, for the first and second specific objectives the sample size was calculated separately and the larger sample size was taken to be used for this study.

### Specific objective 1

For magnitude of discontinuation of Implants.

The sample size was calculated by using single population proportion formula as follows.

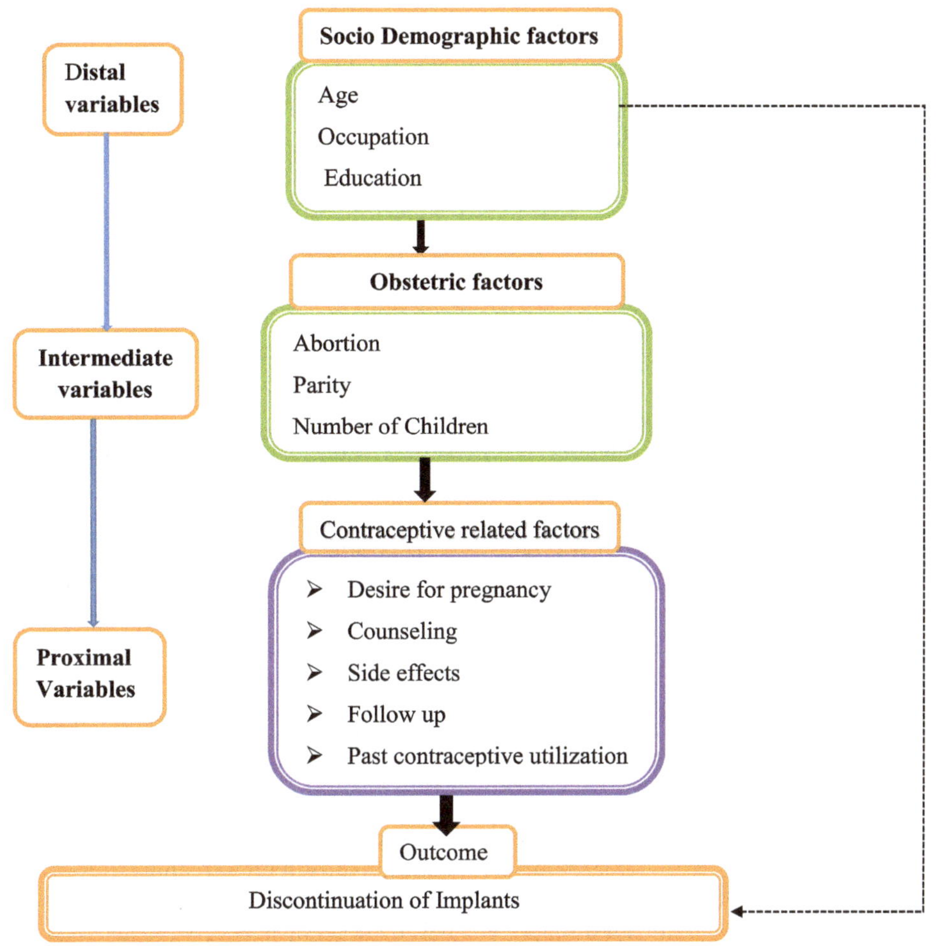


**Fig. 1** Conceptual framework for the study on assessment of discontinuation of Implants and associated factors developed by principal investigator. This conceptual framework is developed from different literature used from a range of cross sectional and case control studies conducted on early discontinuation of use of Implanon and associated factors in Ethiopia [6, 15]

$$n = \frac{(z_{\alpha/2})^2 \times p(1-p)}{d^2}$$

Where $n$ is the minimum sample size required, $p$ is expected proportion of discontinued mothers, $z = 1.96$ (95% CI) and $d = 0.05$ is the margin of error between the sample and the population. For this study $p = 16\%$, from study conducted on Ofla Tigray on the prevalence of discontinuation of implants and associated factors. Thus, applying the formula, by substituting these values into Eq. (1) gives, = 206.5. By adding 10% non-response rate, the final sample size becomes 227 for the first specific objective.

### Specific objective 2

factors associated with discontinuation of Implants.

The sample size of the second specific objective of this study was calculated by considering factors that were significantly associated with the outcome variable, two sided confidence level of 95%, the margin of error of 5%, power by 80% and the ratio of exposed to unexposed 1:1 using Epi-Info Version 7 software.

As it can be seen from Table 1, the calculated sample size of the second objective is larger than that of the first objective. By adding 10% non-response rate, $n = 313*0.1 + 313 = 351$

### Sampling technique / procedure

Out of the 16 health facilities available in Hawassa city administration, both hospitals (i.e. HURH and Adare General Hospital), five HCs, (i.e. Millinium, Adare, Tilite, Tulla and Alamura HCs) and two NGO clinics (i.e. Hawassa family guidance association and Hawassa Marie stops international) were randomly selected for this study using lottery method.

In order to ensure a proportionate allocation of the total sample size determined, the average six-month client flows of each selected health facility were considered prior to the start of data collection. The study subjects were identified based on the information obtained from

**Table 1** Sample size determination for magnitude and associated factors of Implants discontinuation among Implants user women in health facilities of Hawassa city, Southern Ethiopia, 2018/19

| Associated factors | Exposed outcome % | Unexposed outcome % | Sample size | Reference |
|---|---|---|---|---|
| Removal due to side effect | 75.6(side effect faced) | 60.2(side effect not faced) | 313 | [15] |
| Follow up | 35.9(had follow up) | 15.76(hadn't follow up) | 166 | [22] |

the client card. The information obtained from the 6 Months enrollment record (June–December/2018) from the family planning registry books showed that a total of 3500 women were used Implants within 6 months in the selected institutions.

As the result, the average six-months client flow for HURH, AGH, Hawassa family guidance association, Hawassa Marie stops international clinic, Millinium HC, Alamura HC, Adare HC, Tulla HC and Tilite HC was 500, 560, 440, 400, 310, 380, 300, 360, and 250 respectively.

So that, sample was proportionally allocated for each selected institution. Data collectors approached and recruited implants user women who came to the selected clinics due to contraceptives related reasons. Every woman was included in the study until the required sample size was met in each health facility (Fig. 2).

## Data collection methods

### Data collection instruments

The data for this study was collected using pre-tested, structured questionnaire through a face to face interview. The tool for this study is adopted from previous literature of similar studies [6, 15]. The questionnaire contains three main parts. These are; socio-demographic characteristics, Obstetric related factors and contraceptive methods related variables.

### Data collectors

Nine Nurses and Midwives with a qualification of degree were the data collectors. Three supervisors supervised and provided all items necessary for data collection on each data collection day for data collectors.

### Data collection procedure

Data were collected from study subjects using pretested, structured questionnaire through a face-to-face interview. The questionnaire was developed in English and translated into Amharic and then back to English to check for its consistency. The instrument was adopted from different literature developed for similar purposes by different authors [6, 15]. The interviewers were Midwives and Nurses with a qualification of degree. The responsibility of the data collectors was to fill the questionnaire after obtaining informed, voluntary, written and signed consent of the study subjects. The principal investigator and supervisors supervised and provided

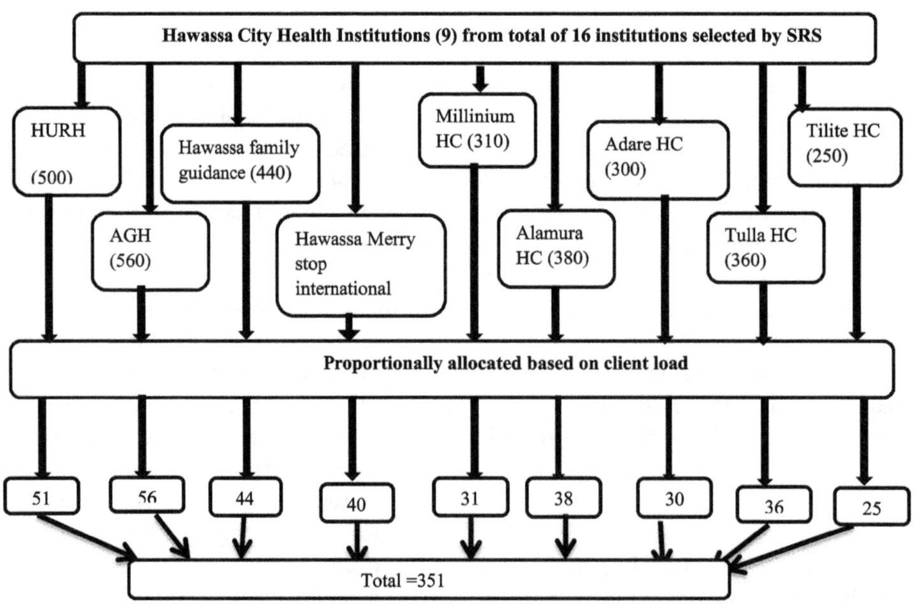


**Fig. 2** Schematic presentation of sampling procedure for the study on discontinuation of implants and associated factors developed by principal investigator. Six months' enrollment in Heath institutions of Hawassa city administration in both public hospitals, five HCs and two NGO clinics from family planning registration book, for sample selection (June–December/2018)

**Table 2** Socio-demographic characteristics of the study participants in health facilities of Hawassa city, Southern Ethiopia, 2019 ($n = 351$)

| Variables | Frequency | Percentage |
|---|---|---|
| **Women's age** | | |
| 19–24 | 100 | 28.5 |
| 25–29 | 164 | 46.7 |
| 30–34 | 69 | 19.7 |
| => 35 | 18 | 5.1 |
| **Marital status** | | |
| Single | 8 | 2.3 |
| Married | 343 | 97.7 |
| **Religion** | | |
| Orthodox | 103 | 29.3 |
| Muslim | 20 | 5.7 |
| Protestant | 218 | 62.1 |
| Catholic | 9 | 2.6 |
| Others | 1 | 3 |
| **Ethnicity** | | |
| Sidama | 146 | 41.6 |
| Wolayta | 82 | 23.4 |
| Amhara | 62 | 17.7 |
| Gurage | 25 | 7.1 |
| Oromo | 14 | 4.0 |
| Others* | 22 | 6.3 |
| **Occupation** | | |
| House wife | 149 | 42.5 |
| Merchant | 62 | 17.7 |
| Private employee | 47 | 13.4 |
| Government employee | 65 | 18.5 |
| Student | 28 | 8.0 |
| **Maternal educational status** | | |
| Unable to read and write | 44 | 12.5 |
| Read and Write | 39 | 11.1 |
| Primary | 99 | 28.2 |
| Secondary | 82 | 23.4 |
| College and above | 87 | 24.8 |
| **Husband educational status ($n = 343$)** | | |
| Unable to read and write | 24 | 7.0 |
| Read and Write | 23 | 6.7 |
| Primary | 55 | 16.0 |
| Secondary | 100 | 29.2 |
| College and above | 141 | 41.1 |
| **Husband's occupation ($n = 343$)** | | |
| Farmer | 21 | 6.1 |
| Merchant | 123 | 35.9 |
| Private employee | 59 | 17.2 |
| Government employee | 123 | 35.9 |
| Student | 7 | 2.0 |
| Others | 10 | 2.9 |

all items necessary for data collection on each data collection day, checking filled questionnaire for completeness and logical consistency and solve problems forwarded during the time of data collection.

### Data quality assurance

To assure the quality of data, properly designed data collection tools were used. Training was given for data collectors and supervisors about research objectives, data collection tools, procedures and interview techniques for 1 day. The principal investigator, together with three supervisors, supervised techniques of data collection and completeness of the tools on the daily basis to give an appropriate feedback accordingly. Data double entry was done to make comparisons of two data clerks and resolved some difference.

### Pre-test

Before the actual data collection period, the questionnaire was tested on 5% of the total sample size (351) on 18 reproductive age women who used implants at none-selected health facilities to check the context of data. After pretest, the questionnaire was revised and amended per necessary.

### *Data processing and analysis*

After data collection, the questionnaire was checked for completeness and data entry was made using EPI DATA V-3.1 and then exported to the Statistical Package for Social Science [SPSS] V-22 computer software for analysis. Descriptive statistics and bivariate analysis were performed. Variables with $p$-value $< 0.25$ in bivariate analysis were planned to be entered in multivariate logistic regression analysis. Multi co-linearity test was carried out to check the linear correlation among independent variables by using standard error and co-linearity statistics. Variance inflation factor > 10 and standard error > 2 were considered as suggestive of the existence of multi co-linearity. Therefore, variables with Variance inflation factor > 10 and/ standard error > 2 were checked to be dropped. Hosmer -Lemeshow goodness- of- fit was used to check model fitness. Omnibus test was significant and Hosmer- Lemeshow's test was found to be insignificant which indicate that the model was fitted. Based on the

**Table 3** Obstetrics related factors for discontinuation of implants among implants user women in health facilities of Hawassa city, Southern Ethiopia, 2019 ($n = 351$)

| Variables | Frequency | Percentage |
|---|---|---|
| **Parity** | | |
| 0 | 28 | 8.0 |
| 1–2 | 207 | 59.0 |
| 3+ | 116 | 33.0 |
| **Number of living children** | | |
| 0 | 29 | 8.3 |
| 1–2 | 226 | 64.4 |
| 3–4 | 86 | 24.5 |
| 5+ | 10 | 2.8 |
| **History of abortion** | | |
| Yes | 107 | 30.5 |
| No | 244 | 69.5 |
| **Desire for pregnancy** | | |
| Yes | 239 | 68.1 |
| No | 112 | 31.9 |
| **When they want to become pregnant($n$ = 239)** | | |
| Within two years | 94 | 39.3 |
| After two years | 145 | 60.7 |

findings of bivariate analysis, variables with $p$-value< 0.25 were entered into multivariate logistic regression analysis with 95% confidence level and 5% significant level. AOR with 95%CI, and level of significant at $p$-value < 0.05 was considered. Variables with $p$-value less than 0.05 in the multivariate logistic regression analysis were considered as statistically significant with implants discontinuation.

## Result

### Socio-demographic characteristics

All study participants had responded to the questionnaire, making a response rate of 100%. The range of study participants' age was between 19 and 44 years with mean (±SD) age 26.6 ± 4.3. Out of the total respondents, 164 (46.7%) of women were in the age range of 25–29. Three hundred forty three (97.7%) of participants were married and about 218 (62.1%) were Protestant followed by Orthodox, 103 (29. 3%) in religion. One hundred forty six (41.6%), of participants were Sidama in Ethnicity.

Among the participants, 149 (42.5%) were housewives and 166 (38.5%) of their husbands were merchants by occupation. Ninety nine (28.2%) of the participants were at primary level and 141 (41.1%) of their husbands were college and above in educational status (Table 2).

### Obstetrics related characteristics

Two hundred and seven (59.0%) respondents had given birth one to two times while 116 (33.0%) of the participants gave birth more than three times. Among the participants who gave birth, 226 (64.4%) women had one to two alive children. Two hundred and forty-four (69.5%) of participants had no history of abortion and 239 (68.1%) women had desire for another pregnancy. Out of those who had desire for another pregnancy, 94 (39.3%) and 145 (60.9%) women desired to become pregnant within two and after two years respectively (Table 3).

### Contraceptive related characteristics

In this study, 261 (74.4%) and 90 (25.6%) of participants were Implanon and Jaddle users respectively. Three hundred and thirty (65.5%) of study participants had ever used contraceptives before the implant they were using during the study period. Out of them 176 (76.5%) had used injectable followed by oral contraceptive pills 83 (36.1%). Of the total participants, 305(87%) women got the implant insertion from government institutions and 252 (71.8%) of them chose the contraceptives by their own.

Three hundred and twenty-seven (93.2%) and 165 (47.0%) of the participants got counseling service about the benefit and side effect of implants during insertion respectively. Two hundred and seventy-five (78.3%) of study participants had an appointment for follow-up during their implant utilization period. One hundred and thirty-six (38.7%) of the study participants had ever faced side effects during their implants utilization period. The suggested reasons for discontinuation of implants were identified that side effect was the major, which accounted 79 (45.7%) followed by 41 (23.7%) of method switching after service end (Table 4).

Among participants who discontinued implants due to non-side effect reasons, method switching after service accounted 41 (23.7%) followed by desire for another pregnancy, 40 (23.1%) and others like husband go abroad, husband's objection, divorce and health concern accounted about 13 (7.5%). Whereas, among women who discontinued implants due to side effects, menstrual disruption accounted 56 (70.0%) followed by 19 (23.8%) weight gain (Fig. 3).

### Magnitude of implants discontinuation

From 351 study participants, 49.3% (95% CI: 44.2, 55.0%) was overall proportion of Implants discontinuation (Fig. 4). The mean (±SD) overall duration of Implants utilization in years was 2.2 ± 1.1.

**Table 4** Contraceptives related characteristics for discontinuation of implants in Health facilities of Hawassa city, Southern Ethiopia, 2019 ($n = 351$)

| Variables | Frequency | Percentage |
|---|---|---|
| **Type of implant used by participants** | | |
| Implanon | 261 | 74.4 |
| Jaddle | 90 | 25.6 |
| **Ever used contraceptives before implant** | | |
| Yes | 230 | 65.5 |
| No | 121 | 34.5 |
| **Type of contraceptive used before implant** | | |
| OCP | 83 | 36.1 |
| Injectable | 176 | 76.5 |
| IUCD | 4 | 1.7 |
| Implants | 34 | 14.8 |
| **Place of insertion of the method** | | |
| Hospital | 162 | 46.2 |
| Health center | 141 | 40.2 |
| Health post | 2 | 0.6 |
| Family guidance | 40 | 11.3 |
| Others* | 6 | 1.7 |
| **Counseling for benefit of implants** | | |
| Yes | 327 | 93.2 |
| No | 24 | 6.8 |
| **Counseling for side effects of implants** | | |
| Yes | 165 | 47.0 |
| No | 186 | 53.0 |
| **Estimation of information participants get during counseling (satisfaction)** | | |
| Yes | 272 | 77.5 |
| No | 79 | 22.5 |
| **Have you ever faced side effects** | | |
| Yes | 136 | 38.7 |
| No | 215 | 61.3 |
| **Who choose implant** | | |
| Own choice | 252 | 71.8 |
| My husband | 31 | 8.8 |
| Health professional | 65 | 18.5 |
| Health extension | 2 | 0.6 |
| My neighbor | 1 | 0.3 |
| **Reasons to choose the method** | | |
| Safety | 70 | 19.9 |
| Long protection | 150 | 42.7 |
| It can remove at any time | 86 | 24.5 |
| Immediate fertility return | 45 | 12.8 |
| **Follow-up** | | |
| Yes | 275 | 78.3 |
| No | 76 | 21.7 |
| **Removal due to side effect**($n = 221$) | | |
| Yes | 79 | 35.7 |
| No | 142 | 64.3 |

Others* Merry stopes international clinic, private hospitals and clinics

### Factors associated with implants discontinuation

Findings from bivariate analysis resulted that, participants' occupational status, maternal educational status, Husband educational status, past contraceptive utilization, lack of counseling about possible benefits, lack of counseling about side effects, lack of appointment for follow-up and developing side effects were associated with discontinuation of implants at $p$-value< 0.25. However, in a multivariate logistic regression analysis, lack of counseling about side effects (AOR = 2.394; 95% CI: 1.422–4.030), lack of appointment for follow up (AOR = 2.241; 95% CI: 1.186–4.234) and developing side effects (AOR = 6.325; 95% CI: 3.719–10.757) were found significantly associated with implants discontinuation (Table 5).

## Discussion

The proportion of implants discontinuation among women who were users of implants was high. Factors such as lack of counseling about side effects, developing side effects and lack of appointment for follow up were significantly associated with discontinuation of implants.

The proportion of implants discontinuation among implants user women was 49.3%. This finding is in line with studies conducted in Netherland, 47% [23], Jordan, 45%(USAID, 2007–2009) and Cambodia, 45% [21]. However, the current proportion is lower than study conducted in Australia, 60% [13] and at Debre Tabor 65% [15]. This result variation might be due to study nature of study participants. In studies conducted in Australia and Debre Tabor, the study participants were both urban and rural, but urban only in this study. As a result, awareness towards the behaviors of contraceptives might be better at urban residents. Moreover, it might be due to efforts made by health providers to improve the retention of utilization.

The current proportion is also higher than studies conducted in the United States, 25.2% [10], Pakistan, 18.0%, Egypt, 36%, Yemen, 43%, [21], Ilorin, Nigeria, 26.5% [4], Abakaliki, southeast Nigeria, 29.6% [14] and at Ofla Tigray, 16%, [6]. The difference might be due to lack of pre-insertion counseling of side effects of the

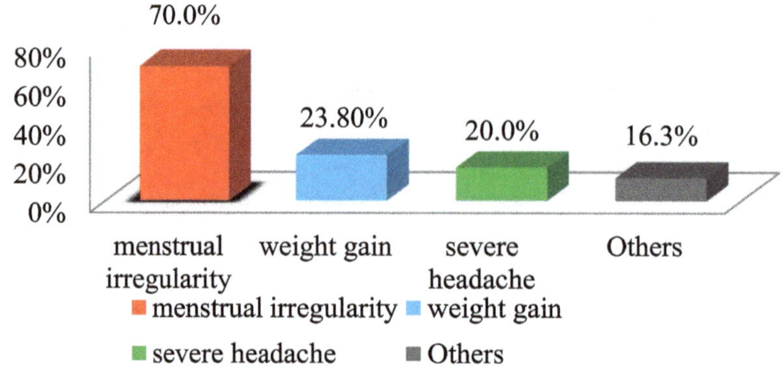


**Fig. 3** The main side effects for discontinuation of implants among implants user women in health facilities of Hawassa city administration, Southern Ethiopia, 2019. Others*: Insertion arm pain, achene, weight reduction and difficult to work

methods as compared to other studies (USAID, 2007–2009). In addition to this, it might be due to lack of appointment for follow up as compared to other studies [4, 10, 21, 23]. The other reason for differences in current proportion might be due to higher sample size of the current study compared to other studies [6, 10, 14]. Another possible reason might be due to sociocultural differences of respondents across the study areas.

This study showed that women who didn't get pre-insertion counseling service about side effects were 2.4 times more likely to discontinue than those who got counseling services. This is consistent with study conducted in Tigray [6], Debre Tabor [15], Jordan, India [5], Diguna Fango [22] and Philippines [20]. Providing counseling about side effects of implants was positively associated with use of the methods [20, 22]. So, the possible justification of this factor might be due to lack of pre-placement counseling and support by the service providers to help women continue on contraception. In addition, sociocultural variations, lack of skilled counselor, outlook and level of understanding of participants towards the contraceptives might be the reasons that made the factor associated with discontinuation of the implants.

According to this study, the likelihood of discontinuing implants among women who developed side effects was 6.3 times higher than those who did not face side effect. This is consistent with studies conducted in Ankara, Turkey, Abakaliki, southeast Nigeria [14], Debre Tabor [15], Arsi, Oromia region [9], Jos, Nigeria [16], Tigray [6], Nepal [24] and Jordan. The possible reasons might be exposing to side effect of the method could contribute for discontinuation of the contraceptives. In addition, respondents who discontinued implants due to side effects may be due to intolerance of side effects and fears that different complications will occur in their health in the future.

This study also revealed that, the odds of discontinuation of implants among women who lacked post insertion follow up were 2.2 times higher than those who had

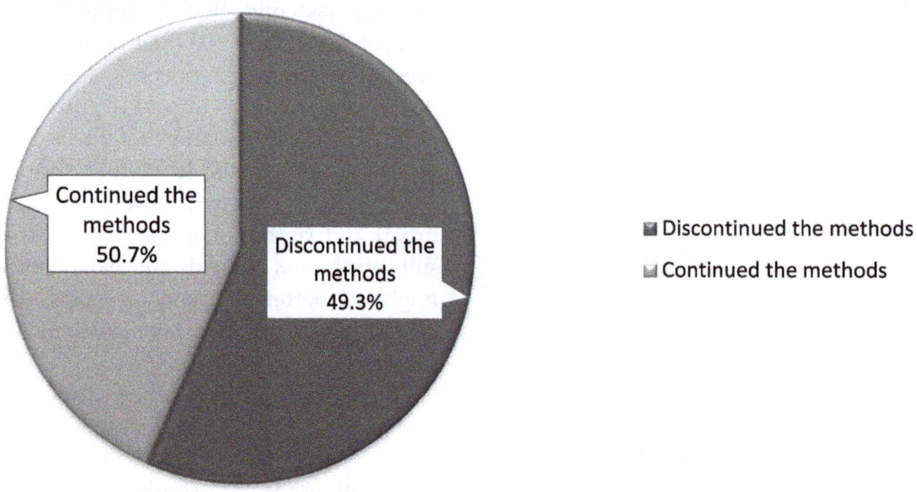


**Fig. 4** Proportion of implants discontinuation among implants user women in health facilities of Hawassa city administration, Southern Ethiopia, 2019

**Table 5** Factors associated with implants discontinuation among implants user women in health facilities of Hawassa city, Southern Ethiopia, 2019 ($n = 351$)

| Variables | LARCs discontinuation Ye s (%) No (%) | | *P*-value | AOR (95% C.I) |
|---|---|---|---|---|
| **Occupation of participant** | | | | |
| House wife | 71 (47.7%) | 78 (52.3%) | **0.110** | 2.622 (0.855–8.041) |
| Merchant | 30 (48.4%) | 32 (51.6%) | **0.164** | 2.613 (0.801–8.529) |
| Private employee | 27 (57.4%) | 20 (42.6%) | 0.559 | 1.531 (0.456–5.141) |
| Government employee | 32 (49.2%) | 33 (50.8%) | **0.184** | 2.337 (0.71–7.694) |
| Student | 18 (64.3%) | 10 (35.7%) | | 1 |
| **Maternal Educational status** | | | | |
| Unable to read and write | 22 (50.0%) | 22 (50.0%) | 0.663 | 1.423 (0.360–5.633) |
| Read and Write | 23 (59.0%) | 16 (41.0%) | 0.605 | 0.798 (0.235–2.712) |
| Primary | 42 (42.4%) | 57 (57.6%) | **0.115** | 2.240 (0.793–6.329) |
| Secondary | 44 (53.7%) | 38 (46.3%) | 0.962 | 1.095 (0.427–2.811) |
| College and above | 47 (54.0%) | 40 (46.0%) | | 1 |
| **Husband's educational level** | | | | |
| Unable to read and write | 13 (48.1%) | 14 (51.9%) | 0.708 | 0.581 (0.159–2.1177) |
| Read and Write | 15 (60.0%) | 10 (40.0%) | 0.465 | 0.351 (0.112–1.118) |
| Primary | 31 (56.4%) | 24 (43.6%) | 0.589 | 0.446 (0.189–1.052) |
| Secondary | 44 (44.0%) | 56 (56.0%) | **0.215** | 0.903 (0.444–1.836) |
| College and above | 75 (52.1%) | 69 (47.9%) | | 1 |
| **Ever used contraceptives before implants** | | | | |
| Yes | 106 (46.1%) | 124 (53.9%) | **0.017** | 1.613 (0.940–2.769) |
| No | 72 (59.5%) | 49 (40.5%) | | 1 |
| **Counseling about side effects of implants** | | | | |
| Yes | 108 (65.5%) | 57 (34.5%) | **< 0.0001** | **2.394 (1.422–4.03) **** |
| No | 70 (37.6%) | 116 (62.4%) | | 1 |
| **Counseling about benefit of implants** | | | | |
| Yes | 171 (52.3%) | 156 (47.7%) | | 1 |
| No | 7 (29.2%) | 17 (70.8%) | **0.034** | 2.312 (0.825–6.480) |
| **Side effects** | | | | |
| Yes | 34 (25.0%) | 102 (75.0%) | **< 0.0001** | **6.33 (3.719–10.76) ***** |
| No | 144 (67.0%) | 71 (33.0%) | | 1 |
| **Follow-up** | | | | |
| Yes | 155 (56.4%) | 120 (43.6%) | | 1 |
| No | 23 (30.3%) | 53 (69.7%) | **< 0.0001** | **2.241 (1.186–4.234) *** |

Significant at ***$p < 0.0001$, **$p = 0.001$, *$p = 0.013$, *AOR* Adjusted odds ratio

appointment for follow up. This is in line with studies conducted in Port, Nigeria [17] and Diguna Fango [22]. It might be due to the fact that post insertion follow-up increases retention of utilization, client trust on health providers, and knowledge about the overall behaviors of the contraceptives via participants.

This study includes nine health facilities (multicenter study) which increase external validity of the study.

Recall bias was not challenging unlike studies conducted on ever used participants.

The study was conducted in an urban health institution setting, though the majority of the population lives in rural setting.

## Conclusion

In this study, the overall proportion of discontinuation of implants was high (49.3%). Out of the overall proportion of discontinuation, reason of side effects and husband objection accounted 23.4%. Factors like lack of counseling about side effects, developing side effects and lack of post insertion follow-up were found statistically significant with implants discontinuation.

## Strengths

Recall bias was not challenging unlike studies conducted on ever used participants.

## Limitation

The study was conducted in an urban health institution setting, though the majority of the population lives in rural setting.

## Recommendations

Health organizations and other stake holders better to work on health care providers at enabling them to give appropriate pre-insertion counseling and post insertion date of follow-up in order to increase the retention of utilization.

Health professionals could give pre-insertion counseling with giving emphasis on possible side effects of implants.

Early side effects management and reassurance is recommended to decrease discontinuation and improve the retention of utilization of implants.

In addition to this, health providers could give post insertion date of follow-up for their clients.

### Abbrivations

AOR: Adjusted odds ratio; BDHS: Bangladesh Demographic Health Survey; COR: Crude odds ratio; CSA: Central Statistical Agency; EDHS: Ethiopia Demographic Health Survey; EFMOH: Ethiopian Federal Ministry of Health; FHI: Family Health International; HURH: Hawassa University Referral Hospital; ICF: International classification of functioning, disability and health; IUCD: Intra uterine contraceptive device; JPFHS: Jordan Population and Family Health survey; MDGs: Millinium development goals; OPDs: Out-Patient Department; SNNPRS: Southern Nation Nationality People's Representative state; SDG: Sustainable development goals; UK: United Kingdom; USAID: United States Agency of International Development; WHO: World Health Organization

### Acknowledgments

First of all, we would like to express our gratitude to the Hawassa City Health Office for giving us the opportunity to study in the city.

Secondly, we would like to express our deepest gratitude to Dr. Bezatu M. for his endless support and constructive comments throughout this paper development.

Finally, we would like to thank those who hold our hands throughout the work (participants, data collectors, supervisors, family and colleagues).

### Authors' contributions

Proposal developments, data collection, analysis, interpretation of results and discussion as well as manuscript preparation were processed by BA. MR had participated in data collection, supervision, analyzed data and advising throughout this paper development. Finally all Authors read and approved the manuscript.

### Author details

[1]Department of Midwifery, College Medicine and Health Sciences, University of Hawassa, PO Box-1560, Hawassa, Ethiopia. [2]Department Statistics, College of Natural and Computational Science, University of Hawassa, PO Box-1560, Hawassa, Ethiopia.

### References

1. Alemayehu M, Belachew T, Tilahun T. Factors associated with utilization of Long acting and permanent contraceptive methods among married women of reproductive age in Mekelle town, Tigray region, North Ethiopia. BMC Pregnancy Childbirth. 2012;12:6.
2. Ali MM, Park MH, Ngo TD. Levels and determinants of switching following intrauterine device discontinuation in 14 developing countries. Contraception. 2014;90:47–53.
3. Ali MM, Sadler RK, Cleland J, Ngo TD, Shah IH. Long-term contraceptive protection discontinuation and switching behavior. Intrauterine device (Iud) use dynamics in 14 developing countries; 2011.
4. Balogun O, Olaomo N, Adeniran A, Fawole A. Implanon sub-dermal implant: an emerging method of contraception in Ilorin, Nigeria. J Med Biomed Sci. 2014;3:1–5.
5. Bhatia P, Nangia S, Aggarwal S, Tewari C. Implanon: subdermal single rod contraceptive implant. J Obstetr Gynecol India. 2011;61:422.
6. Birhane K, Hagos S, Fantahun M. Early discontinuation of Implanon and its associated factors among women who ever used Implanon in Ofla District, Tigray, northern Ethiopia. Int J Pharma Sci Res. 2015;6:544–51.
7. Blumenthal P, Voedisch A, Gemzell-Danielsson K. Strategies to prevent unintended pregnancy: increasing use of Long-acting reversible contraception. Hum Reprod Update. 2010;17:121–37.
8. Bradley SE, Schwandt H, Khan S. Levels, Trends, And Reasons for Contraceptive Discontinuation. Dhs Anal Stud. 2009;20.
9. Burusie A. Reasons for premature removal of Implanon among users in Arsi zone, Oromia region, Ethiopia. Reprod Syst Sex Dis. 2015;4.
10. Casey PM, Long ME, Marnach ML, Bury JE. Bleeding related to Etonogestrel subdermal implant in a us population. Contraception. 2011;83:426–30.
11. EDHS 2016. Contraceptive discontinuation in the 5 years preceding the survey. Retrieved from https://dhsprogram.com/pubs/pdf/FR328/FR328.pdf: Accessed on 15/11/2018.
12. Gebremedhin S. Trend and socio-demographic differentials of caesarean section rate in Addis Ababa, Ethiopia: analysis based on Ethiopia demographic and health surveys data. Reprod Health. 2014;11:14.
13. Harvey C, Seib C, Lucke J. Continuation rates and reasons for removal among Implanon® users accessing two family planning clinics in Queensland, Australia. Contraception. 2009;80:527–32.
14. Igwe N. Intrauterine contraceptive device use in Abakaliki, Southeast Nigeria: a 5-year review. Trop J Med Res. 2016;19:138.
15. Melkamu Asaye M, Syoum Nigussie T, Mequannt Ambaw W. Early Implanon discontinuation and associated factors among Implanon user women in Debre Tabor town, public health facilities, Northwest Ethiopia, 2016. Int J Reprod Med. 2018, 2018.
16. Muthir J, Nyango D. Indications for removal of Etonogestrel implant within two years of use in Jos, Nigeria. East Afr Med J. 2010;87.
17. Ojule J, Oranu E, Enyindah C. Experience with Implanon in southern Nigeria. J Med Med Sci. 2012;3:710–4.
18. Ott, M. A. & Sucato, G. S. 2014. Contraception for adolescents. Pediatrics, Peds 2014–2300.
19. Rademacher, K. H., HL Vahdat, L. & Dorflinger, D. HO., And MJ. Steiner. 2014. "Global Introduction Of A Low-Cost Contraceptive Implant." In Critical Issues In Reproductive Health, Edited By A Kulczycki, . Netherlands: Springer. . 285–306.
20. Ramarao S, Lacuesta M, Costello M, Pangolibay B, Jones H. The link between quality of care and contraceptive use. Int Fam Plan Perspect. 2003:76–83.
21. Staveteig S, Mallick L, Winter R. Uptake and discontinuation of Long-acting reversible contraceptives (Larcs) in low-income countries; 2015.
22. Tadesse, A., Kondale, M., Agedew, E., Gebremeskel, F., Boti, N. & Oumer, B. 2017. Determinant of Implanon discontinuation among women who ever used Implanon in Diguna Fango District, Wolayta Zone, Southern Ethiopia: A Community Based Case Control Study. International Journal of Reproductive Medicine 2017.

23. Teunissen AM, Grimm B, Roumen FJ. Continuation rates of the subdermal contraceptive Implanon® and associated influencing factors. Eur J Contracept Reprod Health Care. 2014;19:15–21.
24. Thapa S. Early discontinuation of intrauterine device in Nepal–a retrospective study. WHO South-East Asia J Public Health. 2012;1:309.
25. WHO 2012. Causes and consequences of contraceptive discontinuation: evidence from 60 Demographic and Health Surveys. Retrieved from https://www.who.int/reproductivehealth/publications/family_planning/9789241504058/en/ : Accessed on 20/11/2018.
26. Yalew SA, Zeleke BM, Tefera AS. Demand for Long acting contraceptive methods and associated factors among family planning service users, Northwest Ethiopia: a health facility based cross sectional study. BMC Res Notes. 2015;8:29.

22

# Use of effective family planning methods and frequency of sex among HIV-infected and HIV-uninfected African women

Jim Aizire[1*], Sufia Dadabhai[1], Frank Taulo[2], Bonus Makanani[2], Luis Gadama[2], Jin Sun[1], Amy Tsui[3] and Taha E. Taha[1,3]

## Abstract

**Background:** Frequency of sex, contraceptive use and HIV infection are key determinants of fertility. Use of an effective family planning (EFP) method (injectable, oral, intra-uterine contraceptive device (IUCD), or Norplant) potentially eliminates women's concerns of unintended pregnancy. We report the association between EFP and frequency of sex among HIV-infected and HIV-uninfected non-pregnant African women.

**Methods:** Prospective fertility intentions study nested within a phase 3 randomized double-masked placebo-controlled trial (2003-2005) to treat genital tract infections in HIV-infected and HIV-uninfected non-pregnant women. Enrollment of study participants was stratified by HIV infection status. Data on demographics, family planning and sexual history were obtained at baseline and at 3, 6, 9 and 12 months. Chi square and Wilcoxon Rank-Sum tests were used to compare categorical and continuous variables, respectively. Generalized Estimating Equations method was used to estimate relative risk (RR) of frequent sex (≥ 2 acts/week) among users of different EFP methods (injectable, oral, implant or intra-uterine contraceptive device).

**Results:** After adjusting for age, current health status, and fertility intentions, EFP use was significantly associated with frequent sex among HIV-infected women (RR 1.32; 95% Confidence Interval [CI] 1.14-1.52); this association was not statistically significant among HIV-uninfected women (RR 1.10; 95% CI 0.96-1.24). Fertility intentions among HIV-infected, and education among HIV-uninfected womenwere independent predictors of sex frequency.

**Conclusion:** These data suggest that the association between EFP use and frequency of sex among women varies by HIV infection status. Service-delivery of diverse EFP methods should be integrated within HIV counseling, testing and treatment facilities.

**Keywords:** Contraception, Sexual behavior, HIV/AIDS, Sub-Saharan Africa

## Background

Previous studies suggest that the choice of a contraceptive method may positively or negatively influence a woman's and/or her male partner's sexual health including sexual desire, arousal and satisfaction [1–6]. Cofactors such as HIV disease are also associated with sexual dysfunction [7–9], and initiation of antiretroviral therapy (ART) has been associated with resumption of sexual libido [9]. However, there appears to be limited data on contraception and sexual health in sub-Saharan Africa, a region with the largest global burden due to unmet contraceptive need and HIV disease, and where scale-up of reproductive health and ART services is ongoing [10–12].

In 2015, with only 10% of the world's population, sub-Saharan Africa was home to more than 60% of new HIV infections and about 70% of the prevalent cases globally, and approximately 60% of the incident and prevalent cases were reproductive-age women [12]. Only one-in-

* Correspondence: jaizire1@jhu.edu
[1]Department of Epidemiology, Johns Hopkins Bloomberg School of Public Health, 615 North Wolfe Street, Baltimore, MD 21205, USA

three of the married women of reproductive age (MWRA) were using some form of contraception, the lowest rate globally [10]. Similarly, the unmet need for family planning (FP) and unintended pregnancy rates are higher in sub-Saharan Africa than in any other region of the world: approximately 19-25% of MWRA had an unmet need for modern or traditional family planning methods [10, 11, 13, 14]; up to 61% of all women regardless of marital status had an unmet need for modern methods [15, 16]; and there were an estimated 108 unintended pregnancies per 1000 women aged 15-44 years [17].

Women are considered to have an unmet need for modern FP methods (sterilization, intrauterine devices (IUD), implants, injectable and oral methods, male condom, vaginal gel and emergency contraception) if they want to avoid pregnancy but are not using any method or are using only traditional methods (withdrawal, rhythm/periodic abstinence, breastfeeding and douching), which are not reliable [10]. Traditional methods are associated with a higher failure rate than modern methods [18]. In sub-Saharan Africa, 87% of unintended pregnancies are attributed to women with a desire to limit or space births who are not using an effective family planning (EFP) method (injectable, oral, intra-uterine contraceptive device (IUCD), or Norplant) [15]. The most commonly reported reasons for not using modern FP by MWRA in sub-Saharan Africa include infrequent sex and safety/side-effects. Others include postpartum/breastfeeding, opposition by the partner, as well as access related reasons [10, 14, 15]. In many countries in the region, one method accounts for 50% or more of all reported FP methods used among MWRA, predominantly injectable (Depo-Provera), a trend attributed to limited varieties of the full range of FP choices and/or unchanged FP messages [10, 19]. In Malawi, the most commonly used methods at the time of this study were injectable contraceptives, and the recent prevalence estimates of the most commonly used methods are: injectable (30%), implants (12%) and 11% female sterilization [20].

Beyond the proximal reproductive health benefits, universal access and utilization of EFP methods has the potential to reduce the high attributable mortality risk among women and children, ameliorate the socioeconomic gender inequities and improve overall health [21–24]. Additionally, EFP scale-up is one of the four prongs adopted by the World Health Organization (WHO) for elimination of mother-to-child transmission of HIV-1 in resource limited settings [25]. The use of EFP methods among women in need of contraception has the potential to increase their self-perceived sub-fecundity and therefore improve their sexual health by disentangling pleasure from the responsibilities of pregnancy.

We report the association between use of EFP methods and frequency of sex among HIV-infected (pre-ART era) and HIV-uninfected post-partum, non-pregnant women in Malawi. In general, while several studies based on African populations previously reported family planning use, the current literature on the specific EFP use and sexual health is limited and no data are available from Malawi. Despite remarkable improvements in the use of modern FP methods (7% (1992); 28% (2004) and 58% (2015-16)), unmet need for FP methods (26% (2010); 19% (2015/6)) and total fertility rate (~ 4.4 children per women) remain high in Malawi [20, 26]. National HIV prevalence was approximaltey 10% in 2010. A national program for the scale-up of ART and injectable contraceptive use among HIV-infected women was implemented in 2011; yet, according to a recent study, the majority (75.0%) of HIV-infected pregnant women on ART reported that their current pregnancy was unintended [27].

## Methods

### Study design and setting

We conducted a prospective cohort study of fertility intentions among HIV-infected and HIV-uninfected women nested within a clinical trial of an intermittent intravaginal antibiotic gel for presumptive treatment of a common genital tract infection - bacterial vaginosis. This trial, known as the METRO study, is registered as trial number NCT00140764 on clinicaltrials.gov. The METRO study was a randomized, double-masked, placebo-controlled, phase 3 trial conducted in Blantyre, Malawi. Overall, 1686 women were enrolled from January 2003 to May 2005: 844 HIV-infected and 842 HIV-uninfected. A detailed description of the study has been previously reported [28, 29]. Briefly, non-pregnant HIV-infected and HIV-uninfected women were recruited via the postnatal care and family planning clinics of the Queen Elizabeth Central Hospital, a tertiary referral hospital in Blantyre, Malawi, and from two nearby health centers. Enrollment of eligible women was stratified by HIV infection status. Women were counseled and provided written informed consent for HIV testing and study enrollment. The criteria for study entry included: age 18 years or older; ability and willingness to give written informed consent; non-pregnant; willingness to return for follow-up visits; willingness to use the intravaginal treatment gel as instructed; willingness to provide specimens at each visit to test for pregnancy and sexually transmitted infections (STIs); and residing in the study area. Exclusion criteria included: inability to provide informed consent; being pregnant; and refusal of any of the enrollment inclusion requirements. The protocol was approved by the College of Medicine Research and Ethics Committee in Malawi and the Johns Hopkins Bloomberg School of Public Health Institutional Review Board in the USA.

### Study procedures

Enrolled women had scheduled visits at enrollment (baseline) and quarterly during follow-up at 3, 6, 9 and 12-months. Demographics, family-planning and sexual history were collected at all study visits using standardized questionnaires by trained study staff. Study participants received standard-of-care counselling on the appropriate family planning methods by trained care providers. Anti-retroviral treatment was not available at the time of the study; however, women received standard-of-care such cotrimoxazole prophylaxis through their respective HIV care programs.

### Measurement

#### *HIV-1 testing*

Women were tested for HIV at trial pre-entry, and at each three-monthly study visit, using a two-tier algorithm including two screening HIV-1 rapid tests or the usual serological tests recommended by the Malawi Ministry of Health. This was followed by a confirmatory Western blot test for those with discordant screening test results and for all new infections.

#### *Pregnancy test*

Real time pregnancy testing was performed at pre-entry and at each follow-up visit; a detailed analysis has already been published. [29] The detection of the Human chorionic gonadotropin (hCG) hormone in the urine followed by a confirmatory ultra-sound scan was used to diagnose pregnancy. A commercial kit (KAT Quick HCG, KAT Medical, http://www.katmedical.com) which was validated against a gold-standard commercial kit called QuickVue, Quidel Corporation, http://www.quidel.com, was used for urine hCG detection.

#### *Exposure – EFP use*

The key independent variable was defined as the proportion of women who self-reported using an EFP method which included an injectable, oral, IUCD or Norplant.

#### *Outcome - sexual frequency*

The outcome in this analysis, sexual frequency, which was assessed at each study visit, was defined as the proportion of women who self-reported 2 or more sexual encounters per week.

### Statistical methods

Data for the METRO trial were entered and cleaned in MS Access. Enrolled women with tubal ligation ($N = 80$) were excluded, while women deaths or losses-to-follow-up, or women with a confirmatory diagnosis of pregnancy during follow-up were censored at that point and therefore did not contribute to this analysis at subsequent follow-up time points. All analyses were conducted separately for the HIV-infected and HIV-uninfected cohorts of women. HIV-uninfected women who seroconverted were classified as HIV-infected at subsequent timepoints. Chi-square and Wilcoxon Rank Sum tests were used to compare categorical and continuous variables, respectively. The Generalized Estimating Equation (GEE) log-binomial model was used to estimate the relative risk (RR) of sex frequency, and the corresponding 95% Confidence Interval (CI),while accounting for within individual correlations from the repeat measures at the multiple visits. To account for key confounding bias, covariates with $p < 0.15$ in the univariate analysis were added to the multivariate GEE model. Fixed variables assessed at baseline included age (in years), education (Form 1-4 and above; Grade 1-8, or no schooling), and number of living children. Time-varying variables included perceived (self-reported) current health status (good/excellent versus poor/fair) and fertility intentions (desire to have another child; not decided/not sure; or no desire to have more children). All statistical tests were two-sided at the alpha = 0.05 level. Statistical analyses were performed using SAS version 9.3, Carey, North Carolina.

## Results

The sample sizes of the data available for the baseline and follow-up visit analyses are shown in Fig. 1a and b and Tables 1 and 2. The vast majority of non-pregnant women enrolled in this study were in marital union; 97.3% of the 809 HIV-infected women and 98.5% of the 797 HIV-uninfected women.

At baseline (enrollment) visit, the reported median frequency of sex per week during the past three months was 2 for both HIV-infected and HIV-uninfected women, and mean frequency of sex per week was 2.2 and 2.7, respectively. Among 1130 women with complete data on type of contraceptive method used at baseline, the commonest contraceptive method was the injectable (79.3%) while the frequency of all other methods was low: oral contraceptive pill 8.9%; Implant 1%; IUCD 1%; condoms 4.9%; all others 4.9% (abstinence, withdrawal and breastfeeding). The relative distribution of reported use of contraceptive methods at baseline was similar to and relatively stable during the study period.

Baseline characteristics at enrolment are summarized by HIV infection status in Table 1. Level of education and the treatment arm (MetroGel versus placebo), were comparable between the HIV-infected and HIV-uninfected women ($p > 0.05$). However, HIV-infected women compared to their HIV-uninfected counterparts were older (63.0% vs. 50.6% were 25 years or older, $p < 0.0001$); less likely to report two or more sexual encounters in the previous week (38.6% vs. 47.3%, $p = 0.0004$); and less likely to be using an EFP method (56.0% vs. 71.3%, $p < 0.0001$). In addition, the median number of living children differed by HIV-status of

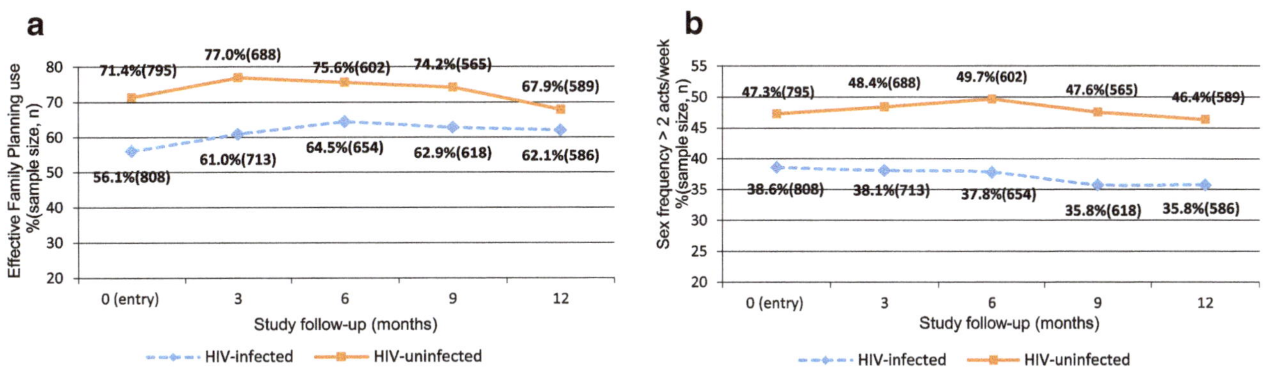


**Fig. 1** Study visit (0) or entry is the enrollment or baseline visit. Effective Family planning methods which were based on self-reported contraceptive use at study entry and during study follow-up include Injectable, oral, Intra-Uterine Contraceptive Device (IUCD), and Norplant and all the other family planning methods are classified as 'other'; self-report sexual frequency assessed at each study visit, was defined as the proportion of women who self-reported 2 or more sexual encounters per week. HIV-infection status was based on HIV test results at study entry (enrollment)

the woman median (IQR) of 2 (2-3) among HIV-infected compared to 3 (2-4) among the HIV-uninfected women, $p < 0.0001$; and less likely to have a desire for another child, 26.6% vs. 58.8%, $p < 0.0001$, respectively.

Differences observed at baseline between HIV-infected and HIV-uninfected women with regard to EFP use and frequency of sex, respectively, were maintained at each of the follow-up visits at 3, 6, 9 and 12-months post enrollment (Fig. 1a and b).

### EFP and sex frequency among HIV-infected women

Baseline characteristics of HIV-infected women by EFP status are summarized in Table 2. Number of living children, fertility intentions, frequency of sex and treatment arm (MetroGel versus placebo), across the EFP use categories were similar ($p > 0.05$). On the other hand, HIV-infected women who reported EFP use versus non-EFP users at baseline were more likely to be younger than 25 years of age (41.3% vs. 31.3%, $p < 0.0001$) and

**Table 1** Baseline characteristics of HIV-infected and HIV-uninfected women, Blantyre, Malawi, 2003-2005.

| Characteristics | level | HIV-infected ($N = 809$) [a] | HIV-uninfected($N = 797$) [a] | *P*-value [b] |
|---|---|---|---|---|
| Age groups, years, n (%) | 30+ | 229 (28.3) | 198 (24.8) | *< 0.0001* |
| | 25-29 | 281 (34.7) | 206 (25.8) | |
| | 20-24 | 271 (33.5) | 328 (41.2) | |
| | < 20 | 28 (3.5) | 65 (8.2) | |
| Education[c], n (%) | Form 1-4 or above | 241 (29.8) | 237 (29.7) | 0.91 |
| | Grade 1-8 | 483 (59.8) | 472 (59.2) | |
| | No Schooling | 84 (10.4) | 88 (11.0) | |
| Number of living children, median [IQR] | | 2 [2-3] | 3 [2-4] | *< 0.0001* |
| Fertility intentions, n (%) | Have another child | 215 (26.6) | 468 (58.7) | *< 0.0001* |
| | Not decided/Not sure or No | 30 (3.7) | 21 (2.6) | |
| | No more children | 564 (69.7) | 307 (38.5) | |
| Family planning methods, n (%) | Effective [d] | 453 (56.0) | 568 (71.4) | *< 0.0001* |
| | No or Other | 356 (44.0) | 229 (28.6) | |
| Frequency of sex, n (%) | ≤ 2 | 496 (61.4) | 419 (52.7) | *0.0004* |
| | > 2 | 312 (38.6) | 376 (47.3) | |
| Treatments, n (%) | Intervention arm | 404 (49.9) | 399 (50.1) | 0.96 |
| | Placebo arm | 405 (50.1) | 398(49.9) | |

[a]Excluded women with tubal ligation ($n = 80$)
[b]*P* values were calculated using Chi-square test for categorical variables, Wilcoxon Rank Sum test for continuous variables. All statistical tests were two-sided at the alpha=0.05 level. Statistically significant differences with a *p*-value equal to or less than 0.05 are italicized
[c]Education (Grade 1-8 of the elementary school; and Form 1-4 of secondary school)
[d]Effective methods include Injectable contraceptives, oral contraceptives, Intra-Uterine Contraceptive Device (IUCD), and norplant; all other methods are classified as 'others'

**Table 2** Baseline characteristics of HIV-infected and HIV-uninfected women by family planning method use, Blantyre, Malawi, 2003-2005

| | | HIV-infected | | | HIV-uninfected | | |
|---|---|---|---|---|---|---|---|
| Characteristics | Level | EFP[a] ($N = 453$) | Non-EFP ($N = 356$) | *P*-value[b] | EFP ($N = 568$) | Non-EFP ($N = 229$) | *P*-value |
| Age groups, *n* (%) | 30+ | 92 (20.3) | 137 (38.5) | *< 0.0001* | 112 (19.7) | 86 (37.6) | *< 0.0001* |
| | 25-29 | 174 (38.4) | 107 (30.1) | | 147 (26.1) | 58 (25.3) | |
| | 20-24 | 169 (37.3) | 102 (28.7) | | 257 (45.2) | 71 (31.0) | |
| | < 20 | 18 (4.0) | 10 (2.8) | | 51 (9.0) | 14 (6.1) | |
| Education[c], *n* (%) | Form 1-4 or above | 154 (34.0) | 87 (24.5) | *0.014* | 179 (31.5) | 58 (25.3) | *0.002* |
| | Grade 1-8 | 254 (56.1) | 229 (64.5) | | 340 (59.9) | 132 (57.6) | |
| | No Schooling | 45 (9.9) | 39 (11.0) | | 49 (8.6) | 39 (17.0) | |
| Number of living children, median [IQR] | | 2 [2-3] | 2 [2-3] | 0.34 | 2 [2-4] | 3 [2-4] | 0.15 |
| Fertility intentions, *n* (%) | Have another child | 108 (23.8) | 107 (30.1) | 0.12 | 347 (61.1) | 121 (53.1) | 0.10 |
| | Not decided/Not sure | 16 (3.5) | 14 (3.9) | | 15 (2.6) | 6 (2.6) | |
| | No more children | 329 (72.6) | 235 (66.0) | | 206(36.3) | 101 (44.3) | |
| Frequency of sex, *n* (%) | ≤ 2 | 265 (58.5) | 231 (65.1) | 0.06 | 299 (52.7) | 120 (52.6) | 0.98 |
| | > 2 | 188 (41.5) | 124 (34.9) | | 268 (47.3) | 108 (47.4) | |
| Treatments, *n* (%) | Intervention arm | 226 (49.9) | 178 (50.0) | 0.98 | 279 (49.1) | 120 (52.4) | 0.40 |
| | Placebo arm | 227 (50.1) | 178 (50.0) | | 289 (50.9) | 109 (47.6) | |

Excluded women with tubal ligation ($n = 80$)
[a]EFP - Effective methods include Injectable contraceptives, oral contraceptives, Intra-Uterine Contraceptive Device (IUCD), and Norplant; all other methods are classified as 'others'
[b]*P* values were calculated using Chi-square test for categorical variables, Wilcoxon Rank Sum test for continuous variables. All statistical tests were two-sided at the alpha=0.05 level. Statistically significant *p*-values equal to or less than 0.05 are italicized
[c]Education (Grade 1-8 of the elementary school; and Form 1-4 of secondary school)

with form 1-4 level of education or higher (34.0% vs. 24. 5%, $p = 0.014$).

The following characteristics were associated with frequent sex (two or more times per week) in the bivariate analyses summarized in Table 3: EFP use versus not, RR (95% CI) =1.30 (1.15-1.46); and fertility intentions - desire to have another child versus no desire, RR (95% CI) =1.19 (1.10-1.33). Education, current health status, and number of living children were not associated with sex frequency. In the multivariate model (Table 3) adjusted for age, fertility intentions, and current health status, EFP use versus not was significantly associated with sex frequency, RR (95% CI) =1.32 (1.14-1.52). Compared to women with no desire for children, those with a desire to have another child, RR (95% CI) =1.19 (1.04-1.36), and those not decided, RR(95% CI) = 1.46 (1.12-1.91), were independently associated with sex frequency (Table 3).

### EFP and sex frequency among HIV-uninfected women

The following baseline characteristics among HIV-uninfected women were homogeneous across the EFP use categories: the number of living children; fertility intentions; frequency of sex; and treatment arm (MetroGel versus placebo), $p > 0.05$ (Table 2). EFP users were more likely to be younger than 25 years of age (54.3% vs. 36.8%, $p < 0.0001$) and with form 1-4 level of education or higher (31.5% vs. 25.3%, $p = 0.002$).

HIV-uninfected women who were using EFP methods compared to those who were not using an EFP method had a 13% higher risk of reporting two or more sexual encounters in the previous week, RR, 95% CI: 1.13(1.01-1.27) (Table 4). However, this association was not statistically significant, OR, 95% CI: 1.10(0.96-1.24) in a multivariate model adjusting for education, number of living children, and fertility intentions(Table 4). A separate multivariate model that included 'treatment arm' showed similar estimates or direction of associations. Higher levels of education attained versus no schooling reported at the baseline visit were independently associated with increased likelihood of self-reporting two or more sex encounters in the previous week: Form 1-4 versus no schooling, RR, 95% CI: 1.32 (1.10-1.65); Grade 1-8 versus no schooling, RR, 95% CI: 1.26 (1.04-1.53).

## Discussion

We assessed the temporal relationship between EFP use and frequency of sex among HIV-infected and HIV-uninfected reproductive-age African women followed for 12 months. Family planning use and other socio-behavioral data were collected prospectively every three months as a part of a large randomized placebo-controlled trial for treatment of a common genital tract infection. There was a statistically significant association between EFP use and increased frequency of sex among HIV-infected women after controlling

**Table 3** Association of family planning method used and other risk factors with the outcome frequency of sex in HIV-infected women, Generalized Estimating Equations (GEE) Log-binomial Regression Model

| Risk factor | | Unadjusted RR[a] (95% CI)[b] | *P*-value[c] | Adjusted RR (95% CI) | *P*-value[c] |
|---|---|---|---|---|---|
| Family planning method | Effective | **1.30 (1.15-1.46)** | *<.0001* | **1.32 (1.14-1.52)** | *0.0002* |
| | No or Other | 1 | . | 1 | . |
| Age (years) | 30+ | **0.77 (0.55-1.06)** | 0.1091 | 0.95 (0.63-1.44) | 0.8200 |
| | 25-29 | 0.99 (0.73-1.36) | 0.9741 | 1.15 (0.78-1.70) | 0.4838 |
| | 20-24 | 0.92 (0.67-1.26) | 0.5934 | 0.97 (0.66-1.44) | 0.8982 |
| | < 20 | 1 | . | 1 | . |
| Education[d] | Form 1-4 or above | 1.00 (0.84-1.23) | 0.9793 | | |
| | Grade 1-8 | 0.96 (0.79-1.16) | 0.6465 | | |
| | No Schooling | 1 | . | 1 | . |
| Number of living children | | 0.98 (0.94-1.03) | 0.4894 | | |
| Fertility intentions | Have another child | **1.19 (1.10-1.33)** | **0.0033** | **1.19 (1.04-1.36)** | **0.0119** |
| | Not decided/Not sure | 1.26 (0.97-1.63) | 0.0852 | **1.46 (1.12-1.91)** | **0.0052** |
| | No more children | 1 | . | 1 | . |
| Current health status | Good or Excellent | 1.15 (0.99-1.34) | 0.0646 | 1.12 (0.96-1.30) | 0.1492 |
| | Poor or Fair | 1 | . | 1 | . |

[a]Relative Risk (RR); [b]Confidence Interval (CI); [c]*P*-value for test of statistical significance of the RR of sex frequency (bold signifies statistically significant);[d] Education (Grade 1-8 of the elementary school; and Form 1-4 of secondary school)
Variables with $p < 0.15$ in the univariate analysis were included in the multivariate model

for potential confounders including age, fertility intentions, and current health status. Among HIV-uninfected women, the adjusted association between EFP use and frequency of sex, which was not statistically significant, was in the expected, same direction. Other factors independently and significantly ($p <$ 0.05 after adjusting for other variables) associated with frequency of sex in this cohort of non-pregnant women who are in union included fertility intentions among HIV-infected women, and level of education among HIV-uninfected women. The differences

**Table 4** Association of family planning method used and other risk factors with the outcome frequency of sex in HIV-uninfected women, Generalized Estimating Equations (GEE) Log-binomial Regression Model

| Risk factor | | Unadjusted RR[a] (95% CI)[b] | *P*-value[c] | Adjusted RR (95% CI) | *P*-value[c] |
|---|---|---|---|---|---|
| Family planning method | Effective | **1.13 (1.01-1.27)** | *0.0356* | 1.10 (0.96-1.24) | 0.1861 |
| | No or Other | 1 | | 1 | |
| Age (years) | 30+ | 1.03 (0.82-1.30) | 0.8137 | | |
| | 25-29 | 1.18 (0.94-1.48) | 0.1533 | | |
| | 20-24 | 1.17 (0.94-1.46) | 0.1524 | | |
| | < 20 | 1 | | 1 | |
| Education[d] | Form 1-4 or above | **1.36 (1.12-1.65)** | *0.0021* | **1.32 (1.10-1.65)** | *0.0131* |
| | Grade 1-8 | **1.26 (1.04-1.51)** | *0.0156* | **1.26 (1.04-1.53)** | *0.0173* |
| | No Schooling | 1 | | 1 | |
| Number of living children | | 0.97 (0.94-1.01) | 0.1390 | 1.00 (0.96-1.04) | 0.9830 |
| Fertility intentions | Have another child | **1.12 (1.01-1.24)** | *0.0251* | 1.10 (0.97-1.22) | 0.1695 |
| | Not decided/Not sure | 1.17 (0.87-1.57) | 0.2976 | 1.20 (0.89-1.63) | 0.2333 |
| | No more children | 1 | | 1 | |
| Current health status | Good or Excellent | 1.08 (0.92-1.26) | 0.3525 | | |
| | Poor or Fair | 1 | | | |

[a]Relative Risk (RR); [b]Confidence Interval (CI);[c]*P*-value for test of statistical significance of the RR of sex frequency (bold signifies statistically significant); [d] Education (Grade 1-8 of the elementary school; and Form 1-4 of secondary school)
Variables with $p < 0.15$ in the univariate analysis were included in the multivariate model

observed in this study based on HIV infection status may reveal the complex biological and behavioral factors that impact the sex behavior and fertility decisions of women in sub-Saharan Africa.

The positive association between EFP use and sexual activity in this analysis is consistent with overall findings from a cross-sectional study that analyzed Demographic and Health Survey (DHS) data of more than 210,000 sexually active women of childbearing age from 47 countries suggesting that couples using contraception compared to non-users were three times more likely to report frequent sex [30]. The DHS data, however, was not stratified by HIV infection status of the woman. Other studies, mostly among non-African populations, that evaluated sexual activity and use of family planning methods [2, 4, 6, 31] tended to have more educated women, and were less likely to have high background biological cofactors and socio-economic and cultural constraints that might influence women's sexual decisions. Women who are more educated and/or reside in settings with less inhibition to openly discuss sex issues may actively consider use of different types of EFP methods to achieve their desires and expectations. Additionally, it is likely that the ability to conceive is valued differently in different settings. For example, in western countries fertility is very low and influenced by economic factors related to the cost of raising and educating a child. In African countries where HIV prevalence is high among women of reproductive age, the impact of HIV on survival of children and their parents is a major determinant of fertility. Successful treatment of HIV with antiretroviral drugs may reverse this health situation and reduce anxieties attributable to concerns of potential vertical transmission in the event of an unintended pregnancy and/or sexual transmission to their HIV-uninfected partners [31].

The heterogeneity of the EFP use and sexual activity measures of association by HIV status observed in this study, is consistent with previous reports of psycho-social, behavioral and biological differences pertaining to sexual function between HIV-infected versus uninfected individuals. A trend towards decreased sexual activity and fertility was observed with advancing HIV disease among Ugandan women in a clinic-based prospective cohort study [7] and a longitudinal study in France showed that the proportion of women who self-reported being sexually active decreased after they discovered that they were HIV-infected [8]. Also, during the convalescent phase after initiating ART, HIV-infected individuals have shown improved sexual desire and resumption of / increased sexual activity [9]. This study predated the introduction of universal ART for all HIV-infected individuals in Malawi, and none of the study women reported ART use. This study enabled a unique opportunity to better understand the sexual benefits of EFP use among HIV-infected women in the absence of ART exposure. In the current era of ART scale-up, an estimated half a million (67%) of HIV-infected individuals and more than 37,000 (73.0%) of the pregnant or breastfeeding women in Malawi were alive on ART through the end of 2014 [26]. This trend towards scale-up of universal ART is consistent across the high HIV burden countries in sub-Saharan Africa, albeit at different paces [12].

At the time the study was conducted, highly sexually active women may have been more motivated to seek and adhere to family planning services including ongoing counseling and utilization of EFP methods. In sub-Saharan Africa, about one in five married women with an unmet need for contraception reported that they were reluctant to use modern contraception methods because of their self-perceived sub-fecundity given their low level of sexual activity [14, 15].

The study was adequately powered (≥ 80.0%) to detect differences in frequent sex among EFP versus non-EFP users, separately for HIV-infected and HIV-uninfected women, respectively. However, the reported measures of association may be biased due to residual-confounding from unmeasured factors, of which intimate-partner violence (IPV) is noteworthy. Previous IPV studies conducted in similar African settings reported a gender-based hierarchy that undermines women's ability to negotiate condom use or refusal to have sex [32]. Similarly, IPV has been associated with unintended pregnancy and HIV acquisition among women [32, 33]. Also, socio-economic dependence on the male partner is pervasive in sub-Saharan African settings and may be a hindrance to women's utilization of reproductive health services and likewise increase their vulnerability to imbalanced sexual relationships [9, 32, 33].

## Conclusion

These study results can be generalized to reproductive-age women in need of contraception in other settings in Malawi and elsewhere in southern Africa with similarly high levels of unmet need for EFP, high HIV burden, and where reproductive health and ART services are being scaled-up. The findings are timely and underscore the call-to-action by the WHO and other stakeholders of an integrated approach for the ongoing country level rapid scale-up of ART and reproductive health services in Africa [11, 25, 31]. Women's sexual health issues will be front-and-center in their decision-making about choice and adherence to family planning methods (in parallel, HIV-infected women are regularly counseled about adherence to their ART use). Avenues should be explored to address women's sex health issues while integrating the counselling messages on family planning and ART during follow-up. It is critical for adherence to family planning that women make a choice for contraception that is effective, convenient and safe.

**Authors' contributions**

JA, contributed to the data analysis plan, and took the lead in writing this manuscript, SD contributed to study implementation and coordination, and edited the manuscript; FT, BM, and LG., were site co-investigators on the trial and edited the manuscript; JS, carried out the statistical analysis and contributed to writing the paper; AT, contributed to the data analysis plan, and edited the manuscript; TT, (Protocol Chair), conceived of the study, contributed to the overall study design and implementation, analysis plan for this substudy, and writing this manuscript. All authors read and approved the final manuscript. The authors acknowledge and thank all the Malawian mothers for their participation in this study, and the study team for their dedicated conduct of the study.

**Author details**

[1]Department of Epidemiology, Johns Hopkins Bloomberg School of Public Health, 615 North Wolfe Street, Baltimore, MD 21205, USA. [2]Department of Obstetrics and Gynecology, College of Medicine, University of Malawi, Blantyre, Malawi. [3]Department of Population, Family and Reproductive Health, Johns Hopkins Bloomberg School of Public Health, Baltimore, MD, USA.

**References**

1. Mohamad Al-Ali B, Shamloul R, Ramsauer J, Bella AJ, Scrinzi U, Treu T, et al. The effect of vasectomy on the sexual life of couples. J Sex Med. 2014;11: 2239–42. https://doi.org/10.1111/jsm.12567.
2. Fataneh G, Marjan MH, Nasrin R, Taraneh T. Sexual function in Iranian women using different methods of contraception. J Clin Nurs. 2013;22: 3016–23. https://doi.org/10.1111/jocn.12289.
3. Davis AR, Castano P. Oral Contraceptives and libido in women. Annu Rev Sex Res. 2004;15:297–320.
4. Wiebe ER, Brotto LA, MacKay J. Characteristics of women who experience mood and sexual side effects with use of hormonal contraception. J Obstet Gynaecol Can. 2011;33:1234–40. https://doi.org/10.1016/S1701-2163(16)35108-8.
5. Wallwiener M, Wallwiener LM, Seeger H, Mueck AO, Zipfel S, Bitzer J, et al. Effects of sex hormones in oral contraceptives on the female sexual function score: a study in German female medical students. Contraception. 2010;82:155–9. https://doi.org/10.1016/j.contraception.2009.12.022.
6. Strufaldi R, Pompei LM, Steiner ML, Cunha EP, Ferreira JAS, Peixoto S, et al. Effects of two combined hormonal contraceptives with the same composition and different doses on female sexual function and plasma androgen levels. Contraception. 2010;82:147–54. https://doi.org/10.1016/j.contraception.2010.02.016.
7. Ross A, Van der Paal L, Lubega R, Mayanja BN, Shafer LA, Whitworth J. HIV-1 disease progression and fertility: the incidence of recognized pregnancy and pregnancy outcome in Uganda. AIDS. 2004;18:799–804. https://doi.org/10.1097/00002030-200403260-00012.
8. De Vincenzi I, Jadand C, Couturier E, Brunet J-B, Gallais H, Gastaut J-A, et al. Pregnancy and contraception in a French cohort of HIV-infected women. AIDS. 1997;11:333–8. https://doi.org/10.1097/00002030-199703110-00011.
9. Homsy J, Bunnell R, Moore D, King R, Malamba S, Nakityo R, et al. Reproductive intentions and outcomes among women on antiretroviral therapy in rural Uganda: a prospective cohort study. PLoS One. 2009;4 https://doi.org/10.1371/journal.pone.0004149.
10. Department of Economic and Social Affairs PDUN. Trends in contraceptive use worldwide 2015. Contraception. 2015:1–70. https://doi.org/10.1016/j.contraception.2012.08.029.
11. UNAIDS. Women need access to dual protection — effective contraceptives and HIV prevention options 2012. http://www.unaids.org/sites/default/files/web_story/20120216_PS_Hormonal_en_0.pdf. Accessed 20 Sept 2016.
12. UNAIDS. HIV/AIDS Fact sheet 2016 2016:8. http://www.unaids.org/sites/default/files/media_asset/UNAIDS_FactSheet_en.pdf Accessed Sept 2016.
13. Alkema L, Kantorova V, Menozzi C, Biddlecom A. National, regional, and global rates and trends in contraceptive prevalence and unmet need for family planning between 1990 and 2015: a systematic and comprehensive analysis. Lancet. 2013;381:1642–52. https://doi.org/10.1016/S0140-6736(12)62204-1.
14. Sedgh G, Hussain R. Reasons for contraceptive nonuse among women having unmet need for contraception in developing countries. Stud Fam Plan. 2014;45:151–69. https://doi.org/10.1111/j.1728-4465.2014.00382.x.
15. Darroch JE, Sedgh G, Ball H. Contraceptive Technologies: Responding to Women's Needs. New York: Guttmacher Institute; 2011. www.guttmacher.org.
16. Darroch JE, Singh S. Trends in contraceptive need and use in developing countries in 2003, 2008, and 2012: an analysis of national surveys. Lancet. 2013;381:1756–62. https://doi.org/10.1016/S0140-6736(13)60597-8.
17. Sedgh G, Singh S, Intended HR. Unintended pregnancies worldwide in 2012 and recent trends. Stud Fam Plan. 2014;45:301–14.
18. Trussell J, Nelson A, Cates W, Kowal D, Policar M. Contracepteive efficacy. Contracept Technol Twent Revis Ed. 2011;9:Table 3-2 https://doi.org/10.1001/archderm.1995.01690210094016.
19. Ross J, Keesbury J, Hardee K. Trends in the contraceptive method mix in low- and middle-income countries: analysis using a new "average deviation" measure. Glob Heal Sci Pract. 2015;3:34–55. https://doi.org/10.9745/GHSP-D-14-00199.
20. Melorose J, Perroy R, Careas S. Demographic and health survey key indicators. Statew Agric L Use Baseline. 2015;1:55. https://doi.org/10.1017/CBO9781107415324.004.
21. Cleland J, Conde-Agudelo A, Peterson H, Ross J, Tsui A. Contraception and health. Lancet. 2012;380:149–56. https://doi.org/10.1016/S0140-6736(12)60609-6.
22. Ahmed S, Li Q, Liu L, Tsui AO. Maternal deaths averted by contraceptive use: an analysis of 172 countries. Lancet. 2012;380:111–25. https://doi.org/10.1016/S0140-6736(12)60478-4.
23. Canning D, Schultz TP. The economic consequences of reproductive health and family planning. Lancet. 2012;380:165–71. https://doi.org/10.1016/S0140-6736(12)60827-7.
24. Singh S, Darroch JE. Adding it up: costs and benefits of contraceptive services estimates for 2012. Guttmacher Inst United Nations Popul Fund (UNFPA). 2012;201:1–28.
25. Who. PMTCT STraTegiC ViSion: Organization. Geneva: WHO Press; 2010. p. 40. http://www.who.int/hiv/pub/mtct/strategic_vision.pdf.
26. Malawi National AIDS Commission. Malawi AIDS Response Progress, vol. 79; 2015.
27. Marston M, Nakiyingi-Miiro J, Hosegood V, Lutalo T, Mtenga B, Zaba B, et al. Reproductive intentions and family planning practices of pregnant HIV-infected Malawian women on antiretroviral therapy. PLoS One. 2015; 212:1–8. https://doi.org/10.1097/QAI.0b013e31825da73f.
28. Taha TE, Kumwenda NI, Kafulafula G, Makanani B, Nikhoma C, Chen S, et al. Intermittent intravaginal antibiotic treatment of bacterial vaginosis in HIV-uninfected and -infected women: a randomized clinical trial. PLoS Clin Trials. 2007;2 https://doi.org/10.1371/journal.pctr.0020010.
29. Taulo F, Berry M, Tsui A, Makanani B, Kafulafula G, Li Q, et al. Fertility intentions of HIV-1 infected and uninfected women in Malawi: a longitudinal study. AIDS Behav. 2009;13:20–7. https://doi.org/10.1007/s10461-009-9547-9.
30. Bell S, Bishai D. Unmet need and sex: investigating the role of coital frequency in fertility control. Stud Fam Plan. n.d.;48:39–53. https://doi.org/10.1111/sifp.12012. Epub 2017 Feb 1.
31. WHO. Hiv Prevention, diagnosis, treatment and care for key populations; 2016. p. 1–8. http://apps.who.int/iris/bitstream/10665/128049/1/WHO_HIV_2014.8_eng.pdf. (Accessed Oct 1, 2016).
32. Fathalla MF, Sinding SW, Rosenfield A, Fathalla MMF. Sexual and reproductive health for all: a call for action. Lancet. 2006;368:2095–100. https://doi.org/10.1016/S0140-6736(06)69483-X.
33. Dunkle KL, Jewkes RK, Brown HC, Gray GE, McIntryre JA, Harlow SD. Gender-based violence, relationship power, and risk of HIV infection in women attending antenatal clinics in South Africa. Lancet. 2004;363:1415–21. https://doi.org/10.1016/S0140-6736(04)16098-4.

23

# Factors that affect the discontinuation of family planning methods in Myanmar: Analysis of the 2015–16 Myanmar Demographic and Health Survey

Khaing Nwe Tin[1*], Thae Maung Maung[2] and Thiri Win[3]

**Abstract**

**Background:** Access to family planning contributes up to a 44% reduction in maternal deaths. Since the majority of unplanned pregnancies and abortions occur in women who were either not using contraception or not using it consistently, greater access to contraception and more consistent use of contraception are crucial in the reduction of unplanned pregnancies and abortions. This study aims to determine which types of contraceptives are most often discontinued, the reasons for discontinuation, and the factors that influence contraceptive discontinuation for women in Myanmar.

**Methods:** This study is a secondary data analysis of calendar data from the 2015–16 Myanmar Demographic Health Survey. The dependent variable is discontinuation of contraception within 12 months among episodes of contraceptive use in the 5 years before the survey among women age 15–49. Multivariable logistic regression was used to identify the predictors of contraceptive discontinuation.

**Results:** The 12-month discontinuation rate for all contraceptive methods was 39%. The discontinuation rates for short-term methods were remarkably high (43% for pills and 42% for injectables), while the rate for long-term methods was very low (7% for intrauterine devices and 0.2% for implants). Discontinuation while still in need of contraception was high (55%) although 28% of those women switched to other modern methods. Multivariable logistic regression showed the factors associated with contraceptive discontinuation were a woman's age, location (state/region), wealth, and number of births within the past 5 years.

**Conclusions:** The high rate of discontinuation while in need is very alarming given goals to reduce the unmet need for family planning in Myanmar. Family planning programs must ensure timely, informed method-switching by women who discontinue contraception, especially among women for whom discontinuation is the highest (age 45–49, middle and richest wealth quintile, regions where high discontinuation and multiparity); increase the availability of long-term contraceptive methods, and improve counseling that ensures clients' informed and voluntary choice of family planning services.

**Keywords:** Contraceptive, Discontinuation, Unmet need, Family planning

* Correspondence: khaingnwetin@gmail.com
[1]Maternal and Reproductive Health Division, Department of Public Health, Ministry of Health and Sports, Naypyitaw, Myanmar

## Introduction

Improving access to family planning (FP) services is fundamental to achieving the Sustainable Development Goals (SDGs) because it is strongly related with women's and children's health, poverty reduction, education, gender equality, and human rights [1]. Access to FP contributes up to a 44% reduction in maternal deaths and a 21% reduction of deaths in children under age 5 [2]. It enhances opportunities for women and girls to attain greater socioeconomic status through education, employment, and empowerment, and accelerates the development of the country by reducing healthcare costs [3].

Myanmar has the second highest maternal mortality ratio (MMR) (178/100,000 live births) among the Association of Southeast Asian Nations (ASEAN[1]) countries [4]. In the 2014 Myanmar Population and Housing Census, the MMR in Myanmar was 282 deaths per 100,000 live births [5]. The pregnancy-related mortality ratio (PRMR) was 227 deaths per 100,000 live births in the 2015–16 Myanmar Demographic and Health Survey (MDHS) [6]. Abortion-related complications were the second leading cause of maternal death [7]. Given these statistics, Myanmar has been working to improve accessibility of modern FP methods to improve maternal and newborn health [8].

Reproductive, maternal, newborn, child, and adolescent health is an explicit public health priority within the Myanmar National Health Plan (2017–2021) [9]. In 2013, Myanmar strongly committed to Family Planning 2020 (FP2020), a global initiative focused on reaching more women with life-saving information and access to contraceptives by the year 2020 and beyond [10].

Myanmar's FP program began in 1991 as a pilot in a single township. Since 2012, the government has increased its health budget, invested additional resources in the FP program, and increased the accessibility of contraceptives at the community level. Myanmar has worked to increase contraceptive use by married couples and unmarried individuals through informed choice. National surveys showed trends toward an increasing modern contraceptive prevalence rate (CPR) from 38 to 51% and decreasing unmet need for FP from 19 to 16% between 2007 and 2016 [6, 11]. However, these gains are inadequate for achieving the FP2020 targets of greater than 60% CPR and less than 10% unmet need [6, 12]. In addition, there are substantional disparities in unmet need for FP among Myanmar's states and regions [6].

The majority of unplanned pregnancies and abortions occur among women who were not using contraception or were using it inconsistently, which can lead to poor maternal and child health outcomes, affecting the development of the country [3]. Therefore, greater access to and consistent use of contraception are crucial in the reduction of unplanned pregnancies and abortions.

Contraceptive dynamics, such as discontinuation, switching, and failure, are important markers of how well public health programs are meeting the FP needs of women and couples [13]. Globally, research has focused on determining the reasons for discontinuation of different methods of contraception. Not all discontinuation is necessarily problematic. Some women discontinue a particular method because it is difficult to use or its use is unacceptable to either the woman or her partner, and subsequently switch to another, more suitable method [14]. Other women discontinue because they no longer have a need for contraception. In contrast, women who discontinue contraception despite their desire to limit or delay childbearing represent an extremely important reproductive health problem [15]. Discontinuation for reasons other than "wanted to become pregnant" can lead to unwanted pregnancies, and some of these pregnancies may be terminated by unsafe methods [14]. In a study of 36 low- and middle-income countries [16], 2 % of unintended pregnancies in the last 5 years were due to discontinuation of traditional methods, 18% were due to discontinuation of short-acting modern methods, and 2 % were due to discontinuation of long-term methods. Therefore, reducing premature discontinuation among women who are currently using contraception can be an effective strategy to reduce unmet need and unintended pregnancies [17].

In a study of 25 low and middle income countries, an average 38% of women discontinued contraceptive use within 12 months, 55% within 24 months, and 64% within 36 months. Twelve-month discontinuation rates were highest among condom users (50%) and lowest among intrauterine device (IUD) users (13%), while around 40% of users of the pill, injectables, periodic abstinence, and withdrawal discontinued within 12 months. Discontinuation due to health concerns /side effects, a method related reason, was the most common reason for discontinuation [13]. Studying contraceptive dynamics can identify problems in contraception use and the gaps in service provision [13]. Understanding the reasons for discontinuation and the characteristics of women who discontinue are necessary to evaluate FP strategy and the resource allocation required to ensure the quality of and equitable access to FP services. Although such information is critical for Myanmar's FP program, there are no prior studies related to contraceptive discontinuation in Myanmar because of a lack of data. The 2015–2016 DHS [6] is the first survey for Myanmar that allows the analysis of contraceptive discontinuation. Thus, this study aims to determine discontinuation rates, the most commonly discontinued

[1]Members of ASEAN countries are Brunei, Cambodia, Indonesia, Laos, Malaysia, Myanmar, Philippines, Singapore, Thailand and Vietnam.

methods, reasons for discontinuation, and factors that affect the discontinuation in Myanmar.

## Methodology

This study is a secondary data analysis of the 2015–16 MDHS, a nationally representative survey providing current information on fertility, reproductive health, and FP [6]. The MDHS included information on 12,885 women age 15–49, across 15 States and Regions and urban and rural areas in Myanmar.

Standard recode data files for the MDHS are freely available for access by the public through The DHS Program website, https://www.dhsprogram.com/data/.

Ethics approval for the MDHS was obtained from the Ethics Review Committee of the Department of Medical Research, and Permission for the secondary data analysis presented in this study was obtained from The DHS Program and the Department of Public Health, Ministry of Health and Sports, Myanmar.

This study included information on women, age 15–49, who used contraception during the 5 years before the survey. The data included socio-demographic characteristics and information on FP such as knowledge of contraception, exposure to FP messages and sources of information, and informed decision making on contraceptive use.

### Variables

The dependent variable in the study was twelve-month contraceptive discontinuation which is defined as women age 15–49 who used contraception in 5 years before the survey and discontinued it within 12 months of use.

The independent variables were 5 year age group, marital status (currently married, never married/widowed/divorced/separated), education (highest level attained), residence (urban or rural), state/regions, household wealth quintile, working status (currently working or not), exposure to FP messages (heard about FP on radio, TV, and newspaper or not), contraceptive knowledge (whether respondent has high or low knowledge of any FP method), contraceptive decision making (who made the decision to use contraception: mainly the woman, mainly the man, or both), informed choice of contraceptive use; measured by the method information index, current use of any contraceptive method, the number of children born in the previous 5 years, and the number of living children.

Contraceptive knowledge was calculated as a combined score of the number of contraceptive methods a woman was able to name and her knowledge of the ovulation cycle. There were 12 items in the knowledge score, with high> = 7 and low< 7. The method information index is a proxy indicator for quality of family planning counseling services and informed choice [18]. It ranges from 0 to 3 based on a woman's "Yes" responses to three variables: 1) the woman was informed about the side effects or problems of the contraceptive method; 2) the woman was informed about what to do if she experienced side effects, and 3) the woman was informed by a health or FP worker of other contraceptive methods that could be used [18].

The selection of variables was guided by a conceptual framework, shown in Fig. 1, and by the availability of data in the MDHS.

### Conceptual framework

The study team developed the conceptual framework to conceptualize a wide range of factors that could influence contraceptive discontinuation, with reference to studies on discontinuation and contraceptive use [15, 19]. It suggests the factors that influence contraceptive discontinuation among women age 15–49 are individual characteristics, community/family characteristics, health system characteristics, and contraceptive method used.

#### *Data management and analysis*

To describe contraceptive dynamics, we used DHS calendar [20] data in the woman's standard recode file, which collected monthly information on contraceptive use and reproductive events retrospectively for the 5 years before the survey. From this data file, the study team created an events file containing 6980 episodes of contraceptive use (the unit of analysis) among women 5431 age 15–49 who used contraception in the 5 years before the survey.

The study used STATA (Version 15 STATA Corp., College Station, TX, USA). All tests were two-sided with a $p$-value of less than 0.05 considered statistically significant. Twelve-month discontinuation rates and reasons for discontinuation are described by frequency and percentages. All possible factors that might influence discontinuation, per the conceptual framework, were included in the bivariate analysis. To identify the factors associated with contraceptive discontinuation, odds ratios (ORs) and their 95% confidence intervals (CIs) were estimated using multivariable logistic regression.

## Results

### Characteristics of contraceptive users

Table 1 shows the socio-demographic characteristics of the sample of women age 15 to 49 who used a contraceptive method within the 5 years before the MDHS. Among contraceptive users ($n = 5431$), 63% were between age 25–39, only 3% were adolescents (age 15–19), and 12% were between age 20–24. Almost all (96%) users were married. Nearly half of the respondents have primary education and only 8% have higher education.

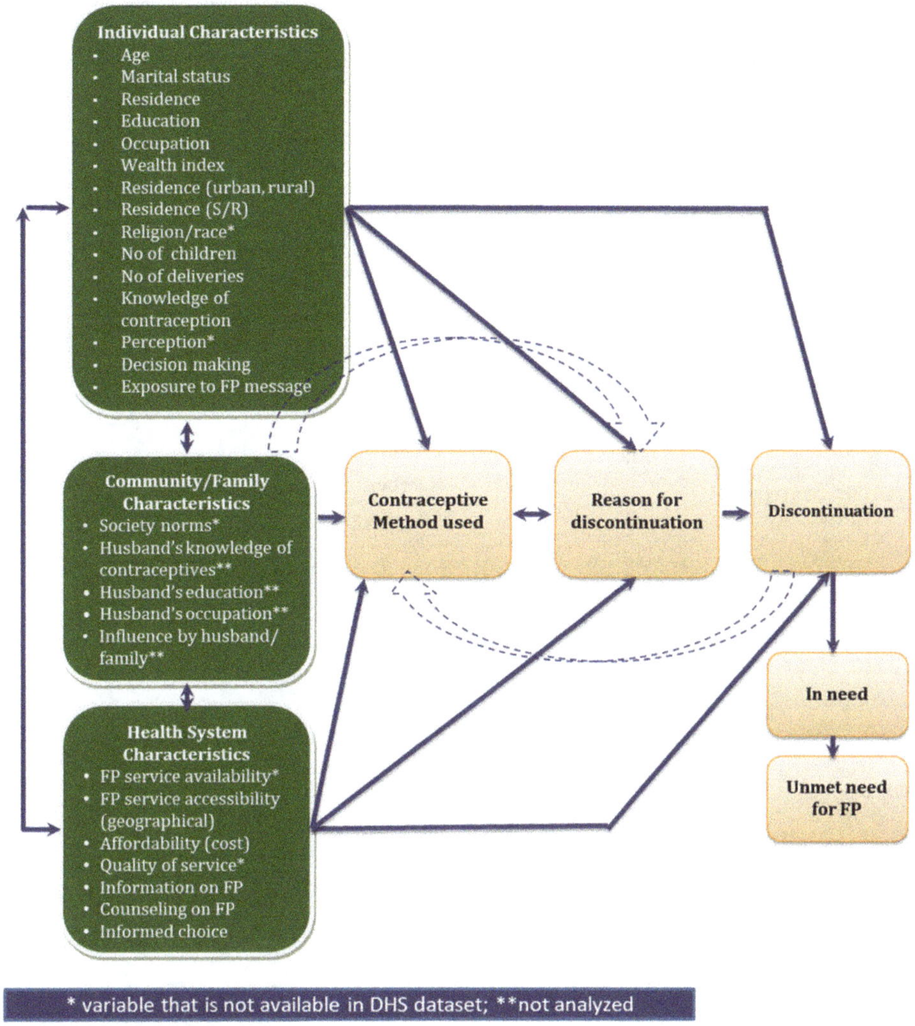


**Fig. 1** Conceptual framework of the factors that influence contraceptive discontinuation among women age 15–49

One-third of the women were not working, and about 70% resided in rural areas.

About half of the women (53%) did not receive FP messages from any source, while 73% had a good contraceptive knowledge score. The method information index; a proxy indicator for quality of counseling services, was 23%, which means that only two in ten of the contraceptive users had informed choice when they used FP methods. About two-thirds (64%) of the women made the decision to use contraception jointly with their partners, while one-third (33%) made the decision themselves.

### 12 month discontinuation rate

As shown in Table 2, the 12-month discontinuation rate for all methods was 39%. Among the different methods, the discontinuation rate for the lactation amenorrhea method (LAM) was the highest. The discontinuation rates for short-term methods were remarkably high, at 43% for pills and 42% for injectables, while the rate for long-term methods was very low, at 7% for the intrauterine device (IUD) and 0.2% for implants.

### Reasons for discontinuation

Table 3 shows the reasons for discontinuation. Health concerns/fear of side effects (31%) was the single most common reason for discontinuing the use of a contraceptive method within 12 months.

These individual reasons can be grouped into *discontinued due to failure,* i.e. became pregnant while using a method; *discontinued due to no need,* such as "wanted to become pregnant" and "other fertility-related" reasons; and *discontinued while in need,* including reasons like "health concerns/side effects" and "wanted a more effective method." As shown in Fig. 2, almost 55% of the contraceptive users discontinued their contraceptive use within 12 months despite still being in need of contraception.

**Table 1** Characteristics of women age 15–49 who used a contraceptive method within 5 years before the 2015–16 MDHS

| Characteristics of contraceptive ever users | (*N*=5,431) n | % |
|---|---|---|
| **Age group** | | |
| 15-19 | 144 | 2.5 |
| 20-24 | 665 | 12.2 |
| 25-29 | 1,058 | 19.3 |
| 30-34 | 1,158 | 21.7 |
| 35-39 | 1,146 | 21.5 |
| 40-44 | 817 | 14.7 |
| 45-49 | 443 | 8.1 |
| **Marital status** | | |
| Married | 5,252 | 96.9 |
| Never married/widowed/divorced/separated | 179 | 3.1 |
| **Education level** | | |
| No formal education | 638 | 12.0 |
| Primary | 2,481 | 46.7 |
| Secondary | 1,842 | 32.6 |
| Higher | 470 | 8.7 |
| **Occupation (*n*=5,417)** | | |
| Not working | 1,626 | 29.1 |
| Professional/technical/managerial | 289 | 4.7 |
| Clerical | 58 | 1.1 |
| Sales | 996 | 18.0 |
| Agricultural-self employed | 442 | 8.7 |
| Agricultural-employee | 301 | 5.5 |
| Household and domestic | 12 | 0.2 |
| Services | 33 | 0.7 |
| Skilled manual | 312 | 6.5 |
| Unskilled manual | 1,348 | 25.5 |
| **Wealth index** | | |
| Poorest | 1,076 | 19.8 |
| Poorer | 1,100 | 20.3 |
| Middle | 1,069 | 19.2 |
| Richer | 1,126 | 20.3 |
| Richest | 1,060 | 20.5 |
| **Residence** | | |
| Urban | 1,551 | 28.0 |
| Rural | 3,880 | 72.0 |
| **Region** | | |
| Kachin | 278 | 2.4 |
| Kayah | 333 | 0.5 |
| Kayin | 303 | 2.2 |
| Chin | 166 | 0.4 |
| Sagaing | 448 | 10.8 |
| Tanintharyi | 321 | 2.3 |

**Table 1** Characteristics of women age 15–49 who used a contraceptive method within 5 years before the 2015–16 MDHS *(Continued)*

| Characteristics of contraceptive ever users | (*N*=5,431) n | % |
|---|---|---|
| Bago | 469 | 11.1 |
| Magway | 362 | 7.4 |
| Mandalay | 393 | 11.1 |
| Mon | 339 | 3.6 |
| Rakhine | 353 | 5.4 |
| Yangon | 454 | 14.4 |
| Shan | 340 | 10.6 |
| Ayeyarwady | 473 | 15.3 |
| Nay Pyi Taw | 399 | 2.8 |
| **Number of births in last 5 years** | | |
| No birth | 2,574 | 49.8 |
| 1 | 2,355 | 42.9 |
| 2 | 451 | 06.5 |
| 3 | 51 | 00.7 |
| **Number of living children** | | |
| 0 | 449 | 9.1 |
| 1 | 1,461 | 28.8 |
| 2 | 1,533 | 28.9 |
| 3 | 1,012 | 18.0 |
| 4+ | 976 | 15.1 |
| **Knowledge on family planning** | | |
| Poor | 1,484 | 27.3 |
| Good | 3,947 | 72.7 |
| **Exposure to FP message/source of information** | | |
| No exposure | 3,047 | 52.5 |
| Exposure from any source | 2,384 | 47.5 |
| **Decision making for contraceptive use** | | |
| Mainly women | 1,215 | 33.0 |
| Mainly husband | 75 | 1.8 |
| Jointly | 2,437 | 64.9 |
| Others | 18 | 0.4 |
| **Informed choice** | | |
| Yes | 806 | 22.6 |
| No | 2,873 | 77.4 |

#### Factors influencing the contraceptive discontinuation

In the bivariate analysis, women who were age 45–49, not currently married, technical and clerical employees, in the richest quintile, and use of any contraceptive method other than LARCs were significantly associated with discontinuation within 12 months (Table 4). Residing in selected states and regions was also associated with discontinuation.

**Table 2** 12-month contraceptive discontinuation rates among episodes of contraceptive use beginning within the 5 years before the 2015–16 MDHS among women age 15–49

| Discontinuation by methods | (*N*=6,980) (%) |
|---|---|
| LAM | 84.9 |
| Pill | 43.0 |
| Injectable | 41.5 |
| All | 39.1 |
| Male condom | 31.0 |
| Withdrawal | 23.0 |
| Periodic abstinence/rhythm | 19.5 |
| IUD | 7.1 |
| Other | 5.4 |
| Implant | 0.2 |

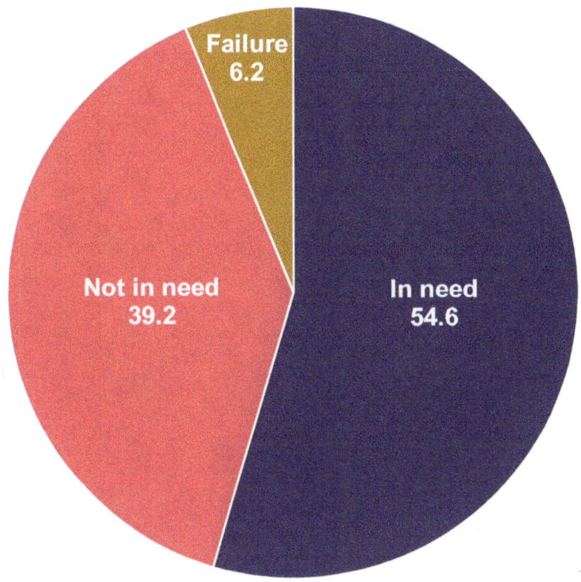


**Fig. 2** Discontinuation rates by need

After controlling for the other factors with multivariable logistic regression, the factors associated with contraceptive discontinuation were the women's age group, location (state/region), wealth quintile, and number of births within 5 years. Women aged 45–49 (OR = 2.68; 95%CI: 1.31 to 5.46) and those from the middle (OR = 1.42; 95%CI: 1.02 to 2.00) and richest quintile group (OR = 1.66; 95%CI: 1.18 to 2.34) were more likely to discontinue contraceptive use. Women with one child (OR = 0.78; 95%CI: 0.62 to 0.98) were 22% less likely to discontinue the contraceptive use. With the exception of Bago and Ayeyarwaddy, residing in any other state or region was found to be significantly and positively associated with discontinuation compared with Yangon. Residents of Tanintharyi had nearly 8 times the odds of discontinuation (OR = 7.8; 95%CI: 4.61 to 13.44) as residents of Yangon (Table 4).

## Discussion

This study was a secondary analysis of the first nationally representative 2015–16 MDHS of 12,885 women age 15–49 from both urban and rural areas in Myanmar. The findings have a number of policy and practical implications for the national FP program because the MDHS was nationally representative. Among the 5431 women used contraception in the preceding 5 years, nearly three-fourths had a good knowledge score, which is the combined score of a woman's ability to name contraceptive methods and to know the fertility period. In the MDHS [6], 97% of all women had heard of a contraceptive method, which was consistent with the 2007 Fertility and Reproductive Health Survey, in which knowledge of FP was 95% [11]. However, in a small Myanmar study, only 20% of married women had a knowledge score that reflected detailed information of contraceptive usage such as eligibility, benefits, side effects, and warning signs of different methods (Tin KN, Mon MM: Task sharing to Auxiliary Midwives for Family Planning Services in selected hard-to-reach areas in Myanmar, unpublished). The MDHS found that about half of women who used contraception in the 5 years before the survey did not receive FP messages from any source [6]. This highlights a high contraceptive knowledge score is not necessarily equated with having comprehensive FP information and the ability to make informed choices regarding contraception. Therefore, it is necessary to strengthen the provision of comprehensive FP information so that women can be more knowledgeable about method choices, and more likely to choose a method satisfactory to them that they can use for a sustained period of time [21].

In this study, the 12-month contraceptive discontinuation rate among women age 15–49 who started an episode of contraceptive use within the 5 years before the MDHS was 39% for all methods., This rate was consistent with the average 12-month discontinuation rate (38%) in 25 other low and middle income countries [13]. The discontinuation rate in this study is similar to the

**Table 3** Reasons for discontinuation among episodes of contraceptive use beginning within the 5 years before the 2015–16 MDHS among women age 15–49

| Reasons for contraceptive discontinuation | (*N*=6,980) (%) |
|---|---|
| Health concerns/side effects | 31.0 |
| Wanted to become pregnant | 26.7 |
| Wanted a more effective method | 12.5 |
| Other fertility-related reason | 12.4 |
| Other method-related | 6.3 |
| Became pregnant while using | 6.2 |
| Don't know | 4.9 |

**Table 4** Factors associated with contraception discontinuation among episodes of contraceptive use beginning within the 5 years before the 2015–16 MDHS among women age 15–49

| Characteristics | Contraceptive Discontinuation % | Crude OR[a] [95% CI] | aOR[b] [95% CI] |
|---|---|---|---|
| **Age group (*n*=4,982)** | | | |
| 15-19 | 23.4 | Ref | Ref |
| 20-24 | 26.33 | 1.16 [.77-1.76] | 1.16 [0.76-1.79] |
| 25-29 | 24.45 | 1.05 [.69-1.59] | 1.04 [0.68-1.59] |
| 30-34 | 24.0 | 1.03 [.67-1.56] | 0.97 [0.63-1.49] |
| 35-39 | 24.1 | 1.03 [.63-1.70] | 0.94 [0.57-1.54] |
| 40-44 | 31.3 | 1.48 [.93-2.36] | 1.29 [0.82-2.05] |
| 45-49 | 5.2 | 3.5* [1.59-7.75] | 2.68* [1.31-5.46] |
| **Marital status (*n*=5,884)** | | | |
| Married | 25.1 | Ref | |
| Never married/widowed/divorced/separated | 95.0 | 5.47* [3.52-8.49] | |
| **Education level (*n*=5,884)** | | | |
| No formal education | 25.5 | Ref | |
| Primary | 25.2 | 0.98 [0.72-1.35] | |
| Secondary | 28.0 | 1.14 [0.77-1.68] | |
| Higher | 25.8 | 1.02 [0.64-1.61] | |
| **Occupation (*n*=4,971)** | | | |
| Not working/dependent | 22.3 | Ref | |
| Professional/technical/managerial | 37.5 | 2.09* [1.01-4.33] | |
| Clerical/sales/services | 28.6 | 1.39* [1.02-1.91] | |
| Agricultural | 27.0 | 1.29 [0.78-2.14] | |
| Manual worker | 26.7 | 1.27 [1.02-1.58] | |
| **Wealth index (*n*=4,982)** | | | |
| Poorest | 23.0 | Ref | Ref |
| Poorer | 25.1 | 1.12 [0.84-1.48] | 1.13 [0.84-1.52] |
| Middle | 30.0 | 1.43 [0.96-2.13] | 1.42* [1.02-2.00] |
| Richer | 24.0 | 1.05 [0.77-1.44] | 1.19 [0.86-1.63] |
| Richest | 29.7 | 1.41* [1.02-1.97] | 1.66* [1.18-2.34] |
| **Residence** | | | |
| Urban | 26.5 | Ref | |
| Rural | 26.1 | 0.98 [0.74-1.29] | |
| **Region (*n*=5,884)** | | | |
| Yangon | 16.4 | Ref | Ref |
| Kachin | 21.8 | 1.41 [0.85-2.36] | 1.62* [1.98-2.67] |
| Kayah | 23.5 | 1.56* [1.05-2.33] | 1.79* [1.19-2.68] |
| Kayin | 37.6 | 3.07* [1.96-4.81] | 3.53* [2.29-5.44] |
| Chin | 28.8 | 2.05* [1.21-3.48] | 2.12* [1.25-3.59] |
| Sagaing | 26.8 | 1.86* [1.23-2.80] | 2.06* [1.38-3.10] |
| Tanintharyi | 56.4 | 6.58* [3.93-11.02] | 7.87* [4.61-13.44] |
| Bago | 15.5 | 0.93 [0.64-1.36] | 1.08 [0.74-1.58] |
| Magway | 36.4 | 2.90* [1.52-5.55] | 3.27* [1.81-5.93] |
| Mandalay | 23.7 | 1.58 [0.98-2.55] | 1.80* [1.11-2.93] |
| Mon | 42.3 | 2.72* [2.35-5.90] | 4.03* [2.54-6.41] |

**Table 4** Factors associated with contraception discontinuation among episodes of contraceptive use beginning within the 5 years before the 2015–16 MDHS among women age 15–49 *(Continued)*

| Characteristics | Contraceptive Discontinuation % | Crude OR[a] [95% CI] | aOR[b] [95% CI] |
|---|---|---|---|
| Rakhine | 34.2 | 2.64* [1.69-4.12] | 3.19* [2.03-5.02] |
| Shan | 32.2 | 2.42* [1.44-4.06] | 2.52* [1.49-4.27] |
| Ayeyarwaddy | 17.5 | 1.08 [0.72-1.61] | 1.35 [0.89-2.02] |
| Nay Pyi Taw | 23.1 | 1.53* [1.03-2.26] | 1.76* [1.17-2.63] |
| **Number of births in last 5 years (*n*=4,982)** | | | |
| No births | 30.3 | Ref | Ref |
| 1 | 23.1 | 0.69* [0.54-0.89] | 0.78* [0.62-0.98] |
| 2 | 28.5 | 0.92 [0.66-1.29] | 1.01 [0.73-1.40] |
| 3 | 37.6 | 1.38 [0.85-2.26] | 1.66 [0.98-2.82] |
| **Number of living children (*n*=4,982)** | | | |
| 0 | 27.7 | Ref | |
| 1 | 27.2 | 0.97 [0.73-1.29] | |
| 2 | 23.5 | 0.80 [0.57-1.14] | |
| 3 | 23.0 | 0.78 [0.55-1.11] | |
| 4+ | 31.4 | 1.19 [0.83-1.72] | |
| **Knowledge on family planning** | | | |
| Poor | 25.8 | Ref | |
| Good | 26.4 | 1.03 [0.84-1.26] | |
| **Exposure to FP message/source of information (*n*=4,982)** | | | |
| No exposure | 26.5 | Ref | |
| Exposure from any source | 25.9 | 0.97 [0.80-1.17] | |
| **Decision making for contraceptive use (*n*=3,494)** | | | |
| Mainly women | 18.0 | Ref | |
| Mainly husband | 12.1 | 0.62 [0.19-2.01] | |
| Jointly | 14.6 | 0.78 [0.54-1.11] | |
| **Informed choice** | | | |
| No | 15.6 | Ref | |
| Yes | 15.9 | 1.02 [0.74-1.40] | |
| **By methods(*n*=1,458)** | | | |
| LARC | 2.0 | Ref | |
| Pills | 31.0 | 22.40* [5.24-95.4] | |
| Injection | 27.3 | 18.74* [4.43-79.18] | |
| Other modern methods including condom | 14.1 | 8.17* [1.70-39.13] | |
| Traditional method | 12.6 | 7.17* [1.30-39.47] | |

*$p<0.05$
[a]crude odds ratios from binomial logistic regression
[b]adjusted odds ratio from multivariate logistic regression

rates of 38% in Bangladesh, 34% in Senegal, 31% in Tanzania and 27% in Ethiopia [22–25], indicating that Myanmar's contraceptive discontinuation magnitude is similarly high as other developing countries.

In addition, discontinuation rates varied by method, with discontinuation of short-term methods being higher than long-term methods. This study found a 12-month discontinuation rate of about 40% for pills or injectables versus 7% for the IUD [6]. These results are similar to the method-specific discontinuation rates found in the 25-country study (40% for pills and injectables versus 13% for IUD) [13]. The MDHS results were also consistent with a study from Senegal, in which discontinuation was lower among long-term methods (6 and 18% for implants and IUD, respectively) than for pills (38%) and injectables (33%) [23]. Likewise in an Ethiopian study, the highest discontinuation rates were found in pill users (38%) while IUD users had the lowest discontinuation rates (14%) [25]. Short-term method users may discontinue at higher rates because they can stop using their method without the assistance of health providers. Additionally, in Myanmar, short-term methods are readily available at both public and private health facilities, pharmacies, drug shops, and retailers in some rural communities. In hard-to-reach areas, untrained community health volunteers provide injections of Depo-Provera, though without providing any comprehensive user information [26]. In the 2015–16 MDHS, the source for pills was the private sector (47%) and other sources (39%), while the source for injectables was mainly the public sector (74%) [6].

In the MDHS, the method information index; an indicator of quality counseling, for all methods was 23%. For short-term methods, the index was quite low (13% for pills and 26% for injectables), compared with long-term methods (64% for implants and 53% for IUD) [6]. This suggests that short-term methods may be given without full counseling and information in both the public and private sectors. This also highlights the critical importance of proper restrictions on selling injections to unskilled individuals, comprehensive information sharing with clients by drug shops and pharmacies, awareness training on FP for drug sellers, as well as quality counseling and adoption of informed choice principles by all healthcare providers.

In this study, the primary reasons for discontinuation were health concerns or fear of side effects. This was similar to the evidence from other studies, which similarly found health concerns/ side effects to be the most common reason and that counseling was inadequate [14, 16]. In a study in Bangladesh, it was also found that the experience of side effects was the main reason for discontinuation [27]. Although the reasons can differ between users of short and long acting methods, this study found that health concerns/side effects was the most common reason for both types of methods. One limitation of this study which uses DHS data, is that we cannot distinguish between discontinuation because women actually experienced health problems and discontinuation due to their fear of side effects. This should be explored with qualitative interviews.

In this study, discontinuation due to method failure was low (6%), which was similar to the findings of a study in Pakistan (8%) [28] but lower than failure rates found in another multi-country study [16]. Because perfect use failure rates are estimated to be less than 1% for all methods [14, 21], the magnitude of method failure in Myanmar might be a result of inadequate counseling or incorrect information on correct and effective use [29].

Discontinuation while still in need of contraception was high in this study (55%). However, 28% of those women reported switching to other modern methods. High discontinuation while still need of contraception is alarming in light of the country's efforts to reduce unmet need for family planning and to prevent unwanted pregnancies. Family planning programs must ensure timely, accurate information on alternative methods to those women who discontinue contraception in order to prevent unintended pregnancies and unsafe abortion [14].

According to the MDHS, unmet need for FP in Myanmar was 16%, comprised of 11% who had an unmet need for limiting and 5% who had an unmet need for spacing. There is considerably high use (68.4%) of short-term methods (pills or injectables) in Myanmar, given the large proportion of women who want to limit births [6]. This reliance on short-term methods may be unsustainable and contribute to discontinuation, indicating a need to improve service availability, quality and counseling to help women make an informed choice.

When identifying the factors that influence discontinuation, women age 45–49, from the middle and richest wealth quintile, location (all states and regions except Bago and Ayeyarwaddy) were positively associated and having one birth in the past 5 years was negatively associated with discontinuation after controlling for other possible confounding factors. It is worth exploring the reasons for the high discontinuation rates found in the Taninthari region. In a similar analysis of the 2013 Nigeria DHS, the predictors for discontinuation were women's age, residence, education, number of children under age 5, marital duration, women's occupation, men's occupation, and wealth [19]. Family size and number of children were associated with discontinuation in a Pakistan study [28].

Among the factors associated with contraceptive discontinuation in bivariate regression, the method used was the most important factor; it could not be included in multivariate analysis due to the small sample size of IUD users. In this study, women who used short-term methods and traditional methods were more likely to discontinue than long-term methods users, which is consistent with studies in other countries [13, 14]. Thus, information and counseling should be more focused to short-term method users to prevent discontinuation while in need. In addition, there might be other potential family/community and health service factors that might influence contraceptive discontinuation which could not be identified in this study. Further qualitative research could explore these gaps.

The method information index was high for long-term method users but quite low for short-term method users. It is possible that long-term contraceptives are provided by trained medical personnel who provide professional counseling. Although there was not a significant association between discontinuation and the method information index, after controlling for the method used, FP programs should promote the availability of long-term methods through effective counseling to make informed choice that assure sustained contraception. Long-term methods are cost-effective methods as compared with short-term contraceptives, and align with Myanmar FP2020 commitments to increase access to and consistent use of contraception in Myanmar [12, 30].

### Strengths and limitations

This study utilized data from the 2015–16 MDHS, the first nationwide representative survey conducted in Myanmar. The study used DHS-standardized data collection tools, data management strategies, and data analysis techniques, which generate nationally representative data that can be compared with data from other countries where DHS were conducted. The study had some limitations. Husband/family/community factors and some health system factors (service availability, accessibility, and quality of services) were not assessed in the study because this information was not available in the MDHS. Since this study was based on cross-sectional data, possible causal associations with some factors is limited, which limits our understanding of individuals' and couples' experiences that contribute to contraceptive discontinuation.

## Conclusion

The 12-month discontinuation rate for all methods was high, primarily due to discontinuation of short-term methods. Discontinuation while in need was also considerably high, with health concerns/fear of side effects cited as the most common reason. While women's age group, location (state/region), wealth, and number of births within 5 years were significantly associated with discontinuation, the method information index was not statistically significant in this study. Timely and accurate information on method alternatives should be promoted to reduce contraceptive discontinuation while women are in need and promote informed choice, especially among older (age 45–49) women and women with multiple births, and in regions which have high discontinuation rates. The Myanmar FP program must also improve the availability of contraception including long-term methods to ensure clients can choose their preferred method from a range of choices through effective counseling and voluntary FP services.

### Abbreviations

ASEAN: Association of Southeast Asian Nations; CPR: Contraceptive prevalence rate; CI: Confidence intervals; DHS: Demographic and Health Survey; FP: Family planning; FP2020: Family Planning 2020; IUD: Intrauterine device; LAM: Lactation amenorrhea method; MDHS: Myanmar Demographic Health Survey; MII: Method information index; MMR: Maternal mortality ratio; OR: Odds ratio; PRMR: Pregnancy related mortality ratio; SDGs: Sustainable Development Goals

### Acknowledgements

The authors thank The Demographic and Health Surveys Program for the data used in this study. We also would like to thank the U.S. Agency for International Development for funding support for the research through the Myanmar DHS Fellows Program, which is implemented by The DHS Program. We also thank ICF for their technical support of the DHS Fellows Program in Myanmar, and especially Dr. Kerry L. D. MacQuarrie for her technical assistance with developing the decomposition command used in the analysis and preparing the manuscript.

### Authors' contributions

The work was conceived and designed by KNT, TMM and TRW. KNT and TMM contributed to the study conceptualization. TMM advised on data analysis and helped to draft the manuscript. KNT and TRW contributed to writing the paper. All authors read and approved the final manuscript.

### Author details

[1]Maternal and Reproductive Health Division, Department of Public Health, Ministry of Health and Sports, Naypyitaw, Myanmar. [2]Department of Medical Research, Ministry of Health and Sports, Yangon, Myanmar. [3]Department of Public Health, Ministry of Health and Sports, Naypyitaw, Myanmar.

### References

1. New JR, Cahill N, Stover J, Gupta YP, Alkema L. Levels and trends in contraceptive prevalence, unmet need, and demand for family planning for 29 states and union territories in India: a modelling study using the family planning estimation tool. Lancet Glob Health. 2017;5:e350–8.
2. Starbird E, Norton M, Marcus R Investing in Family Planning: Key to Achieving the Sustainable Development Goals doi: https://doi.org/10.9745/GHSP-D-15-00374.
3. Kaye K, Gootman JA, Ng AS, Finley C. The benefits of birth control in America: getting the facts straight. The National Campaign to prevent teen and unplanned Pregnanc. Washington, DC: The National Campaign to Prevent Teen and Unplanned Pregnancy; 2014.
4. WHO Global Health Observatory data repository | By category | Maternal mortality - Data by country. In: WHO. http://apps.who.int/gho/data/node.main.15. Accessed 12 Aug 2018.
5. Department of Population; Ministry of Labour Immigration; Ministry of Health and Sports. The 2014 Myanmar population and housing census. Naypyitaw: Republic of Union of Myanmar; 2015.
6. Ministry of Health and Sports. Myanmar demographic and health survey 2015–16. Nay Pyi Taw: Ministry of Health and Sports, The Republic of the Union of Myanmar; 2017.
7. Department of Public Health M of H and S. Maternal death surveillance and response 2017. Nay Pyi Taw: The Republic of the Union of Myanmar; 2019.
8. Ministry of Health and Sports. Five-year strategic plan for reproductive health (2014–2018). Nay Pyi Taw: The Republic of the Union of Myanmar; 2013.
9. Ministry of Health and Sports. Myanmar National Health Plan (2017–2021). Nay Pyi Taw: Republic of Union of Myanmar; 2016.
10. Department of Public Health. Costed implementation to meet FP2020 commitments Myanmar 2014. Nay Pyi Taw: The Republic of the Union of Myanmar; 2015.
11. Department of Population and UNFPA. Country report on 2007 fertility and reproductive health survey. Nay Pyi Taw: The Republic of the Union of Myanmar; 2009.
12. Myanmar Commitment Maker since 2013. http://www.familyplanning2020.org/MYANMAR. Accessed 30 Sep 2019.
13. Ali MM, Cleland J, Shah IH. Causes and consequences of contraceptive discontinuation: evidence from 60 demographic and health surveys; 2012.
14. Castle S, Askew I. Contraceptive Discontinuatin: reasons, challenges and solutions; 2015.

15. Azuike EC, Ikeako LC, Ezeobi I, Ezebialu IU, Umeobika JC, Obi KN, Anene JO, Azuike ED. Predictors of discontinuation of contraceptive use among Nigerian women: results of 2013 Nigeria demographic and health surveys. J Sci Res Stud. 2017;4(7):6.
16. Bellizzi S, Mannava P, Nagai M, Sobel HL. Reasons for discontinuation of contraception among women with a current unintended pregnancy in 36 low and middle-income countries. Contraception. 2020;101:26–33.
17. Jain AK, Obare F, RamaRao S, Askew I. Reducing unmet need by supporting women with met need. Int Perspect Sex Reprod Health. 2013;39:133–41.
18. Track20. http://www.track20.org/pages/data_analysis/in_depth/opportunities/quality.php. Accessed 3 Aug 2020.
19. Ejembi CL, Tukur D, Ajhaji A. Contextual factors influencing modern contraceptive use in Nigeria. DHS Work. Pap; 2015.
20. The Demographic and Health Surveys Program. DHS contraceptive calendar tutorial the demographic and health surveys program. Rockville: the United States Agency for International Development (USAID); 2018.
21. World Health Organization and Johns Hopkins Bloomberg School of Public Health. Family planning: a global handbook for providers. Geneva: World Health Organization and Johns Hopkins Bloomberg School of Public Health/Center for CommunicationPrograms; 2018.
22. Mahumud RA, Hossain G, Sarkar AR, Islam N, Hossain R, Saw Aik S, Khan J. Prevalence and associated factors of contraceptive discontinuation and switching among Bangladeshi married women of reproductive age. Open Access J Contracept. 2015;6:13.
23. Barden-O'Fallon J, Speizer IS, Calhoun LM, Corroon M. Women's contraceptive discontinuation and switching behavior in urban Senegal, 2010-2015. BMC Womens Health. 2018;18:1–9.
24. Safari W, Urassa M, Mtenga B, Changalucha J, Beard J, Church K, Zaba B, Todd J. Contraceptive use and discontinuation among women in rural north-West Tanzania. Contracept Reprod Med. 2019;4:18.
25. Belete N, Zemene A, Hagos H, Yekoye A. Prevalence and factors associated with modern contraceptive discontinuation among reproductive age group women, a community based cross-sectional study in Humera town, northern Ethiopia. BMC Womens Health. 2018;18:190.
26. Population Service International . Myanmar 2016 FPwatch Survey: Findings from a contraceptive commodity and service assessment among private sectoroutlets. http://www.actwatch.info/sites/default/files/content/publications/attachments/Myanmar. Accessed 12 Aug 2018.
27. Mitra, Ajita, The Reasons of Discontinuing the Use of Contraceptive Methods (June 30, 2016). OIDA International Journal of Sustainable Development. 2016;9(6):19–26. Available at SSRN: https://ssrn.com/abstract=2810594.
28. Rizvi F, Irfan G. Reasons for Discontinuation of Contraceptive Methods among Couples with Different Family Size and Educational Status. J Ayub Med Coll Abbottabad. 2012;24.
29. Haq I, Sakib S, Talukder A. Sociodemographic factors on contraceptive use among ever-married women of reproductive age: evidence from three demographic and health surveys in Bangladesh. Med Sci (Basel). 2017. https://doi.org/10.3390/medsci5040031.
30. Mavranezouli I. Health economics of contraception. Best Pract Res Clin Obstet Gynaecol. 2009;23:187–98.

# 24

# Prevalence and factors influencing modern contraceptive use among HIV-positive women in Kilimanjaro region, northern Tanzania

Damian J. Damian[1,2*], Johnston M. George[3,4], Erick Martin[3], Beatrice Temba[3] and Sia E. Msuya[1,2,4]

## Abstract

**Background:** Mother-to-Child-Transmission (MTCT) of HIV is still a public health problem in sub-Saharan Africa. The region has a high unmet need for family planning and high unplanned pregnancy rates among HIV-positive women. Most efforts to prevent MTCT of HIV have focused on the third prong, a strategy which offers antiretroviral (ARV) drugs to HIV-infected pregnant women and their exposed infants. However, the effective use of contraceptives to prevent unplanned pregnancies among women living with HIV is more effective in reducing HIV MTCT. This study aimed at determining the prevalence and factors influencing modern contraceptive use among HIV-positive women in northern Tanzania.

**Methods:** This was a cross-sectional study conducted between January and June 2014 in three selected districts of Kilimanjaro region, Tanzania. Data were collected during face-to-face interviews with HIV-positive women attending Care and Treatment Clinics (CTC) in the selected districts. Multivariate logistic regression analysis was used to determine independent predictors of modern contraceptive use.

**Results:** In total 672 HIV-positive women were enrolled. Their mean age was 36.4 years (±7.7). Fifty four percent (362) were currently using modern contraceptives, and the most common method used was male condoms 76% (275) followed by Depo-Provera 28% (101). A total of 33% (121) of the users reported dual contraceptive use. Women with primary education [Adjusted Odds Ratio (AOR) = 7.54, 95% Confidence Interval (CI): 1.51–17.48, $P = 0.014$]; post-secondary [AOR = 6.23, 95% CI: 1.14–14.07, $P = 0.035$]; not currently on ARVs [AOR = 11.29, 95% CI: 2.60–19.94, $P = 0.001$]; currently sexually active [AOR = 8.40, 95% CI: 4.47–15.78, $P < 0.001$]; ever discussed contraceptive use with partner [AOR = 3.68, 95% CI: 1.67–8.11, $P = 0.001$]; and being counseled on dual contraceptive use at CTC [AOR = 2.94, 95% CI: 1.66–5.23, $P < 0.001$]; had significantly higher odds of currently using modern contraceptive methods.

**Conclusions:** Given the population studied, the prevalence of modern contraceptive use was low. Strategies are required to increase the use of dual and long-term contraceptive methods among women who do not want more children in order to reduce MTCT, and to improve maternal and child health in the region. Programme managers and health care providers need to identify counseling strategies that are specific to HIV-positive women that not only impart knowledge on contraceptives, but also address the issue of responsibility for influencing HIV transmission in the community.

**Keywords:** Modern contraceptives, Contraceptive use, HIV-positive, CTC, Kilimanjaro, Tanzania

* Correspondence: d_jeremy5@yahoo.com
[1]Department of Community Medicine, Kilimanjaro Christian Medical Centre (KCMC), Moshi, Tanzania
[2]Department of Epidemiology & Biostatistics, Institute of Public Health, KCMUCo, P. O. Box 2240, Moshi, Tanzania

## Background

Since the 1960s, family planning (FP) programmes have helped women worldwide to avoid millions of unintended pregnancies often associated with high risk abortions and with maternal, newborn and child morbidity and mortality [1]. Globally, about 220 million women have an unmet need for FP and 80 million unplanned pregnancies occur each year [2, 3]. In sub-Saharan Africa (SSA), around 14 million unintended pregnancies occur yearly [4]. Investing in FP to prevent unwanted pregnancies has the potential of averting 13% of maternal, newborn and child deaths [5].

Recently, the use of FP has been seen to be of high benefit to women living with HIV [1, 6]. As compared to women in the general population, HIV-positive women have high unwanted pregnancy rates (51–90%), especially in SSA region [7]. Prevention of unintended pregnancies among HIV-infected women has a vital role in the prevention of mother-to-child-transmission (MTCT) of HIV. Reducing unintended pregnancies among HIV-positive women through FP reduces the number of HIV-exposed infants born from HIV-positive women and ultimately decreases MTCT [1, 6]. Prevention of unwanted pregnancies also reduces the vulnerability of women and infants to morbidity and mortality related to pregnancies [6, 8]. FP has also proven to be a cost-effective strategy for the prevention of HIV transmission, as contraception costs are less than the cost of drugs used in the Prevention of Mother-To-Child Transmission (PMTCT) [8, 9].

For the elimination of MTCT of HIV, WHO recommends a comprehensive PMTCT strategy with the 4 prongs: 1) Primary prevention of HIV infection among women of childbearing age; 2) FP for preventing unintended pregnancies among HIV-infected women; 3) preventing HIV transmission from HIV-infected women to their infants; and 4) treatment, care and support for HIV-infected women and their children [10]. However, PMTCT of HIV in most SSA countries including Tanzania is based on the third prong which is usually complex, labour and resource intensive [11]. This has led to the second prong gaining recognition as having a vital role in PMTCT.

The mathematical projection from 2009 on the burden of paediatric HIV indicated the synergistic effect of FP on reducing the number of HIV-positive pregnancies. The model showed that while HIV services to prevent mother-to-child transmission averted an estimated 8.1% of vertical infections, FP had the potential to avert 19.7% [7]. According to the model, unintended pregnancies accounted for 21.3% of new paediatric infections [6]. If all women wanting to avoid pregnancy used modern contraceptive methods, unintended pregnancies would decline by 71% [12]. There is therefore the need to improve strategies to raise FP use among HIV-positive women.

Despite the benefits, the unmet need for FP in most SSA countries is high both in general population [13–16] and among HIV-positive women [16–21]. In Tanzania, the unmet need for FP has remained unchanged over the past two decades (22–24%) [14]. In 2015–16, the Contraceptive Prevalence Rate (CPR) among currently married women (15–49 years) was 32%, while the national target by the end of 2015 was 60% [14]. The consequence of low CPR and a high unmet need for FP in this context is a high number of unwanted/unplanned pregnancies. High unwanted pregnancy rates among people living with HIV can further be linked with risk of exposing children to HIV infection unnecessarily [10].

While there is data on trends and current levels of CPR, unmet need, fertility rates and HIV prevalence from various surveys in Tanzania; there is limited information on FP use in HIV-positive women. Understanding the prevalence, patterns and factors influencing modern contraceptive use among HIV-positive women of reproductive age is critical to the expansion of comprehensive HIV prevention programmes, targeted at achieving a reduction in unwanted pregnancies and decreasing the incidence of HIV-infected children.

## Methods

### Study design and site

This was a facility-based cross-sectional study conducted between January and June 2014 among HIV-positive women aged 15–49 in three districts of the Kilimanjaro region, northern Tanzania. The Kilimanjaro region is located in the northern zone of the country and is the home of Africa's highest mountain, Mt. Kilimanjaro. The region has a population of 1,640,087 people, which is 3. 6% of Tanzania's population [22]. The region has seven districts from which Hai, Moshi urban and Mwanga districts were selected for this study. During the study period, the national HIV prevalence was estimated to be 5.1% [23]. Prior to this study, the regional HIV prevalence was estimated to be 3.8%; with Hai district 5.6%, Mwanga 4.2% and Moshi urban 3.6% respectively [23].

### Study population and enrolment procedures

Three districts with a high HIV prevalence in the region were selected, i.e. Hai, Mwanga and Moshi urban. A simple random sampling technique was used to select health facilities with Care and Treatment Clinics (CTCs) from the three districts. Eight, six and five facilities were selected from Moshi urban, Hai and Mwanga districts respectively. All HIV-positive women aged 15–49 attending a CTC who were eligible to participate and those meeting the inclusion criteria were invited to participate. We excluded HIV-positive women aged 15–49 who had a hysterectomy or did not consent to participate in the study. After obtaining participants' informed consent, a trained research assistant administered a questionnaire during face-to-face interviews. The collected information included: socio-demographic information (age, education level, marital status, occupation); individual health (time since diagnosed with HIV, current CD4 count, whether was on ART drugs); sexual and reproductive health history (parity, sexual activity, condom use); and methods and pattern of FP use (ever heard of FP, ever used FP, currently using FP). Information on facility factors, partner communication and FP challenges was also collected.

### Variables and outcome measures

In this study, modern contraceptive use was the main study outcome and was defined as using any of the following methods to delay pregnancy i.e. female sterilization, intra-uterine device, injectables (depo-provera), implants, pills, condoms and emergency contraception.

### Statistical analysis

Data were entered, cleaned and analysed using Statistical Package for Social Science (SPSS) version 23.0 (SPSS, Chicago, IL, USA). Descriptive statistics were used to summarise data. Bivariate logistic regression analysis was used to examine the association between current modern contraceptive use and predictors of interest. Multivariate logistic regression analysis was used to determine independent predictors of current modern contraceptive use. *P*-value was considered statistically significant at 5% level. In a multivariate logistic regression analyses, the results were adjusted for marital status, income, intention to have more children, ever discussed with partner on the number of children, ever received counseling on modern contraceptive in CTC and disclosure of HIV status to partner.

**Table 1** Socio-demographic and economic characteristics of participants ($N = 672$)

| Characteristic | *n* (%) |
|---|---|
| Age category (years): | |
| 15–24 | 56 (8.3) |
| 25–34 | 201 (29.9) |
| 35+ | 415 (61.8) |
| Current marital status: | |
| Currently in union | 305 (45.4) |
| Never in union | 127 (18.9) |
| Formerly in union | 240 (35.7) |
| Education level: | |
| No formal education | 22 (3.3) |
| Primary education | 517 (76.9) |
| Secondary or higher education | 133 (19.8) |
| Average daily income ($n = 511$): | |
| ≤ $1 per day | 192 (37.6) |
| > $1 per day | 319 (62.4) |
| Employed and receive regular salary: | |
| Yes | 82 (12.2) |
| No | 590 (87.8) |
| District: | |
| Moshi urban | 305 (45.4) |
| Hai | 187 (27.8) |
| Mwanga | 180 (26.8) |
| Living arrangements: | |
| Living together with the partner | 270 (87.4) |
| Visits | 35 (11.3) |
| Living apart for more than 6 months | 4 (1.3) |

## Results

### General characteristics of the study participants

#### *Socio-demographic and economic characteristics of the participants*

Out of 680 HIV-positive women approached to participate in this study, 672 gave consent, giving a response rate of 98.8%. The mean (±standard deviation) age of participants at enrolment was 36.4 (±7.7) years. More than half of the study participants were aged between 35 and 49 years (61.8%), not currently married (54.6%), had primary education (76.9%), were in informal employment (88%) and living together with partner (87.3%). Table 1 shows the socio-demographic and economic characteristics of participants.

#### *Clinical, sexual and reproductive health, couple communications and counseling*

Almost half of study participants (49.0%) were diagnosed with HIV between 1 and 4 years prior to enrolment in the study. The majority of participants were on ARVs (89.1%), sexually active (60.4%), and 76.8% had multiple lifetime sexual partners. The vast majority of women (90.3%) reported to have had a child and nearly one quarter (23.8%) were intending to have more children in future. Less than half of the study participants (45.5%) reported to have ever discussed modern contraceptive use with their partners and the number of children they both wanted (42.3%). More than half (55.5%) of the study participants reported having ever received counseling on modern contraceptive use at their respective CTCs, and among those counseled, 64.9% were counseled on dual contraceptive use. Table 2 depicts clinical, sexual and reproductive health, and couple communications characteristics of participants.

### Prevalence of modern contraceptive use

The majority of participants (84%) reported that they had ever used modern contraceptive methods. The prevalence of current modern contraceptive use was 53.9% ($n = 362$). Of the 362 users, 121 (33.4%) reported using dual contraceptives (i.e. condoms and any modern contraceptive method). Of those who reported current modern

**Table 2** Clinical, sexual and reproductive health, couple communication and counseling characteristics ($N = 672$)

| Characteristics | n (%) |
|---|---|
| Duration since diagnosed with HIV: | |
| < 1 year | 35 (5.3) |
| 1–4 years | 325 (49.0) |
| 5 years or more | 303 (45.7) |
| Currently on ARVs: | |
| Yes | 599 (89.1) |
| No | 73 (10.9) |
| Duration on ARVs: | |
| < 1 year | 166 (27.7) |
| 1–4 years | 210 (35.1) |
| 5 years or more | 223 (37.2) |
| Currently sexually active: | |
| No | 266 (39.6) |
| Yes | 406 (60.4) |
| Number of lifetime sexual partner(s): | |
| Single | 156 (23.2) |
| Multiple | 516 (76.8) |
| Number of sexual partner(s) in past 12 months: | |
| Single | 625 (93.0) |
| Multiple | 47 (7.0) |
| Have children: | |
| No | 65 (9.7) |
| Yes | 607 (90.3) |
| Intend to have more children: | |
| No | 512 (76.2) |
| Yes | 160 (23.8) |
| Ever discussed with partner on number of children: | |
| No | 388 (57.7) |
| Yes | 284 (42.3) |
| Ever discussed with partner on modern contraceptive use: | |
| No | 366 (54.5) |
| Yes | 306 (45.5) |
| Ever received counseling on modern contraceptives at CTC: | |
| No | 299 (44.5) |
| Yes | 373 (55.5) |
| Ever counseled on dual contraceptives at CTC: | |
| No | 131 (35.1) |
| Yes | 242 (64.9) |
| Ever given modern contraceptives at CTC: | |
| No | 368 (54.8) |
| Yes | 304 (45.2) |

contraceptive use, more than one quarter 98 (27.1%) reported that their partners were not aware of it.

### Types of modern contraceptive methods used

The most common used modern contraceptives methods among the 362 women were male condoms (76.0%), Depo-Provera (28.2%) and implants (13.3%). Figure 1 shows types of modern contraceptive methods used by the study participants.

### Factors influencing current modern contraceptive use

Table 3 shows the results of logistic regression analysis of the independent predictors of current modern contraceptive use. In a multivariate analysis woman with primary education had a 8-fold increase in odds of current modern contraceptive use compared to those who never attended school (AOR = 7.54, 95% CI: 1.51–17.48), $P = 0.014$). Those with secondary or higher education, the odds of current modern contraceptive use was 6 times higher than those who never attended school (AOR = 6.23, 95% CI: 1. 14–14.07), $P = 0.035$). Not currently on ARVs (AOR = 11. 29, 95% CI: 2.60–19.94, $P = 0.001$); currently sexually active (AOR = 8.40, 95% CI: 4.47–15.78, $P < 0.001$); discussed modern contraceptive use with a partner (AOR = 3.68, 95% CI: 1.67–8.11, P = 0.001) and being counseled on dual contraceptive methods at a CTC (AOR = 2.94, 95% CI: 1. 66–5.23, $P < 0.001$) had significantly higher odds of current modern contraceptive use. For brevity, the common reasons for modern contraceptive non-use among study participants are presented in Fig. 2.

## Discussion

The results of this study showed that slightly more than half (54%) of the HIV-positive women between the ages of 15 and 49 were currently using modern contraceptive methods. The prevalence of current modern contraceptive use among HIV-positive women in Kilimanjaro was higher than the national (32%) and the regional (47.8% - Kilimanjaro region) prevalence in the general population [14]. It is also higher than that observed among HIV-positive women in Ethiopia (46%) [24], Rwanda (43%) [25], Ghana (43%) [26], Lesotho (35%) [17] and Uganda (28%) [27] but lower than that in women on ART in Zambia (69%) [18] and among women attending CTC care in Dar es Salaam (68.5%) [28]. A higher contraceptive use among HIV-positive women than in the general population may be due to comprehensive counseling and guidance these women receive in various HIV interventions e.g. PMTCT and CTC programmes. A facility-based study conducted in Thailand showed that the vast majority (92%) of women on a PMTCT programme were currently using modern contraceptive methods. This was higher than among those who were referred to HIV CTCs [29]. In Tanzania, most of the women attending a

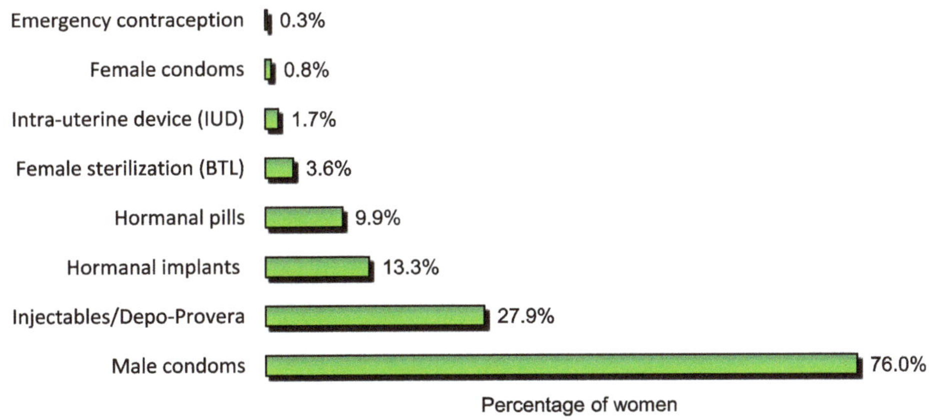


**Fig. 1** Types of modern contraceptive methods used by study participants ($n = 362$)

CTC have been referred through PMTCT programmes [30]. Through this programme (PMTCT), counseling on prevention of vertical and horizontal HIV transmission is strongly emphasised. In addition, the majority of women in this study (89%) were currently on ARVs. This group receives intensive counseling on ARV adherence and pregnancy preventions. This might have influenced the high prevalence (as compared to the general population) of current modern contraceptive use in this study.

The use of dual contraceptive methods included correct and consistent use of condoms in conjunction with another type of modern contraceptive method. Evidence from literature has shown its effectiveness (dual methods) in preventing both horizontal and vertical HIV transmission, STIs and pregnancy [5, 6, 8]. The prevalence of dual contraceptive use in this study (33%) is an increase from 19% reported by Antelman et al. among women living with HIV attending HIV clinical care in Dar es Salaam Tanzania in 2001 [19]. The prevalence of dual contraceptive use among women who reported using modern contraceptive methods was relatively higher compared to data from USA (7%) [31], Cambodia (17%) [32], Zambia (25%) [18] and Uganda (4%) [33]; but lower than that reported in Ethiopia (60%) [24] and similar to the recent reports in Dar Es Salaam, Tanzania (32.7%) [28]. The finding that only a third of those using modern contraceptives are using dual methods was in the background that most women (65%) reported to have received counseling on dual contraceptive methods in a CTC. It can be argued that counseling alone is probably not sufficient to improve dual contraceptive use, other novel interventions needs to be developed and tested.

This study showed male condoms to be the most common method of modern contraceptive used (76%) followed by Depo-Provera (28%) and implants (13%). Despite condoms being effective in preventing HIV transmission, the use of alternative effective contraceptive methods to prevent pregnancy was low in this setting. These findings are consistent with data obtained in Ghana, Nigeria, Zambia, Rwanda, Kenya and Dar Es Salaam, Tanzania where male condoms were the most common method of contraceptive used (80%, 53%, 60%, 30%, 20% and 43% respectively) [18, 26, 28, 34, 35]. However, these results are contrary to the results from the Tanzania Demographic and Health Survey whereby in Kilimanjaro region, injectables (21%) followed by implants (10%) were the most common contraceptive methods used by currently married women aged 15–49 [36]. Other results contrary to our findings were observed from Malawi whereas injectables (20%) followed by condoms (13%) [20] were the most common methods of contraceptive used, and in Ethiopia where injectables (71%) were followed by male condoms (48%) [37]. It seems possible that the male condom is a method of contraceptive used frequently by most study participants, as they are more easily available and accessible in the society than other long-term contraceptive methods. In this setting, condoms are obtainable in drug dispensing units, clinics, supermarkets and other marketing areas. Also, the fact that 16% of women who did not use certain modern contraceptive methods due to their fear of side effects, might have favoured the use of the male condom.

Couple communication was a strong predictor of modern contraceptive use in this study. HIV-positive women who reported of ever discussing with the partner on any of the Sexual and Reproductive Health (SRH) issues such as: number of children they wanted, contraceptive use or HIV testing, had significantly higher odds of using modern contraceptives than others. There is a need to introduce couple-communication interventions and interventions that increase the skills of women in negotiating and communicating with partners on SRH issues. Couple communication has not only shown to increase modern contraceptive use in India, Zambia and Malawi [38, 39], but it has also known to improve other maternal and child health indicators like adherence to ART and PMTCT interventions, minimizing loss to

**Table 3** Factors influencing current modern contraceptive use ($N = 672$)

| Characteristics | Modern contraceptive use (%) | COR¥ (95% CI) | AOR[a] (95% CI) |
|---|---|---|---|
| *Education level* | | | |
| Never attended to school | 31.8 | 1 | 1 |
| Primary education | 52.6 | 2.38 (0.95–5.93) | 23.83 (2.84–331.45)* |
| Secondary/higher education | 62.4 | 3.56 (1.36–9.32) | 13.35 (1.50–187.80)* |
| *Marital status* | | | |
| Never in union | 53.5 | 1 | |
| Currently in union | 71.8 | 2.21 (1.44–3.39)* | |
| Formerly union | 31.3 | 0.39 (0.25–0.61)* | |
| *Level of daily income (n = 511)* | | | |
| ≤ $1 | 49.5 | 1 | |
| > $1 | 58.6 | 1.45 (1.01–2.07)* | |
| *Current on ARV* | | | |
| Yes | 52.3 | 1 | 1 |
| No | 67.1 | 1.87 (1.12–3.12)* | 19.21 (2.60–141.75)** |
| *Intend to have more children* | | | |
| No | 59.4 | 1 | |
| Yes | 68.1 | 2.18 (1.50–3.18)* | |
| *Currently sexually active* | | | |
| No | 19.2 | 1 | 1 |
| Yes | 76.6 | 13.80 (9.42–20.22)** | 12.29 (5.62–26.89)** |
| *Ever discussed with partner on modern contraceptive use* | | | |
| No | 39.1 | 1 | 1 |
| Yes | 71.6 | 3.93 (2.84–5.43) ** | 5.26 (1.94–14.26)* |
| *Ever discussed with partner on number of children* | | | |
| No | 45.6 | 1 | |
| Yes | 65.1 | 2.23 (1.63–3.05) ** | |
| *Received counseling on contraceptives at CTC* | | | |
| No | 36.8 | 1 | |
| Yes | 67.6 | 3.58 (2.60–4.93) ** | |
| *Counseled on dual contraceptives at CTC (n = 373)* | | | |
| No | 50.4 | 1 | 1 |
| Yes | 76.9 | 3.27 (2.08–5.15) ** | 2.72 (1.29–5.76)** |
| *Disclosed HIV status to partner* | | | |
| No | 40.8 | 1 | |
| Yes | 62.8 | 2.44 (1.78–3.35) ** | |

¥*COR* Crude odds ratio, *AOR* Adjusted Odds Ratio
*Indicates $p$-value < 0.05, **Indicates $p$-value < 0.001
[a]The results are adjusted for marital status, income, intention to have more children, ever discussed with partner on the number of children, ever received counseling on modern contraceptive in CTC and disclosure of HIV status to partner

follow up in ART/PMTCT programs as well as improving HIV disclosure [40].

Report of receiving counseling on contraceptives and on dual methods, as well as availability of contraceptive methods at CTC were the health facility factors associated with modern contraceptive use in this study. These findings were consistent with report by Polisi et al. in the Western Ethiopia in 2014 [21]. Tanzania developed guidelines on integration of FP services into HIV CTC in 2013. Adherence to this recommendation is not known, but evidence of this work highlight the need to have a 'supermarket' approach in that all the centres offering HIV care and treatment

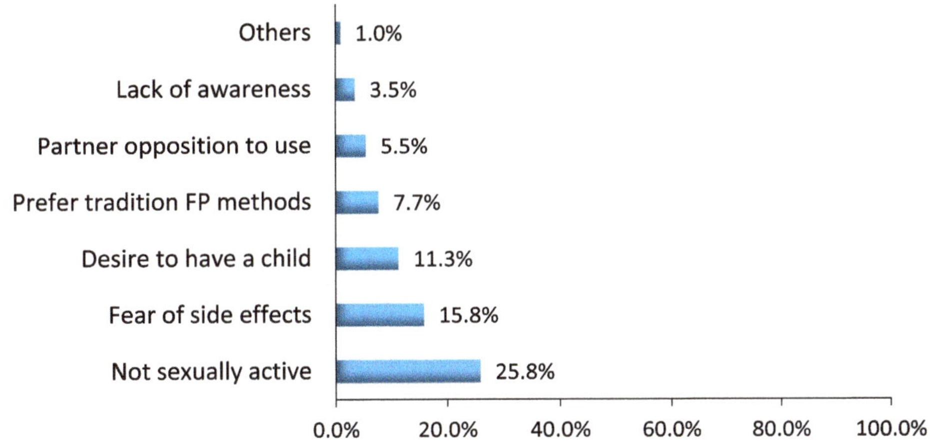


**Fig. 2** Common reasons for not using modern contraceptive methods ($n = 310$)

services should also offer FP services in the same setting to minimise referrals. Integration of FP services and counseling in CTC improve contraceptive uptakes as evidenced by both experimental and observational studies in different settings [41–44].

The generalisability of these results is subject to certain limitations. For instance, contraceptive use was based on self-report by the women i.e. no method was available to confirm the reported information. However, women might have reported what they thought research assistants wanted to hear, or what was perceived as socially correct, which would have underestimated or overestimated the prevalence obtained in this study. The major strength of this study lies in the population studied which represent both rural and urban settings. The information can fairly represent HIV-positive women in Kilimanjaro region. Another key strength is the high response rate by the study participants.

## Conclusion

Almost one in two women in this study who knew their HIV status were not using any barrier or hormonal methods to prevent unwanted pregnancies or HIV transmission to uninfected partners. The consequence of low CPR in this context and a high unmet need for FP is a high number of unwanted/unplanned pregnancies which can further be linked with risk of exposing children to HIV infection unnecessarily. Programme managers and health care providers need to identify counseling strategies that are specific to HIV-positive women that not only impart knowledge on contraceptives, but also address the issue of responsibility for influencing HIV transmission in the community. Planners need to come up with strategies involving couple communications so as to increase the use of adequate and effective contraceptives methods in preventing unwanted pregnancies in this population.

### Abbreviations

AOR: Adjusted odds ratio; CI: Confidence interval; COR: Crude odds ratio; CPR: Contraceptive prevalence rate; CTC: Care and treatment clinics; FP: Family planning; MTCT: Mother-to-child-transmission; PMTCT: Prevention of mother-to-child transmission; SSA: Sub-Saharan Africa

### Acknowledgements

The authors thank the Regional Medical Officer, Medical Officers and clinics in charge in Moshi urban, Hai and Mwanga districts for giving permission to conduct this study in their facilities. We also thank the study participants for their valuable participation in this study. Furthermore, we would like to thank the research assistants for their positive participation and involvement in this study.

### Authors' contributions

DJD, BT and SEM designed the study. DJD, JG and EM collected data. DJD, JG and SEM analysed the data and drafted the manuscript. DJD, JG, BT and SEM contributed to the final draft of the manuscript. All authors gave their final approval to the manuscript.

### Author details

[1]Department of Community Medicine, Kilimanjaro Christian Medical Centre (KCMC), Moshi, Tanzania. [2]Department of Epidemiology & Biostatistics, Institute of Public Health, KCMUCo, P. O. Box 2240, Moshi, Tanzania. [3]Kilimanjaro Christian Medical University College (KCMUCo), Moshi, Tanzania. [4]Department of Community Health, Institute of Public Health, KCMUCo, Moshi, Tanzania.

### References

1. WHO. Sexual and reproductive health of women living with HIV/AIDS: guidelines on care, Treatment and support for women living with HIV/AIDS and their children in resource-constrained settings. 2006.
2. Darroch JE, Sedgh G, Ball H. Contraceptive technologies: responding to Women's needs. New York: Guttmacher Institute; 2011. p. 1–51.
3. Singh S, Sedgh G, Hussain R. Unintended pregnancy: worldwide levels, trends, and outcomes. Stud Fam Plan. 2010;41:241–50. https://doi.org/10.1111/j.1728-4465.2010.00250.x.
4. Hubacher D, Mavranezouli I, McGinn E. Unintended pregnancy in sub-Saharan Africa: magnitude of the problem and potential role of contraceptive implants to alleviate it. Contraception. 2008;78:73–8. https://doi.org/10.1016/j.contraception.2008.03.002.
5. Bongaarts J, Cleland J, Townsend JW, Betrand JT, Gupta M. Family planning programs for the 21st century: Rationale and design. New York: The Population Council; 2012.
6. Rutenberg N, Baek C. Field experiences integrating family planning into programs to prevent mother-to-child transmission of HIV. Stud Fam Plan. 2005;36:235–45.

7. Souza JP, Cecatti JG, Haddad SM, Parpinelli MA, Costa ML, Katz L, et al. The WHO maternal near-miss approach and the maternal severity index model (MSI): tools for assessing the Management of Severe Maternal Morbidity. PLoS One 2012;7. doi:https://doi.org/10.1371/journal.pone.0044129.
8. Halperin DT, Stover J, Reynolds HW. Benefits and costs of expanding access to family planning programs to women living with HIV. AIDS. 2009;23(Suppl 1):S123–30. https://doi.org/10.1097/01.aids.0000363785.73450.5a.
9. Reynolds HW, Steiner MJ, Cates W. Contraception's proved potential to fight HIV. Sex Transm Infect. 2005;81:184–5. https://doi.org/10.1136/sti.2004.012013.
10. WHO. Guidance on global scale-up of the prevention of mother-child transmission of HIV: towards universal access for women, infants and young children and eliminating HIV and AIDS among children. Geneva: WHO; 2007.
11. WHO. PMTCT strategic vision 2010–2015. Geneva: World Health Organization; 2011.
12. UNAIDS. The gap report: children and pregnant women living with HIV. Geneva: UNAIDS; 2014.
13. Sedgh G, Hussain R, Ashfordand LS. Unmet need for contraception in developing countries: examining Women's reasons for not using a method. New York: Guttmacher Institute; 2016.
14. Ministry of Health, Community Development, Gender, Elderly and Children (MoHCDGEC) [TanzaniaMainland], Ministry of Health (MoH) [Zanzibar], National Bureau of Statistics (NBS), Office of the Chief Government Statistician (OCGS), and ICF. Tanzania Demographic and Health Survey and Malaria Indicator Survey (TDHS-MIS) 2015-16. Dar es Salaam, Tanzania, and Rockville, Maryland, USA: MoHCDGEC, MoH, NBS, OCGS, and ICF, 2016.
15. Gebre G, Birhan N, Gebreslasie K. Prevalence and factors associated with unmet need for family planning among the currently married reproductive age women in Shire-Enda- Slassie, northern west of Tigray, Ethiopia 2015: a community based cross-sectional study. Pan Afr Med J. 2016;23:195. https://doi.org/10.11604/pamj.2016.23.195.8386.
16. Kassebaum NJ, Bertozzi-Villa A, Coggeshall MS, Shackelford KA, Steiner C, Heuton KR, et al. Saving mothers in South Africa. South African Med J. 2014; 10:1–9. https://doi.org/10.1086/605027.
17. Adair T. Desire for children and unmet need for contraception among HIV-positive women in Lesotho. Maryland, USA: Calverton; 2007.
18. Hancock NL, Chibwesha CJ, Bosomprah S, Newman J, Mubiana-Mbewe M, Sitali ES, et al. Contraceptive use among HIV-infected women and men receiving antiretroviral therapy in Lusaka, Zambia: a cross-sectional survey. BMC Public Health. 2016;16:392. https://doi.org/10.1186/s12889-016-3070-5.
19. Antelman G, Medley A, Mbatia R, Pals S, Arthur G, Haberlen S, et al. Pregnancy desire and dual method contraceptive use among people living with HIV attending clinical care in Kenya, Namibia and Tanzania. J Fam Plan Reprod Heal Care. 2015;41:e1. https://doi.org/10.1136/jfprhc-2013-100784.
20. Habte D, Namasasu J. Family planning use among women living with HIV: knowing HIV positive status helps - results from a national survey. Reprod Health. 2015;12:41. https://doi.org/10.1186/s12978-015-0035-6.
21. Polisi A, Gebrehanna E, Tesfaye G, Asefa F. Modern contraceptive utilization among female ART attendees in health facilities of Gimbie town, West Ethiopia. Reprod Health. 2014;11:30. https://doi.org/10.1186/1742-4755-11-30.
22. National Bureau of Statistics. Population distribution by age and sex. Dar Es Salaam/Tanzania: NBS & OCGS; 2013.
23. Tanzania Commission for AIDS (TACAIDS), Zanzibar AIDS Commission (ZAC), National Bureau of Statistics (NBS), Office of the Chief Government Statistician (OCGS), and ICF International. Tanzania HIV/AIDS and Malaria Indicator Survey 2011-12. Dar es Salaam, Tanzania: TACAIDS, ZAC, NBS, OCGS and ICF International; 2013.
24. Berhane Y, Berhe H, Abera GB, Berhe H. Utilization of modern contraceptives among HIV positive reproductive age women in Tigray, Ethiopia: a cross sectional study. Isrn Aids. 2013;2013:319724. https://doi.org/10.1155/2013/319724.
25. Elul B, Delvaux T, Munyana E, Lahuerta M, Horowitz D, Ndagije F, et al. Pregnancy desires, and contraceptive knowledge and use among prevention of mother-to-child transmission clients in Rwanda. AIDS. 2009; 23(Suppl 1):S19–26. https://doi.org/10.1097/01.aids.0000363774.91376.dc.
26. Laryea DO, Amoako YA, Spangenberg K, Frimpong E, Kyei-Ansong J. Contraceptive use and unmet need for family planning among HIV positive women on antiretroviral therapy in Kumasi, Ghana. BMC Womens Health. 2014;14:126. https://doi.org/10.1186/1472-6874-14-126.
27. Muyindike W, Fatch R, Steinfield R, Matthews LT, Musinguzi N, Emenyonu NI, et al. Contraceptive use and associated factors among women enrolling into HIV care in southwestern Uganda. Infect Dis Obstet Gynecol 2012;2012. doi:https://doi.org/10.1155/2012/340782.
28. Kashagam E, Ngocho JS. Prevalence of modern contraceptive methods use among women living with HIV attending care and treatment clinic at Amana Hospital Dar Es Salaam, Tanzania. Int J Soc Sci Humanit Invent. 2015; 2:1740–6. https://doi.org/10.18535/ijsshi/v2i12.04.
29. Delvaux T, Nöstlinger C. Reproductive choice for women and men living with HIV: contraception, abortion and fertility. Reprod Health Matters. 2007; 15:46–66. https://doi.org/10.1016/S0968-8080(07)29031-7.
30. MoHSW. Tanzania Elimination of Mother To Child Transmission of HIV Plan, 2012–2015. Dar Es Salaam, Tanzania: MoHSW; 2013.
31. Chakrapani V, Kershaw T, Shunmugam M, Newman PA, Cornman DH, Dubrow R. Prevalence of and barriers to dual-contraceptive methods use among married men and women living with HIV in India. Infect Dis Obstet Gynecol 2011;2011. doi:https://doi.org/10.1155/2011/376432.
32. Nakaie N, Tuon S, Nozaki I, Yamaguchi F, Sasaki Y, Kakimoto K. Family planning practice and predictors of risk of inconsistent condom use among HIV-positive women on anti-retroviral therapy in Cambodia. BMC Public Health. 2014;14:170. https://doi.org/10.1186/1471-2458-14-170.
33. Homsy J, Bunnell R, Moore D, King R, Malamba S, Nakityo R, et al. Reproductive intentions and outcomes among women on antiretroviral therapy in rural Uganda: a prospective cohort study. PLoS One. 2009;4: e4149. https://doi.org/10.1371/journal.pone.0004149.
34. Imbuki K, Todd CS, Stibich M a, Shaffer DN, Sinei SK. Factors influencing contraceptive choice and discontinuation among HIV-positive women in Kericho, Kenya. Afr J Reprod Health 2010;14:98–109. doi:https://doi.org/10.2307/41329759.
35. Ezechi OC. Contraceptive behavior, practices and associated factors among Nigerian women living with human immunodeficiency virus infection. J HIV Hum Reprod. 2013;1:30.
36. Ministry of Health CDGE and C-MM, MoH/Zanzibar M of H-, NBS/Tanzania NB of S-, OCGS/Zanzibar O of CGS-, ICF Tanzania Demographic and Health Survey and Malaria Indicator Survey 2015–2016 2016.
37. Melaku YA, Zeleke EG. Contraceptive utilization and associated factors among HIV positive women on chronic follow up care in Tigray region, northern Ethiopia: a cross sectional study. PLoS One. 2014;9:e94682. https://doi.org/10.1371/journal.pone.0094682.
38. Chakrapani V, Kershaw T, Shunmugam M, Newman PA, Cornman DH, Dubrow R. Prevalence of and barriers to dual-contraceptive methods use among married men and women living with HIV in India. Infect Dis Obstet Gynecol. 2011;2011:376432. https://doi.org/10.1155/2011/376432.
39. Grabbe K, Stephenson R, Vwalika B, Ahmed Y, Vwalika C, Chomba E, et al. Knowledge, use, and concerns about contraceptive methods among sero-discordant couples in Rwanda and Zambia. J Women's Health (Larchmt). 2009;18:1449–56. https://doi.org/10.1089/jwh.2008.1160.
40. Msuya SE, Mbizvo EM, Hussain A, Uriyo J, Sam NE, Stray-Pedersen B. Low male partner participation in antenatal HIV counselling and testing in northern Tanzania: implications for preventive programs. AIDS Care. 2008;20: 700–9. https://doi.org/10.1080/09540120701687059.
41. King R, Khana K, Nakayiwa S, Katuntu D, Homsy J, Lindkvist P, et al. "Pregnancy comes accidentally–like it did with me": reproductive decisions among women on ART and their partners in rural Uganda. BMC Public Health. 2011;11:530. https://doi.org/10.1186/1471-2458-11-530.
42. Schwartz SR, Rees H, Mehta S, Venter WDF, Taha TE, Black V. High incidence of unplanned pregnancy after antiretroviral therapy initiation: findings from a prospective cohort study in South Africa. PLoS One. 2012;7:e36039. https://doi.org/10.1371/journal.pone.0036039.
43. Cohen CR, Grossman D, Onono M, Blat C, Newmann SJ, Burger RL, et al. Integration of family planning services into HIV care clinics: Results one year after a cluster randomized controlled trial in Kenya. PLoS One. 2017;12: e0172992. https://doi.org/10.1371/journal.pone.0172992.
44. Lopez LM, Hilgenberg D, Chen M, Denison J, Stuart G. Behavioral interventions for improving contraceptive use among women living with HIV. Cochrane Database Syst Rev. 2013:8–11. https://doi.org/10.1002/14651858.CD010243.pub2.

# Contraceptive use among HIV-positive and negative women: Implication to end unintended pregnancy

Amanual Getnet Mersha[1], Daniel Asfaw Erku[2], Sewunet Admasu Belachew[3], Asnakew Achaw Ayele[3], Begashaw Melaku Gebresillassie[3] and Tadesse Melaku Abegaz[3*]

## Abstract

**Background:** With the advancement of antiretroviral therapy and improved life expectancy, women living with HIV/AIDS are enjoying a better sexual life. Yet, the consistent utilization of contraceptive in such patients is highly recommended. There is paucity of data regarding contraceptive use among HIV-positive and negative women in Ethiopia. The present study aimed at examining the use of contraceptives among HIV-positive and HIV-negative women in Ethiopia.

**Methods:** A comparative cross-sectional study was conducted among HIV-positive and HIV-negative women attending family planning Clinic of Gondar university referral hospital between January 2016 and August 2017. Descriptive statistics were used to present categorical data and Pearson's chi-square test was done to examine differences in the utilization of contraceptives between HIV-positive and HIV-negative women. Kaplan Meier test was also carried out to determine the incidence of unintended pregnancy. A *p*-value of 0.05 was deemed significant with corresponding 95% confidence intervals.

**Results:** A total of 894 participants consisting of 314 HIV-positive and 580 HIV-negative women were included in the study. The rate of previous unintended pregnancy was 280 (31.3%) in HIV-negative women and 115 (12.9%) in HIV-infected women. Women who routinely utilized contraceptives were more likely to avoid unintended pregnancy [log rank: 2.89, $p < 0.05$]. Unlike HIV-negative women (2.9%), HIV-positive (28.4%) women reported a higher rate of intrauterine device use. Male condom was used more commonly in HIV-infected women (26.7%) as compared to HIV negative (3.9%) women (*p-value* < *0.05*).

**Conclusions:** Intrauterine contraceptive device was reported to be the most commonly used contraceptive method in HIV patients. Further, unintended pregnancy was relatively common in women with low contraceptive practice. The use of dual contraceptives should be advocated for HIV-positive women so as to protect unintended pregnancy and curtail the transmission of HIV.

**Keywords:** Contraceptive use, Ethiopia, HIV-positive women, Unintended pregnancy

* Correspondence: abegaztadesse981@gmail.com
[3]Department of Clinical Pharmacy, School of Pharmacy, College of Medicine and Health Sciences, University of Gondar, Gondar, Ethiopia

## Background

Globally, 36.7 million people were living with HIV/AIDS at the end of 2016 and 50% of all adults with HIV infection were women [1]. Approximately, 70% of HIV infected individuals are located in sub-Saharan Africa. In Ethiopia, an estimate number of 1.1 million people are supposed to live with HIV at the end of 2010 and the prevalence is higher in females (1.9%) than males (1.2%) [2–5].

According to the 2016 Ethiopia demographic and health survey report, one in every three currently married women used a method of contraception mostly modern methods [2]. In addition, nearly one fourth of the current users (23%) were on injectable contraceptive method; 8% were using long acting or permanent methods; and, 4% of them were utilizing condom [2, 6].

HIV-infected women are at substantial risk of unintended pregnancy and other sexually transmitted infections (STIs). Hence, the recommended method of contraceptive is dual contraceptive method. Dual contraception is a utilization of one of the highly effective modern contraception coupled with condom to ensure protection from unintended pregnancy as well as STIs [9, 10].

A 2010 study conducted in Zambia reported the rate of dual contraceptive use to be 17.7% among all clients living with HIV/AIDS [7]. A comparative study conducted in Uganda reported that as compared to HIV negative individuals, sexually active HIV infected young counter people are less likely to use contraception and condoms [8] that make them vulnerable for other sexually transmitted infections, unintended pregnancy and its complications.

One of the most effective approaches to prevent mother to child HIV transmission is decreasing the rate of unintended pregnancy [9]. Irrespective of HIV status unintended pregnancy and unprotected sexual intercourse causes a major morbidity and mortality. In contrast to HIV none infected women, HIV infected women should consider multiple conditions including, the risk of having severe form of other sexually transmitted infections, resistant strains of HIV and greater risk of morbidity and mortality during pregnancy as well as motherhood period. Furthermore, HIV infected individuals are at risk of transmitting HIV to their uninfected partners. [10–12].

Irrespective of the HIV status of a woman, the inappropriate utilization of contraceptive leads to unintended pregnancy. All around the globe an estimated 80 million unintended pregnancies occur each year and the majority ended up in unsafe abortion [13, 14]. Unplanned pregnancy and unprotected sex may lead to many complications including but not limited to unsafe abortion, transmission of STIs, delayed or no prenatal care, poor maternal mental health, reduced quality of mother/child relationship, physical abuse and violence against women, poor developmental outcomes for children, increased risk of low birth weight as well as increased morbidity and mortality. The complications of unintended pregnancy were found to be significantly higher in HIV infected individuals [10–12].

There is paucity of data regarding the use of contraceptives among HIV-positive and negative women in Ethiopia. Evaluating current contraceptive use will enable clinicians to properly select and allocate appropriate contraceptive for both HIV infected and non-infected mothers. The current study aimed to determine the pattern of contraceptive use among HIV-positive and HIV-negative women. In addition, we intended to estimate unintended pregnancy in the set-up. It intends to help policymakers, service providers and program coordinators in Ethiopia to identify the difference that being HIV infected imposes on the choice of contraceptive methods as such evidence is an essential part to improve the reproductive health service delivery to HIV positive individuals.

## Methods

### Study design and setting

A comparative cross-sectional study was conducted to assess pattern of contraceptive use among HIV positive and HIV negative women attending family planning Clinic of Gondar university referral hospital (GURH), Northwest Ethiopia from January 2016 to August 2017. GURH is a teaching and referral hospital with more than 1000 beds and a range of specialties including internal medicine, pediatrics, surgery, gynecology, psychiatry, HIV/AIDS care and outpatient clinics.

### Study population and sampling technique

Sample size was determined using single population proportion formula considering the following assumptions: prevalence of unplanned pregnancy = 34% [21], confidence level of 95%, and a 5% degree of precision. Taking non-respondent rate = 10%, the final minimum sample size was 378. A convenience sample of HIV-negative and HIV-positive women who visited the family planning clinic of GURH during the study period was included in the study. Women who were unable to give the required information due to serious illness were excluded.

### Data collection procedure

Data was collected using an interviewer administered questionnaire. The data collection tool was created by modifying items from previously used instruments regarding contraceptive use among HIV-positive and HIV-negative women [7]. All items were thoroughly reviewed for relevance and content validity by a team of experts. The survey instrument was further validated by pre-testing on 20 participants who were not included in the final analysis. After the pretest, appropriate modifications were taken to the final questionnaire.

### Data analysis

Data were entered into and analyzed using Statistical Package for the Social Sciences (SPSS) software version 21.0 for windows. Descriptive data was presented as mean, standard deviation and percentages. Pearson's chi-square test was used to examine the differences in contraceptive use between the study groups. Kaplan Meier test was carried out to examine the incidence of unintended pregnancy. A *p*-value of 0.05 was deemed significant with a corresponding 95% confidence interval (CI).

### Ethical considerations

This study was approved by the Institutional review board of University of Gondar. Informed written consent was obtained from each participant before starting the interview and participants were also told their right to stop the interview at anytime. The participants were also told that participation is based on their willingness. The obtained information was kept anonymous and recorded in such a way that the respondent could never be known.

## Results

### Socio demographic and clinical characteristics of participants

A total of 894 women were approached for the study that consist of 314 HIV-positive and 580 HIV-negative women. All of the invited women responded for the interview. The mean age of participants was 35 ± 3.21 years for HIV positive women and 33 ± 4.33 years for HIV-negative women. Nearly half of the respondents (49.7%) were urban residents and one third of the participants (32.5%) never went to school in both groups. Detailed socio-demographic characteristics of participants are presented in Table 1.

**Table 1** Socio demographic characteristic of participants, ($n = 894$)

| Variables | HIV Positive ($N = 314$) | HIV Negative ($N = 580$) | *P* - value |
|---|---|---|---|
| Age | | | 0.56 |
| Mean ± SD | 35 ± 3.21 | 33 ± 4.33 | |
| 16–24 | 16(4.2%) | 144(24.8%) | |
| 25–34 | 143(45.5%) | 258(44.4%) | |
| ≥35 | 155(49.3%) | 178(30.7%) | |
| Residency | | | 0.36 |
| Urban | 156(49.7%) | 281(48.5%) | |
| Rural | 158(50.3%) | 299(51.5%) | |
| Education | | | 0.38 |
| Never went to school | 102(32.5%) | 193(33.3%) | |
| Primary school | 100(31.8%) | 178(30.7%) | |
| High school | 86(27.4%) | 151(26%) | |
| College and above | 26(8.3%) | 58(10.1%) | |
| Employment status | | | 0.27 |
| Government employed | 112(35.7%) | 214(36.9%) | |
| Unemployed | 202(64.3%) | 366(63.1%) | |
| Monthly household income | | | 0.67 |
| < 500 birrs | 8(2.5%) | 133(22.9%) | |
| 500–1000 birrs | 198(63.1%) | 364(62.7%) | |
| > 1000 birrs | 108(34.4) | 83(14.4) | |
| Mean ± SD | 981 ± 102 | 952 ± 123 | 0.09 |
| Marital status | | | 0.81 |
| Single | 14(4.5%) | 106(18.3%) | |
| Married | 192(61.1%) | 394(67.9%) | |
| Separated | 52(16.6%) | 54(9.3%) | |
| Widowed | 56(17.8%) | 26(4.5%) | |

**Table 2** Reproductive and clinical characteristics of clients attending Gondar university hospital, $n = 894$

| Variables | HIV Positive ($N = 314$) | HIV Negative ($N = 580$) | Chi-square test ($\times^2$), *p- value* |
|---|---|---|---|
| Number of previous pregnancies | | | 0.71, 4.93 |
| None | 19(6.1%) | 41(7%) | |
| Once times | 86(27.3%) | 159(27.4%) | |
| Twice times | 114(36.3%) | 204(35.2%) | |
| Three or more times | 95(30.2%) | 176(30.3%) | |
| Pregnancy intention | | | 0.04, $\times^2$, 3.18 |
| Intended pregnancy | 199(63.4%) | 300(33.6%) | |
| Unintended pregnancy | 115 (36.6%) | 280 (31.3%) | |
| Mean ± SD | 2.4 ± 1.1 | 2.6 ± 1.3 | 0.4, $\times^2$,6.75 |
| Number of living children | | | 0.60, $\times^2$,1.49 |
| None | 26(8.3%) | 44(7.6%) | |
| One child | 92(29.3%) | 172(29.6%) | |
| Two children | 112(35.6%) | 201(34.6%) | |
| Three or more children | 84(26.7%) | 163(28.1%) | |
| Mean ± SD | 2.2 ± 1.2 | 2.1 ± 1.3 | 0.07, $\times^2$,1.85 |
| Desired number of children | | | |
| None | 13(4.1%) | 16(2.75) | |
| One child | 65(20.7%) | 93(16%) | |
| Two children | 158(50.3%) | 313(53.9%) | |
| Three or more children | 78(24.8%) | 158(27.2%) | |
| Mean ± SD | 2 ± 1.1 | 2.4 ± 1.4 | 0.06, $\times^2$,0.98 |
| Number of sex partners in last 12 months | | | 0.10, $\times^2$,1.63 |
| One | 198(63.1%) | 389(67.1%) | |
| Two | 109(34.7%) | 174(30%) | |
| Three or more | 7(2.2) | 17(2.9%) | |
| Mean ± SD | 1.8 ± 1.3 | 1.6 ± 0.9 | 0.52, $\times^2$,0.59 |
| Menstrual irregularity | | | 0.51, $\times^2$,5.2 |
| Yes | 47(14.9%) | 88(15.2%) | |
| No | 267(85.1%) | 492(84.8%) | |
| Chronic illness other than HIV/AIDS | | | 0.93, $\times^2$,2.6 |
| Yes | 19(6.1%) | 19(3.3%) | |
| No | 295(93.9%) | 561(96.7%) | |
| Knowledge of partner's HIV status | | | 0.31, $\times^2$,0.74 |
| Yes | 255(81.2%) | 521(89.8%) | |
| No | 59(18.8%) | 59(10.2%) | |
| Desired number of childrenfulfilled | | | 0.75, $\times^2$, 1.8 |
| Yes | 205(65.3%) | 434(74.8%) | |
| No | 109(34.7%) | 146(25.2%) | |
| Partner desires same number children | | | 0.06, $\times^2$, 1.3 |
| Yes | 202(64.3%) | 437(75.3%) | |
| No | 98(3.2%) | 37(6.4%) | |
| Has no partner | 14(4.5) | 106(18.3%) | |
| Feeling if unexpectedly pregnant today | | | $P < 0.05$, $X^2$,1.7 |
| I would feel sad | 223(71.1%) | 192(33.1%) | |

**Table 2** Reproductive and clinical characteristics of clients attending Gondar university hospital, $n = 894$ *(Continued)*

| Variables | HIV Positive ($N = 314$) | HIV Negative ($N = 580$) | Chi-square test ($\times^2$), *p- value* |
|---|---|---|---|
| I would feel happy | 64(20.4%) | 294(50.7%) | |
| Indifferent | 27(8.5%) | 94(16.2%) | |
| History of STI within one year | | | 0.01, $X^2$ =2.9 |
| Yes | 146(46.5%) | 52(8.9%) | |
| No | 168(53.5%) | 528(91.1%) | |
| Partner with previous STI | | | 0.04, $X^2$ =1.3 |
| Yes | 101(32.2%) | 49(8.4%) | |
| No | 213(67.8%) | 531(91.6%) | |

**Reproductive and clinical characteristics of participants**

About 63.1% of HIV positive and 67.1% of HIV negative women reported to have only one sexual partner in the last 12 months period, and over a quarter of participants knew the sero-status of their partner. About 146(46.5%) of clients in the HIV infected group reported history of STI in the last 12 months as compared to 52(8.9%) with ($p = 0.01$, $\times^2 = 2.9$) in non HIV infected women. Furthermore, 101(32.2%) of HIV positive women had partner history of STI as compared to 49(8.4%) in the HIV negative women. The rate of unintended pregnancy was 31.32% in HIV-negative women versus 12.86% in HIV-infected women (Table 2).

**HIV and HAART characteristics of HIV positive women**

From a total of 314 HIV infected women, 153 (48.7%) were one HAART with a mean duration of HAART use of $10 \pm 2.34$ months. The mean duration of time since the diagnosis of HIV/AIDS was $2.7 \pm 1.21$ with a mean CD4 count of $692 \pm 102.4$ cells/m$^3$. Approximately, three fourth 229 (73%) of women know the sero-status of their current partner and 233(74.2%) had disclosed their HIV status to their partner. Around 107 (34.1%) of clients had experienced stigmatization at least once in their life since acquisition of HIV (Table 3).

**Contraceptive method utilization**

Intrauterine contraceptive device (IUCD) was reported to be used in 28.4% of HIV patients as compared to only 2.9% among HIV negative clients. Male condom was used more frequently in HIV patients (26.7%) as compared to HIV negative women (3.9%). Around 6.4% of HIV-positive women used dual contraceptive methods. Nearly a half of HIV-negative clients (50.1%) used injectable contraceptive method as compared to 25.8% of HIV positive women (Table 4).

**The effect of contraceptive use on the rate of unintended pregnancy**

When women are followed for a mean period of three years for the trend of their past contraceptive use, those who routinely utilize contraceptive tended to avoid unintended pregnancy, [log rank: 2.89, $p$ - *value* $<$ 0.05].(Fig. 1).

## Discussion

Evaluation of contraceptive use among HIV sero-positive patients is essential so as to achieve effective control of unintended pregnancy and mother to child transmission of the retrovirus. Unintended pregnancy remained a major problem in developing nations particularly among HIV-positive women [4]. The current study aimed to compare the pattern of contraceptive use among HIV-positive and negative women.

In the present study, the use of at least one method of contraception was reported to be higher both in HIV infected 93.63% and HIV negative women (73.1%). However, previous studies reported low rate of contraceptive

**Table 3** HIV and HAART characteristics of HIV positive women ($n = 314$)

| Variables | Frequency N (%) |
|---|---|
| HAART | |
| Yes | 153(48.7%) |
| No | 161(51.3%) |
| HIV status of current partner | |
| HIV Positive | 229(73%) |
| HIV Negative | 49(15.6%) |
| I don't know | 36(11.4%) |
| Time since HIV diagnosis years | $2.7 \pm 1.21$ |
| Duration of HAART use in months (Mean ± SD) | $10 \pm 2.34$ |
| Ever been stigma | |
| Stigmatized | 207(65.9%) |
| Non- Stigmatized | 107(34.1%) |
| Disclosed for the partner' | |
| Yes | 233(74.2%) |
| No | 81(25.8%) |
| CD4 count(mean ± SD) | $692 \pm 102.4$ cells/m$^3$ |

**Table 4** Types of contraceptive method used among HIV- positive and HIV-negative individuals

| Method preference | HIV- Positive (294,93.63) | HIV-Negative (424, 73.1) | $X^2$ -test, *p-value* |
|---|---|---|---|
| Oral contraceptive pills (OCP) of available type | 22(7%) | 48(12.1%) | 2.6,p < 0.05 |
| Injectable (Depot) | 81(25.8%) | 294(50.1%) | 1.03, p < 0.05 |
| Implant (Jadelle or Implanon) | 16(5.1%) | 40(6.9%) | 4.01, p < 0.05 |
| Intra uterine contraceptive device (IUCD) | 89(28.4%) | 17(2.9%) | 1.9, p < 0.05 |
| Consistent male condom use | 84(26.7%) | 23(3.9%) | 2.8. p < 0.05 |
| Consistent female condom use | 2(0.6%) | 2(0.3%) | 2.7, p < 0.05 |
| Dual contraceptive methods (condom and hormonal methods) | 20(6.4%) | 0(0%) | 1.56, p < 0.05 |

use in the same set-up. This discrepancy might be due to the changing attitude of clients towards family planning and the decline of risk of HIV transmission through interventions at antenatal care units and HIV follow-up clinics. Comparative study has been obtained from Addis Ababa, Ethiopia, in which about three-fourth of HIV infected women and nearly two-third of HIV non-infected women utilize contraceptive [15]. Contraceptive use was reported to be 34 and 59% among HIV-positive and negative individuals respectively among Ugandan population respectively [8]. Whereas, 42.6% of HIV -infected women were found to utilize a contraception method in Ghanaian society [16].

Our study revealed that, HIV positive patients usually utilized Intrauterine contraceptive device (IUCD) as compared to HIV negative clients who instead preferred hormonal contraceptives.. This might be due to the fact that hormonal contraceptives are expected to have untoward possible pharmacokinetic interactions between antiretroviral drugs which directs the preference to intrauterine device and condom use for HIV- positive clients on HAART [17]. In addition, the proportion of male condom use was significantly higher among HIV-positive women 84(26.7%) than HIV-negative ladies 23(3.9%). This finding is consistent with a study conducted in Malawi [18]. Condom is supposed to play dual purpose to protect both unintended pregnancy and STI. HIV-positive couples are advised to use this backup method as long as they decide to have sexual intercourse which by far increases the rate of utilization of condom as compared to HIV-negative mothers.

The utilization of dual contraceptive methods found to be frequently observed among HIV-positive patients. None of the respondents reported dual contraceptive

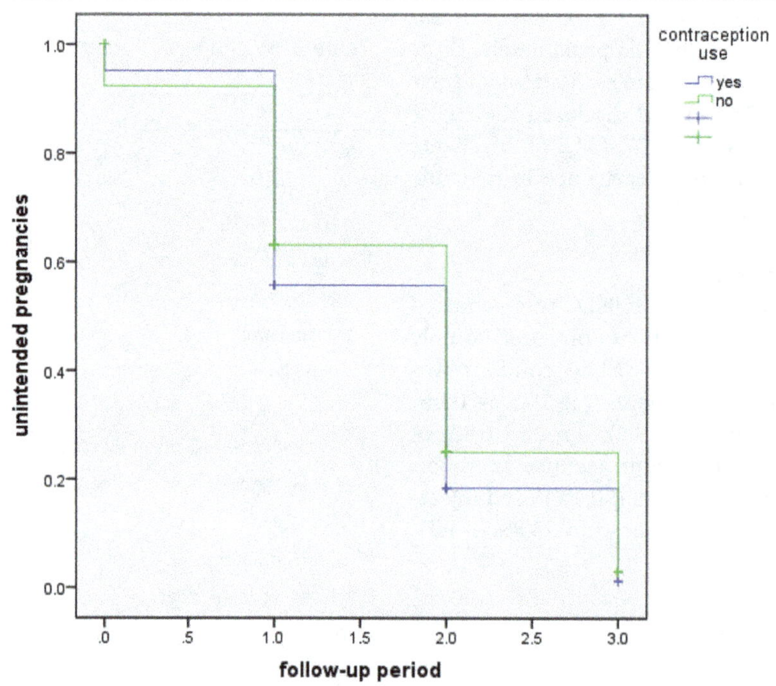


**Fig. 1** The effect of contraceptive use on the rate of unintended pregnancy

use in the HIV non-infected group. The parallel application of condom use along with other methods is warranted to reduce the risk of unwanted pregnancy, transmission of HIV to a non-infected couple, to minimize transmission of drug resistant virus to an individual with HIV infection [19, 20]. Although, all HIV infected women are expected to use dual protection, the current study revealed that only limited number of patients (6.4%) applied dual contraception. Only small number of respondents (17.7%) reported dual method use in Zambia [7]. Poor utilization of dual contraception might contribute for higher incidence of STI in the sero-positive group 101(32.2%) versus 49(8.4%), in HIV negative clients. Further, under utilization of combination of methods could be due to high level of illiteracy 102(32.5%) of participants. A hospital based cross-sectional study also stated that low educational status was found to be associated with inadequate use of contraceptives among sexually active HIV positive individuals in the same set-up.

This study also illustrated that women who had unintended pregnancy used contraceptive methods occasionally. Even though Ethiopia has a promising achievement on contraceptive coverage, it is still difficult to control unintended pregnancies. This might be due to the lack persistence with the modern contraception. In addition, the low literacy and the high level of unemployment complicate the odds of unintended pregnancy in developing countries.

### Limitations

In general, the present study provided a comparative evidence regarding the pattern of contraceptive use among HIV-infected and non-infected women. However, its findings are only interpreted in the light of the following limitations. First of all the study is limited to single center and qualitative data on the reasons to choose a certain type of contraceptive is not included. Therefore, we recommend a multicenter study including large number of subjects and mixed type of study design to incorporate qualitative aspects. Further, the present study also highlighted that significant number of patients were not on HARRT. The reason for low consumption of the HARRT should be investigated.

## Conclusion

Intrauterine contraceptive device was reported to be the most commonly used contraceptive method in HIV patients as compared to HIV negative counter parts. Male condom use was found to be higher among HIV positive patients as compared to HIV negative women. Nearly, one-half of HIV negative clients use injectable contraceptive methods as compared to around a quarter in the HIV positive women. Further, unintended pregnancy was relatively common in women with low contraceptive practice. The use of dual contraceptives condom use in particular, should be advocated for HIV-positive women so as to protect unintended pregnancy, HIV transmission to partner, other strain and sub type HIV infections. Education and Communication campaigns should be strengthened in the community about reproductive health services in general and family planning services in particular. Access to quality contraceptive methods should be scaled up in community.

### Abbreviations

GURH: Gondar University Referral Hospital; HAART: Highly Active Antiretroviral Therapy; HIV: Human Immune Virus; IUCD: Intrauterine Contraceptive Device; STI: Sexually Transmitted Diseases; WHO: World Health Organization

### Acknowledgments

Our gratitude goes to university of Gondar, data collectors and participants of the study.

### Authors' contributions

AGM and TMA conceived the study, involve in acquisition of data, analyze the data and write the final part of the manuscript. DAE, SAB, AAA, BMG interpret and analyzed the data and wrote the initial draft of manuscript. All the authors read, approved the final manuscript and agreed to be accountable for all aspects of the work.

### Author details

[1]Department of Gynecology and Obstetrics, School of Medicine, College of Medicine and Health Sciences, University of Gondar, Gondar, Ethiopia. [2]Department of Medicinal Chemistry, School of Pharmacy, College of Medicine and Health Sciences, University of Gondar, Gondar, Ethiopia. [3]Department of Clinical Pharmacy, School of Pharmacy, College of Medicine and Health Sciences, University of Gondar, Gondar, Ethiopia.

### References

1. UNAIDS/WHO. AIDS epidemic Update. UNAIDS/17, September 2017. Available: http://www.unaids.org/sites/default/files/media_asset/AIDS-by-the-numbers-2016_en.pdf
2. 2016 Central Statistical Agency [Ethiopia] and ICF International. Ethiopia Demographic and Health Survey 2016. Addis Ababa, Ethiopia and Calverton, Maryland, USA: Central Statistical Agency and ICF International.
3. FHAPCO: Monthly HIV Care and ART update February 2010. In. Addis Ababa: Federal HIV AIDS Prevention and Control Secreteriate;2010.
4. World Health Organization. HIV/AIDS 2015. Available: http://www.who.int/mediacentre/factsheets/fs360/en/.
5. Simon V, Ho DD, Karim QA. HIV/AIDS epidemiology, pathogenesis, prevention, and treatment. The Lancet. 2006;368(9534):489–504).
6. Megabiaw B. Awareness and utilization of modern contraceptives among street women in north-West Ethiopia. BMC Womens Health. 2012;12(1):31.
7. Carla J. Chibwesha et al. Modern contraceptive and DualMethod use among HIV-infected women in Lusaka, Zambia, infectious diseases in obstetrics and gynecology volume 2011, Article ID 261453, 2011, 8 pages doi:https://doi.org/10.1155/2011/261453.
8. Beyeza-Kashesya J, Kaharuza F, Ekström AM, Neema S, Kulane A, Mirembe F. To use or not to use a condom: a prospective cohort study comparing contraceptive practices among HIV-infected and HIV-negative youth in Uganda. BMC Infect Dis. 2011;11(1):144.
9. Wilcher R, Cates W. Reproductive choices for women with HIV. Bull World Health Organ. 2009;87:833–839. [PMC free article][PubMed].
10. Luchters SM, VandenBroeck D, Chersich MF, et al. Association of HIV infection with distribution and viral load of HPV types in Kenya: a survey with 820 female sex workers. BMC Infect Dis. 2010;10:18. [PMC free article][PubMed].
11. Jamieson DJ, Duerr A, Klein RS, et al. Longitudinal analysis of bacterial vaginosis: findings from the HIV epidemiology research study. Obstet Gynecol. 2001;98:656–63. PubMed

12. Kissinger P, Amedee A, Clark RA, et al. Trichomonas vaginalis treatment reduces vaginal HIV-1 shedding. Sex Transm Dis. 2009;36:11–16. [PMC free article][PubMed]).
13. World Health Organization: Unsafe Abortion: Global and Regional Estimates of the Incidence of Unsafe Abortion and Associated Mortality in 2008. 2011, Geneva: World Health Organization.
14. World Health Organization: Information sheet. Unsafe abortion incidence and mortality Global and regional levels in 2008 and trends during 1990–2008. 2012, Geneva: World Health Organization.
15. Worke MD, Bezabih LM, Woldetasdik MA. Utilization of contraception among sexually active HIV positive women attending art clinic in University of Gondar Hospital: a hospital based cross-sectional study. BMC Women's Health. 2016;16:67. doi:https://doi.org/10.1186/s12905-016-0348-9
16. Asfaw HM, Gashe FE. Contraceptive use and method preference among HIV positive women in Addis Ababa, Ethiopia: a cross sectional survey. BMC Public Health. 2014;14:566. Published 2014 Jun 6. doi:https://doi.org/10.1186/1471-2458-14-566
17. Laryea DO, Amoako YA, Spangenberg K, Frimpong E, Kyei-Ansong J. Contraceptive use and unmet need for family planning among HIV positive women on antiretroviral therapy in Kumasi. Ghana BMC Women's Health. 2014;14(1):126.
18. Taiwo OO, Hassan Z. The impact of highly active antiretroviral therapy (HAART) on the clinical features of HIV - related oral lesions in Nigeria. AIDS Res Ther. 2010;7(1):19.
19. Petruney, T. (January 01, 2008). Contraception is the best kept secret for prevention of mother-to-child HIV transmission. Bulletin of the World Health Organization. Bulletin De L'organisationMondiale De La Santé, *86,* 6, 495.).
20. Mitchell HS, Stephens E Contraception choice for HIV positive women Sexually Transmitted Infections 2004;80:167–173.).
21. Mulat S, Fekadu M, Abera H, Bekele G, Bedaso A. Prevalence of unplanned pregnancy and associated factors among mothers attending antenatal Care at Hawassa City Public Hospitals, Hawassa, SNNPR. Ethiopia J Women's Health Care. 2017;6(387):2167–0420.

# Permissions

All chapters in this book were first published by BioMed Central; hereby published with permission under the Creative Commons Attribution License or equivalent. Every chapter published in this book has been scrutinized by our experts. Their significance has been extensively debated. The topics covered herein carry significant findings which will fuel the growth of the discipline. They may even be implemented as practical applications or may be referred to as a beginning point for another development.

The contributors of this book come from diverse backgrounds, making this book a truly international effort. This book will bring forth new frontiers with its revolutionizing research information and detailed analysis of the nascent developments around the world.

We would like to thank all the contributing authors for lending their expertise to make the book truly unique. They have played a crucial role in the development of this book. Without their invaluable contributions this book wouldn't have been possible. They have made vital efforts to compile up to date information on the varied aspects of this subject to make this book a valuable addition to the collection of many professionals and students.

This book was conceptualized with the vision of imparting up-to-date information and advanced data in this field. To ensure the same, a matchless editorial board was set up. Every individual on the board went through rigorous rounds of assessment to prove their worth. After which they invested a large part of their time researching and compiling the most relevant data for our readers.

The editorial board has been involved in producing this book since its inception. They have spent rigorous hours researching and exploring the diverse topics which have resulted in the successful publishing of this book. They have passed on their knowledge of decades through this book. To expedite this challenging task, the publisher supported the team at every step. A small team of assistant editors was also appointed to further simplify the editing procedure and attain best results for the readers.

Apart from the editorial board, the designing team has also invested a significant amount of their time in understanding the subject and creating the most relevant covers. They scrutinized every image to scout for the most suitable representation of the subject and create an appropriate cover for the book.

The publishing team has been an ardent support to the editorial, designing and production team. Their endless efforts to recruit the best for this project, has resulted in the accomplishment of this book. They are a veteran in the field of academics and their pool of knowledge is as vast as their experience in printing. Their expertise and guidance has proved useful at every step. Their uncompromising quality standards have made this book an exceptional effort. Their encouragement from time to time has been an inspiration for everyone.

The publisher and the editorial board hope that this book will prove to be a valuable piece of knowledge for researchers, students, practitioners and scholars across the globe.

# List of Contributors

**Afework Tadele and Rahma Ali**
Population and family health, Jimma University, Jimma, Ethiopia

**Dessie Abebaw**
Epidemiology, Jimma University, Jimma, Ethiopia

**Pranta Das**
Department of Statistics, University of Dhaka, Dhaka, Bangladesh

**Nandeeta Samad**
Department of Public Health, North South University, Dhaka, Bangladesh

**Hasan Al Banna**
Institute of Social Welfare and Research, University of Dhaka, Dhaka, Bangladesh

**Temitayo Eniola Sodunke**
Bachelor of Science in Anatomy, University of Ilorin, Ilorin, Nigeria

**John Elvis Hagan Jr**
Department of Health, Physical Education, and Recreation, University of Cape Coast, Cape Coast, Ghana
Neurocognition and Action-Biomechanics-Research Group, Faculty of Psychology and Sport Sciences, Bielefeld University, Bielefeld, Germany

**Bright Opoku Ahinkorah**
School of Public Health, Faculty of Health, University of Technology Sydney, Ultimo, Australia

**Abdul-Aziz Seidu**
Department of Population and Health, University of Cape Coast, Cape Coast, Ghana
College of Public Health, Medical and Veterinary Sciences, James Cook University, Townsville, Queensland, Australia

**Alemu Degu Ayele, Bekalu Getnet Kassa, Dagne Addisu Sewyew and Gedefaye Nibret Mihretie**
Department of Midwifery, College of Health Sciences, Debre Tabor University, Debre Tabor, Ethiopia

**Fentahun Yenealem Beyene**
Department of Midwifery, College of Medicine and Health Sciences, Bahir Dar University, Bahir Dar, Ethiopia

**Aklilu Tilahun**
Adare General Hospital, Maternal and Child Health service case team, Hawassa, Ethiopia

**Amanuel Yoseph and Mesay Hailu Dangisso**
School of Public Health, College of Medicine and Health Sciences, Hawassa University, Hawassa, Ethiopia

**Sena Belina Kitila, Yonas Biratu Terfa and Adugna Olani Akuma**
Faculty of Health Sciences, School of Nursing and Midwifery, Jimma University Institute of Health Science, Addis Abeba, Ethiopia

**Ayantu Kebede Olika**
Department of Epidemiology, Faculty of Public Health, Jimma University Institute of Health, Addis Abeba, Ethiopia

**Alemi Kebede Olika**
Population and Family Health Department, Faculty of Public Health, Jimma University Institute of Health Science, Addis Abeba, Ethiopia

**Sara Dokuhaki**
Community Based Psychiatric Care Research Center, Department of Midwifery, School of Nursing and Midwifery, Shiraz University of Medical Sciences, Shiraz, Iran

**Fateme Dokuhaki**
Department of Psychology, Islamic Azad University of Marvdasht, Marvdasht, Iran

**Marzieh Akbarzadeh**
Maternal-fetal Medicine Research Center, Department of Midwifery, School of Nursing and Midwifery, Shiraz University of Medical Sciences, Shiraz, Iran

**Beena Joshi, Siddesh Shetty, Ragini Kulkarni and Shahina Begum**
Indian Council of Medical Research- National Institute for Research in Reproductive Health (NIRRH), Mumbai, Maharashtra, India

**Bhushan Girase**
Indian Council of Medical Research- National Institute for Research in Reproductive Health (NIRRH), Mumbai, Maharashtra, India
Family Health Department, PATH India, New Delhi, India

**Vinita Verma**
National AIDS Control Organization, New Delhi, India

**Shrikala Acharya**
Mumbai District AIDS Control Society, Mumbai, Maharashtra, India

**Pramod Deoraj**
Maharashtra State AIDS Control Society, Mumbai, Maharashtra, India

**Gurmessa Daba**
Ambo University College of Medicine and Health Science, Ambo, Ethiopia

**Jembere Tesfaye Deressa and Workinesh Sinishaw**
Addis Ababa University College of Health Science, School of Nursing & Midwifery, Addis Ababa, Ethiopia

**Abel Nzabona and Richard Tuyiragize**
School of Statistics and Planning, Makerere University, Kampala, Uganda

**Paula Anita**
School of Statistics and Planning, Makerere University, Kampala, Uganda
Marie Stopes Uganda, Kampala, Uganda

**Joseph Ngonzi, Musa Kayondo and Godfrey Mugyenyi**
Department of Obstetrics and Gynecology, Mbarara University of Science and Technology, Mbarara, Uganda

**Joy Muhumuza**
Department of Obstetrics and Gynecology, Mbarara University of Science and Technology, Mbarara, Uganda
Department of Obstetrics and Gynecology, Kampala International University, Kampala, Uganda

**Richard Migisha**
Department of Physiology, Mbarara University of Science and Technology, Mbarara, Uganda

**Gemechu Kejela, Tariku Tesfaye and Ebisa Turi**
Department of Public Health, Institute of Health Sciences, Wollega University, Nekemte, Ethiopia

**Aga Wakgari, Moa Adugna, Netsanet Alemu and Latera Jebessa**
School of Medicine, Institute of Health Sciences, Wollega University, Nekemte, Ethiopia

**Ifeyinwa Chizoba Akamike, Ijeoma Nkem Okedo-Alex and Irene Ifeyinwa Eze**
Department of Community Medicine, Alex Ekwueme Federal University Teaching Hospital, Abakaliki, Nigeria
African Institute for Health Policy and Health Systems, Ebonyi State University, Abakaliki, Nigeria

**Chigozie Jesse Uneke**
African Institute for Health Policy and Health Systems, Ebonyi State University, Abakaliki, Nigeria

**Obumneme Benaiah Ezeanosike**
Department of Paediatrics, Alex Ekwueme Federal University Teaching Hospital, Abakaliki, Nigeria

**Robinah Nalwanga, Afra Nuwasiima, Janet U. Babigumira and Francis T. Asiimwe**
GHE Consulting, Kampala, Uganda

**Vitalis P. Ngambouk**
Department of Community Medicine and Public Health, Sahlgrenska Academy, University of Gothenburg, 40530, Gothenburg, Sweden

**Elly Nuwamanya**
GHE Consulting, Kampala, Uganda
Department of Community Medicine and Public Health, Sahlgrenska Academy, University of Gothenburg, 40530, Gothenburg, Sweden

**Joseph B. Babigumira**
Global Medicines Program, Department of Global Health, University of Washington, Seattle, WA 98195, USA

**Woineshet Asrat**
Amhara Regional Health Office, Bahir Dar, Ethiopia

**Teferi Mekonnen**
Public Health Nutrition department, School of Public Health, Bahir Dar University, Bahir Dar, Ethiopia

**Melkamu Bedimo**
Department of Epidemiology and Biostatistics', School of Public Health, Bahir Dar University, Bahir Dar, Ethiopia

**Gedefaw Abeje Fekadu**
Pan African University, Institute of Life and Earth Sciences (including health and Agriculture), University of Ibadan, Ibadan, Nigeria
College of Medicine and Health Sciences, School of Public Health, Bahir Dar University, Bahir Dar, Ethiopia

**Akinyinka O. Omigbodun and Olumuyiwa A. Roberts**
University College Hospital, University of Ibadan, Ibadan, Nigeria

**Alemayehu Worku Yalew**
School of Public health, College of Medicine, Addis Ababa University, Addis Ababa, Ethiopia

**Jonathan Ian Coomson**
M&C Health System, LG DTD 10081, East Legon, Accra, Ghana

**Abubakar Manu**
Department of Population, Family and Reproductive Health, School of Public Health, University of Ghana, Accra, Ghana

**Birye Dessalegn Mekonnen**
Department of Nursing, Teda health Science College, Gondar, Ethiopia

**Rima Mourtada**
Department of Epidemiology and Population Health, London School of Hygiene and Tropical Medicine, Keppel St, Bloomsbury, London WC1E 7HT, UK
Faculty of Health Sciences, American University of Beirut, Bliss Street, Beirut, Lebanon

**Hyam Bashour**
Faculty of Medicine, University of Damascus, Damascus, Syria

**Fiona Houben**
Faculty of Health and Wellbeing, Canterbury Christ Church University, North Holmes Road, Canterbury, Kent CT1 1QU, UK

**Michele Troutman**
Department of Obstetrics and Gynecology, Beth Israel Deaconess Medical Center, Boston, MA, USA

**Saima Rafique**
Advantia Ob/Gyn Shady Grove, Rockville, MD, USA

**Torie Comeaux Plowden**
Department of Obstetrics and Gynecology, Womack Army Medical Center, Ft Bragg, NC, USA

**Karina M. Shreffler and Stacy Tiemeyer**
Oklahoma State University, 700 N. Greenwood Ave, Tulsa, OK 74106, USA

**Jameca R. Price**
University of Oklahoma Health Sciences Center, 4502 E. 41st St, Tulsa, OK 74135, USA

**Lance T. Frye**
Oklahoma State University Center for Health Sciences, 1111 W. 17th St, Tulsa, OK 74107, USA

**Belay Amare Abebe**
Department of Midwifery, College Medicine and Health Sciences, University of Hawassa, Hawassa, Ethiopia

**Mulu Reda Terefe**
Department Statistics, College of Natural and Computational Science, University of Hawassa, Hawassa, Ethiopia

**Jim Aizire, Sufia Dadabhai and Jin Sun**
Department of Epidemiology, Johns Hopkins Bloomberg School of Public Health, 615 North Wolfe Street, Baltimore, MD 21205, USA

**Frank Taulo, Bonus Makanani and Luis Gadama**
Department of Obstetrics and Gynecology, College of Medicine, University of Malawi, Blantyre, Malawi

**Amy Tsui**
Department of Population, Family and Reproductive Health, Johns Hopkins Bloomberg School of Public Health, Baltimore, MD, USA

**Taha E. Taha**
Department of Epidemiology, Johns Hopkins Bloomberg School of Public Health, 615 North Wolfe Street, Baltimore, MD 21205, USA
Department of Population, Family and Reproductive Health, Johns Hopkins Bloomberg School of Public Health, Baltimore, MD, USA

**Khaing Nwe Tin**
Maternal and Reproductive Health Division, Department of Public Health, Ministry of Health and Sports, Naypyitaw, Myanmar

**Thae Maung Maung**
Department of Medical Research, Ministry of Health and Sports, Yangon, Myanmar

**Thiri Win**
Department of Public Health, Ministry of Health and Sports, Naypyitaw, Myanmar

**Damian J. Damian**
Department of Community Medicine, Kilimanjaro Christian Medical Centre (KCMC), Moshi, Tanzania
Department of Epidemiology & Biostatistics, Institute of Public Health, KCMUCo, Moshi, Tanzania

**Erick Martin and Beatrice Temba**
Kilimanjaro Christian Medical University College (KCMUCo), Moshi, Tanzania

**Johnston M. George**
Kilimanjaro Christian Medical University College (KCMUCo), Moshi, Tanzania
Department of Community Health, Institute of Public Health, KCMUCo, Moshi, Tanzania

**Sia E. Msuya**
Department of Community Medicine, Kilimanjaro Christian Medical Centre (KCMC), Moshi, Tanzania
Department of Epidemiology & Biostatistics, Institute of Public Health, KCMUCo, Moshi, Tanzania
Department of Community Health, Institute of Public Health, KCMUCo, Moshi, Tanzania

**Amanual Getnet Mersha**
Department of Gynecology and Obstetrics, School of Medicine, College of Medicine and Health Sciences, University of Gondar, Gondar, Ethiopia

**Daniel Asfaw Erku**
Department of Medicinal Chemistry, School of Pharmacy, College of Medicine and Health Sciences, University of Gondar, Gondar, Ethiopia

**Sewunet Admasu Belachew, Asnakew Achaw Ayele, Begashaw Melaku Gebresillassie and Tadesse Melaku Abegaz**
Department of Clinical Pharmacy, School of Pharmacy, College of Medicine and Health Sciences, University of Gondar, Gondar, Ethiopia

# Index

## O



## P



## R



## S



## T



## U



## W

www.ingramcontent.com/pod-product-compliance
Lightning Source LLC
LaVergne TN
LVHW082141200926
848484LV00008B/2090